# Assessment in Behavioral Medicine

# BIOBEHAVIOURAL PERSPECTIVES ON HEALTH AND DISEASE PREVENTION

From the perspective of behavioural science, the series examines current research, including clinical and policy implications, on health, illness prevention, and biomedical issues. The series is international in scope, and aims to address the culturally specific, as well as the universally applicable.

Series Editor: Lydia R. Temoshok, PhD, Institute of Human Virology, Division of Clinical Research, University of Maryland Biotechnology Center, 725 West Lombard Street, Room N548, Baltimore, Maryland 21201, USA

# Assessment in Behavioral Medicine

Edited by

## Ad Vingerhoets
*Department of Psychology, Tilburg University, The Netherlands*

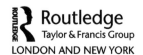

Routledge
Taylor & Francis Group
LONDON AND NEW YORK

First published by Brunner-Routledge 2001

This edition published in 2012 by Routledge
27 Church Road, Hove, East Sussex BN3 2FA
711 Third Avenue, New York, NY 10017, USA
*Routledge is an imprint of the Taylor & Francis Group, an informa business*

*British Library Cataloguing in Publication Data*
A catalogue record for this book is available from the British Library

*Library of Congress Cataloging in Publication Data*
A catalog record for this book is available from the British Library

ISBN - 978 01 5839 1227 0

To Louwrens J. Menges, my major source of inspiration

# Contents

# List of Figures

# List of Tables

# List of Boxes

# Preface

Over the past two decades, behavioral scientists and clinicians have played an increasing role in medical research and practice. They have also carved out and defined areas of research in which behavioral factors are paramount: the effects of psychosocial factors and life style on the onset and course of disease, how patients and those in their social environment cope with illness, and how illness affects well-being and quality of life. Much of the appeal of behavioral medicine lies in its attempt to integrate knowledge from the behavioral and biomedical sciences to reach solutions to practical problems of physical health and illness. What psychologists can contribute to medicine is, in particular, the theory and technology of assessment, model building, and theory construction, in addition to interventions capable of remediating or preventing the psychosocial antecedents or consequences of disease. Those interested in establishing the role of psychosocial factors in health and disease face the challenge of precise and valid measurement of their concepts: clarity in the definition of the different psychosocial concepts and in the expression of those definitions in adequate measures is crucial when doing research.

It is instructive to recall that in 1943, Halliday had already formulated four central questions pertinent to disease etiology, and that behavioral issues dominated these questions: (1) what kind of person is the patient? (2) why did (s)he take ill, when (s)he did? (3) why did (s)he develop this specific disease? and (4) what is the patient getting at, and toward what end or purpose is this behavior directed? Additional information that behavioral medicine researchers have emphasized more recently include how patients cope with their disease, hospitalization, and medical procedures, and how patients interact with medical providers, the medical system, and their social environments.

With the increasing demands of evidence-based medicine, it is becoming more critical to evaluate all interventions, including those in behavioral medicine, with respect to their impact on both physical and mental well-being. The foundation, as well as the first step in evaluation, is assessment, which is the focus of this volume. Measurement is the process by which concepts are operationalized and quantified. It is axiomatic that assessment tools in behavioral medicine and health psychology need to have adequate psychometric qualities. Perhaps more important, however, is their conceptual validity: to what extent they can "capture," measure, and predict important constructs, which are then translated into predictive and outcome variables. Maintaining rigor in defining and measuring both independent and dependent variables and in the execution of intervention strategies is paramount. Attempts to clarify diagnostic, definitional, and other conceptual issues in relation to the problem area covered are crucial. Measurement of these concepts serves many functions, mainly to help in diagnosis, to predict or evaluate the response to treatment and to monitor change. Adequate assessment leads to an enhanced understanding of the clinical status of the patient and his/her relationship to the psychosocial environment. The process of theorizing, developing, and refining such core behavioral medicine constructs as stress, coping, social support, and quality of life, has been accompanied by a rapid proliferation of measures designed to assess these constructs, their subconstructs, and related constructs.

The aim of the present volume is to advance the state of measurement in the multidisciplinary fields of behavioral medicine and health psychology by bringing together state-of-the-art theory and research on assessment issues in these areas. In selecting topics to be included, I was guided by the generally accepted stress-and-coping model of mental and physical disease development and progression. In addition to self reports (questionnaires and interviews), attention is given to observational measures and, if appropriate, 'objective' indicators of health behaviors, as well as psychobiological measures.

The volume opens with an overview of assessment in the clinical context (Chapter 1), the theoretical foundations of methodology in assessing etiological linkages (Chapter 2), and the impact of psychosocial interventions (Chapter 3). To address the need for assessing specific health-related attitudes and opinions, for which few standardized measures exist, I have incorporated contributions on the theoretical and practical aspects of assessment (Chapters 4 and 5). Particularly relevant to the stress-and-coping model are the chapters on assessment of stressors (Chapter 6), coping (Chapter 7), and social support (Chapter 8). Of further relevance as moderating variables are illness cognitions (Chapter 9) and personality (Chapter 10), as well as compliance (Chapter 11) and life style variables (Chapter 12) which are particularly significant as control variables, but also as outcome measures for health promotion and intervention programs. There are several chapters which concentrate on critical outcome measures: pain

(Chapter 13), fatigue (Chapter 14), health status (Chapter 15), and quality of life (Chapters 16 and 17). In terms of psychobiological assessment, there are three chapters which focus on, respectively, cardiovascular (Chapter 18), endocrine (Chapter 19), and immunologic (Chapter 20) measures.

I am delighted that so many eminent researchers were willing to share their experience, knowledge, and perspectives in this volume. I hope that both researchers and clinicians will benefit from their contributions. Finally, I would like to acknowledge Rinus Verkooyen, whose humor, help and assistance was invaluable when preparing the manuscript.

## Reference

Halliday, J.L. (1943). Principles of aetiology. *British Journal of Medical Psychology, 19*, 367–380.

# List of Contributors

**Maurice Alberts**
Department of Medical Psychology, University Hospital Radboud, Nijmegen, The Netherlands

**David Almeida**
Division of Family Studies, University of Arizona, Tucson AZ, USA

**Gayle Baker**
Department of Medical and Clinical Psychology, Uniformed Services University of the Health Sciences, Bethesda MD, USA

**Andrew Baum**
Department of Psychiatry and Pittsburgh Cancer Institute, University of Pittsburgh, Pittsburgh PA, USA

**Cynthia D. Belar**
American Psychological Association, Education Directorate, Washington DC, USA

**Gijs Bleijenberg**
Department of Medical Psychology, University Hospital Radboud, Nijmegen, The Netherlands

**Sally Brotman**
Frontier Science and Technology Research Foundation, Inc., Chestnut Hill MA, USA

**George W. Brown**
Department of Social Policy and Social Science, Royal Holloway and Bedford College, University of London, London, UK

**Geert Crombez**
Department of Psychology, University of Ghent, Ghent, Belgium

**Norman S. Endler**
Department of Psychology, York University, North York, Ontario, Canada

**Julie D. Fox**
Department of Medical Microbiology, University of Wales, College of Medicine, Heath Park, Cardiff, UK

**Ellen Frank**
Western Psychiatric Institute and Clinic, University of Pittsburgh, Pittsburgh PA, USA

**Howard S. Friedman**
Department of Psychology, University of California, Riverside CA, USA

**Joop W. Furer**
Department of General Practice and Social Medicine, University of Nijmegen, Nijmegen, The Netherlands

**Larry W. Hawk, Jr.**
Department of Psychology, State University of New York at Buffalo, Buffalo NY, USA

**Michael Irwin**
Department of Psychiatry, University of California, San Diego and VA Medical Centre, San Diego CA, USA

**Evguenia Jilinskaia**
Frontier Science and Technology Research Foundation, Inc., Chestnut Hill MA, USA

**Judith M. Johnson**
Department of Psychology, York University, Ontario, Canada

**Beth A. Jones**
Department of Epidemiology and Public Health, Yale University School of Medicine, New Haven CT, USA

**Robert M. Kaplan**
Department of Family and Prevention Medicine, University of California, San Diego, La Jolla CA, USA

**Adrian A. Kaptein**
Department of Medical Psychology, University of Leiden, Oegstgeest, The Netherlands

**Stanislav V. Kasl**
Department of Epidemiology and Public Health, Yale University School of Medicine, New Haven CT, USA

**Ronald C. Kessler**
Department of Sociology and Institute of Social Research, University of Michigan, Ann Arbor MI, USA

**Erik de Klerk**
AARDEX Ltd., Maastricht, The Netherlands

**Christiane König-Zahn**
Department of General Practice and Social Medicine, University of Nijmegen, Nijmegen, The Netherlands

**Willem J. Kop**
Department of Medical and Clinical Psychology, Uniformed Services University of the Health Sciences, Bethesda MD, USA

**David S. Krantz**
Department of Medical and Clinical Psychology, Uniformed Services University of the Health Sciences, Bethesda MD, USA

**Leslie R. Martin**
Department of Psychology, La Sierra University, Riverside CA, USA

**Jane Ogden**
Department of General Practice and Primary Care, Guy's, Kings and St Thomas' School of Medicine, London, UK

**Tricia L. Park**
Department of Clinical and Health Psychology, University of Florida Health Science Center, Gainesville FL, USA

**Robbert Sanderman**
Northern Centre for Healthcare Research, University of Groningen, Groningen, The Netherlands

**Margreet Scharloo**
Unit of Psychology, Leiden University Medical Centre, Oegstgeest, The Netherlands

**Carolyn E. Schwartz**
Family Medicine and Community Health, University of Massachusetts Medical School, Worcester MA, USA

**William J. Sieber**
University of California at San Diego, Health Outcomes Assessment Program, La Jolla CA, USA

**Jan Snel**
Department of Psychology, University of Amsterdam, Amsterdam, The Netherlands

**Eric van Sonderen**
Northern Centre for Healthcare Research, University of Groningen, Groningen, The Netherlands

**Bert Tax**
Department of General Practice and Social Medicine, University of Nijmegen, Nijmegen, The Netherlands

**Fred Tudiver**
Center for Evidence Based Practice, Department of Family Medicine, SUNY Health Science Center, Syracuse NY, USA

**Jos Twisk**
Institute for Extramural Medicine, Vrije Universiteit Amsterdam, Amsterdam, The Netherlands

**Kav Vedhara**
Department of Medicine, Dorothy Crowfoot Hodgkin Laboratories, University of Bristol, Marlborough Street, Bristol, UK

**Jan H.M.M. Vercoulen**
Department of Medical Psychology, University Hospital Radboud, Nijmegen, The Netherlands

**Ad Vingerhoets**
Department of Clinical Health Psychology, Tilburg University, Tilburg, The Netherlands

**Johan W.S. Vlaeyen**
Institute for Rehabilitation Research, Hoensbroek, The Netherlands

**Jolanda de Vries**
Department of Clinical Health Psychology, Tilburg University, Tilburg, The Netherlands

**Edward C.Y. Wang**
Department of Medicine, University of Wales, College of Medicine, Cardiff, UK

**John A. Weinman**
Unit of Psychology, United Medical and Dental School of Guy's and St Thomas Hospitals, London, UK

**Elaine Wethington**
Department of Human Development and Family Studies, Cornell University, Ithaca NY, USA

# 1 PSYCHOLOGICAL ASSESSMENT IN THE MEDICAL SETTING

Cynthia D. Belar and Tricia L. Park

In contrast to traditional psychological assessment which focuses on personality and defense mechanisms for the purpose of treatment of mental health problems, psychological assessment in the medical setting involves the integration of information regarding cognitive, affective and behavioral functioning vis à vis physiological health, illness and disability. While seemingly broad in nature, health psychology assessment is necessarily focal, driven by the clinical question and context of the assessment. Although an integral component in the design of psychological treatments, a major use of this specific type of assessment is to solve problems for other health professionals in providing care for their patients. Thus, consultation activities are often an integral part of the assessment process.

The assessment issues addressed in the present chapter are relevant for health promotion, primary and secondary prevention, tertiary care, and rehabilitation. Assessment recipients include the normal population undergoing risk assessment, the "worried well" seeking to promote health, and identified patients in both acute and chronic phases of illness or injury/disability. As noted elsewhere (e.g., Belar, 1997; Belar & Deardorff, 1995), there are many purposes of assessment, including differential diagnosis, treatment planning, and outcome assessment. For example, specific assessment can help clarify diagnostic issues associated with: (a) psychological presentations of organic disease (e.g., depression in hypothyroidism, delusional thinking in HIV+ dementia); (b) psychological problems secondary to disease (e.g., post cardiotomy delirium, body image problems subsequent to amputation, post myocardial infarction depression, post-traumatic stress disorder resulting from accidental burn); (c) somatic effects of psychological distress (e.g., angina, headache, decreased pain tolerance); and (d) somatic presentations of psychological disorder (e.g., masked depression, somatization, chest pain in panic attack).

Assessment for treatment planning includes that associated with the treatment of psychophysiological disorders, interventions for psychological reactions to illness/disability, cessation of deleterious health habits, and development of health-promoting behaviors. Assessment is also used in planning psychological interventions that have been successful in producing changes in actual physical symptoms (e.g., vasospasms) and health status indicators such as length of hospital stay.

It is important to emphasize that in addition to planning for psychological interventions, psychological assessment is as important for the planning of many medical, surgical and rehabilitative treatments. Many clinical health psychologists provide assessments related to readiness for treatment such as organ transplantation, competence to make decisions regarding termination of life support systems, informed consent for participation in elective procedures such as oocyte donation, and issues of adherence to medical regimens. Clinical health psychology assessment is used post-treatment to identify progress with respect to intervention targets, and to assess sequelae of various medical-surgical treatments.

Psychologists who use assessment in medical treatment planning often work as a member of a multidisciplinary team, providing case-centered consultation as well as leadership in team-building processes. Thus another use of assessment is to understand problems of health care providers and health care systems, with a focus on such issues as provider-patient relationships, staff burnout, design of delivery systems and organizational culture.

Clinical health psychology assessment can occur in a variety of settings, e.g., private practice office, emergency room, inpatient unit, outpatient clinic, primary care setting, tertiary care center, rehabilitation hospital, nursing home, or patient's home. Population assessments often occur in public settings such as shopping malls, exercise centers and community facilities. However, this chapter will focus primarily on assessment of patients in clinical settings.

No one clinical health psychologist has expertise in each and every area of possible practice. The kinds of assessments conducted will be determined by the characteristics of the clinical problems addressed and the nature of the referral sources. Thus training of referral sources is an important part of practice. To facilitate the health psychologists' learning, we provide with materials that describe both criteria for referral and examples of physician-patient communications that can facilitate the referral process.

In brief, clinical health psychology assessment involves evaluating assessment needs, choosing appropriate methods, gathering information, formulating impressions, and concisely communicating results.

The remainder of this chapter will describe a particular model for understanding the assessment needs of patients, discuss methods of data collection, address issues in case conceptualization and communication of results, and examine specific pitfalls to be avoided in the process. The attempt is to be comprehensive, but not exhaustive in scope.

## A model for assessment

Clinical health psychology assessment varies widely depending on the referral question, patient status, illness/disability, referral source, and treatment setting. For case conceptualization and treatment planning purposes, it is useful to have a model to help direct assessment efforts and to ensure a thorough appraisal of pertinent medical, biological, psychological, and social information. In earlier work (Belar et al., 1987), the senior author proposed a model based on an extension of work by Engel (1977) and Leigh and Reiser (1980) who advocate for a biopsychosocial model in health care. Our model articulates targets of assessment by domain of information (biological or physical, affective, cognitive, behavioral) and unit of assessment or source of data (patient, family environment, health care system and sociocultural context), all of which are the building blocks of the assessment process (see Table 1.1). Each block also has a developmental and historical perspective.

Although portrayed as categorical blocks of information, information in these blocks is interrelated in complex ways and we encourage the reader not to think in a compartmentalized fashion when evaluating its meaningfulness. This model is appropriate for the assessment of any clinical problem, although depending on the issues addressed, some blocks may be more pertinent than others. While it is briefly summarized below, other chapters in this text provide greater detail about specific content and methods pertinent to selected clinical problems or issues.

### BIOLOGICAL TARGETS

Basic biological parameters such as age, gender, and race have immediate and long-term implications for medical and psychological care. Rozensky et al. (1997) underscore the need to consider life stage in the assessment of medical patients, particularly in terms of understanding the impact of chronic illness on interpersonal relationships, independence and dependence, body image, existential concerns, and goals

Table 1.1. Targets of Assessment

| Domain of Information | Patient | Environment | | |
| --- | --- | --- | --- | --- |
| | | Family | Health care system | Sociocultural context |
| *Biological or physical* | Age, sex, race<br>Physical appearance<br>Symptoms, health status<br>Physical examination<br>Vital signs, lab data<br>Medications, drugs<br>Psychophysiological data<br>Constitutional factors<br>Genetics<br>History of injury, disease, and surgery | Characteristics of the home setting<br>Economic resources<br>Size of the family<br>Familial patterning (e.g., headache history)<br>Other illness in family | Characteristics of the treatment setting<br>Characteristics of medical procedures and treatment regimens<br>Availability of prosthetic aids | Social services<br>Financial resources<br>Occupational setting<br>Physical job requirements<br>Health hazards |
| *Affective* | Mood<br>Affect<br>Feelings about illness, treatment, health care, providers, self, family, job, and social network<br>History of affective disturbance | Members' feelings about patient, illness, and treatment | Providers' feelings about patient, illness, and treatment | Sentiments of culture regarding patient, illness, and treatment |

Table 1.1. (*continued*)

| Domain of Information | Patient | Environment | | |
| --- | --- | --- | --- | --- |
| | | Family | Health care system | Sociocultural context |
| *Cognitive* | Cognitive style<br>Thought content<br>Intelligence<br>Education<br>Knowledge about diseases<br>Health beliefs<br>Attitudes and expectations regarding illness, treatment, health care, and providers<br>Perceived meaning of the illness<br>Philosophy of life<br>Religious beliefs | Knowledge about illness and treatment<br>Attitudes and expectations about patient, illness, and treatment<br>Intellectual resources | Providers' knowledge<br>Providers' attitude toward patient, illness, and treatment | Current state of knowledge<br>Cultural attitudes towards patient and illness |
| *Behavioral* | Activity level<br>Interactions with family, friends, and co-workers<br>Health habits<br>Health care utilization (previous medications and psychological treatment)<br>Compliance<br>Ability to control physical symptoms | Participation in patient care<br>Reinforcement contingencies for health and illness | Providers' skills in education and training patients<br>Reinforcement contingencies for health and illness | Employment policies<br>Laws regulating health care practice, disability, provision of care, health habits<br>Handicapped access<br>Customs in symptom reporting and help seeking |

(p. 67). The psychologist also seeks to understand the potential impact on behavior of ongoing medical problems and their treatments (e.g., uremia associated with kidney failure, impact of high dose cortico-steroids). With this information the clinician can more sensitively tailor the assessment as well as better understand the patient's current presentation. Clinicians also need to know about previous illnesses, injuries, surgeries, number and length of hospitalizations, plus history of substance use.

Research has found many sociodemographic factors to be pertinent to a number of psychological assessment issues (Robinson & Klesges, 1997; Rodrigue, 1997; Weidner et al., 1997). For example, geriatric patients often present with decreased visual/auditory acuity, as well as slowed information processing and response speed (Andersen & Haley, 1997). Varying behavior and attention patterns of males and females with insulin dependent diabetes mellitus (IDDM) may be explained by differences in glycemic control (Eriksson & Rosenquist, 1993; La Greca et al., 1995). Verbal fluency and manual dexterity have been shown to vary by age and gender (Benton et al., 1983; Bornstein, 1985). Moreover, race has been demonstrated to have significant relationships with physiologic and behavioral risk factors as well as health care utilization and access (Raczynski & Lewis, 1992).

Potentially crucial to the emerging clinical picture are data from the physician's examination and laboratory assessments. Although technical in nature and sometimes difficult to interpret without consultation, this information can enhance the clinician's understanding of the quality and severity of a patient's past or present medical problem(s), including factors that may affect the behavioral presentation. According to Piotrowski and Lubin (1990), nearly half of clinical health psychologists surveyed utilized such data in the assessment process.

Finally, it may also be important to gather psychophysiological data such as electromyographic levels for tension headache and polysomnography for sleep disorders.

## AFFECTIVE TARGETS

Critical in the evaluation of medical patients is the assessment of current emotional status as well as patients' feelings about illness, health care, family, friends, anticipated future and, of course, self. However, equally important is material pertaining to a patient's past emotional functioning, both in general and under conditions of stress. In gathering information about affect, it is important to consider the timing, context, and sources of information. When assessing affect in inpatients, it is naive to believe that a one-shot consultation, often requested at a time of crisis, can reveal the more stable clinical picture. Repeat visits are often required.

## COGNITIVE TARGETS

In assessing cognitive aspects, the clinician focuses on thoughts, beliefs, and attitudes as well as intellectual capacity. Intellectual, memory, and language tests are often used to elicit information about information processing style and capacity. To interpret findings, consideration of both medical and affective status is imperative since these factors can directly affect motivation and functional ability.

In addition to estimating patients' intellectual capacity and ability to comprehend medical terminology and concepts, patients' knowledge of their own disease should be understood. An analysis of these factors can promote an understanding of problems in adherence to medical regimens and suggest relevant interventions. For example, a highly anxious surgical patient with a low verbal intelligence may benefit from recommendations highlighting the need for concrete/simplistic language, repetition of information, visual presentations, and follow-up contacts for questions. While seemingly rudimentary in nature, such interventions may facilitate physician/patient communication as well as promote quality of care.

Clinical health psychologists also consider patients' guiding philosophies in the areas of health (e.g., their specific health belief model), personal relationships, medical care, and world view, including religious beliefs. For those coming from different cultural backgrounds it is important to assess degree of acculturation. This information can help clarify current functioning, health behaviors, compliance patterns, and relationships with medical staff.

## BEHAVIORAL TARGETS

Clinicians strive to understand patients' overall behavioral patterns in areas of interpersonal, occupational, and recreational functioning. Focal targets include self-care and behaviors related to the reason for referral, including interactions with health care providers. Of special interest is whether the patient can exert voluntary control over any physical symptoms.

Integral to assessment of behavioral targets is information about lifestyle behaviors (e.g., use of alcohol, drugs, and tobacco; dietary habits; exercise patterns), health promoting behaviors (e.g., sleep, use of vitamins and relaxation methods) and illness-specific behaviors (e.g., adherence to medical regimens, health care utilization patterns). Rewards and consequences and existing contingencies in the various domains of functioning (e.g., home, work, doctor's office, hospital) are also carefully weighed. Given that future behavior is often predicted by past behavior, inquiry about past hospitalizations, response to illness, and ability to cope with illness and treatment is necessary.

ENVIRONMENTAL TARGETS

To complete a biopsychosocial assessment, the psychologist must understand the various environments within which the patient functions: (1) the family unit; (2) the health care system; and (3) his or her sociocultural context. Psychologists must also assess the demands, limitations, and supports that these environments provide in the physical, affective, cognitive and behavioral domains of functioning.

(1). *Family environment*. Information pertaining to role functioning and the dynamics of intra-familial relationships should be obtained, with special inquiry concerning changes in family roles from illness onset and the role of each family member with respect to the patient's illness. Obtaining developmental history about the patient and family, the birth of children, major stressors, and family reactions can help clarify these issues.

Also vital is consideration of family members' feelings about a patient's illness, limitations, and treatment in the context of their understanding and attitude regarding the specific health issue. It is crucial to screen for beliefs and behaviors that may impair a patient's recovery or prevent institution of healthy lifestyles (e.g., overprotectiveness, secondary smoke). Additional areas for exploration are more concrete aspects of the home environment, including available financial resources and perhaps physical characteristics of the home (e.g., accessibility), depending upon the problem being assessed.

(2). *Health care environment*. Before proceeding with an evaluation in the hospital setting, examination of environmental characteristics such as room size and privacy level, noisiness, and level of care is recommended so that special accommodations for interview or testing can be anticipated. Particularly important in working with the chronically and/or severely ill is an understanding of environments which in and of themselves can affect physical and emotional features (e.g., the doctor's office and "white coat hypertension", a bone marrow transplant unit and feelings of isolation). One must have knowledge of the nature of various medical procedures and the special issues associated with various health care sites.

The clinician must also pay attention to the quantity and quality of the interactions between patients and staff. Patient care can be jeopardized by staff attitudes, beliefs and behaviors that are influenced by worry or limited understanding and skill. For example, staff may silently fear working with persons who are HIV+. Unique staff issues can arise for victims and perpetrators of crimes as well as younger patients with severe illnesses who decline medical treatments. Consideration of the interpersonal dynamics among those receiving and giving treatment can be crucial for understanding referral questions and safeguarding the quality of care and rights of patients. Also important to assessment is the awareness of relevant hospital policies (e.g., rules about infection control and visitation), and health care system resources such as available treatment options covered by insurance.

(3). *Sociocultural context.* Essential in the assessment of patients is the understanding of sociocultural factors in health, illness, disability and treatment. Knowledge of race-related risk factors, minority group health care utilization patterns, and culturally based health practices is important in understanding different clinical presentations and potentials for intervention. Sociocultural information can also help with interpretation of unusual somatic complaints. Furthermore, information concerning base rates of health behaviors in different groups can facilitate understanding of social influences on behavior.

For treatment planning purposes, it is also important to consider the availability of social services (e.g., securing a home health aide, obtaining disability benefits), the nuances of a patient's social support network (quality, closeness, proximity), and the presence of any ecological hazards in the patient's environment (e.g., overcrowding, noise, pollution).

Cultural factors may also present special challenges during the assessment process itself. For example, it is problematic for a strict Muslim woman to be interviewed by a male in a room with the door closed. And the report of intra familial conflict could be very shameful for some Asians. Moreover, individuals from traditional, non-Western societies may report symptoms which seem bizarre or pathological outside of known spiritual or religious contexts (e.g., mind control by a dead person; Keh-Ming, 1996).

Individuals may also have difficulty understanding test directions due to language barriers. Although an individual may appear to speak the clinician's language well, he/she may have difficulty translating test questions and instructions, or describing specific medical and psychological symptoms, particularly during stressful situations (Jewell,

1989). In scoring tests, findings should be compared with the most appropriate normative sample, keeping the patient's cultural context in mind. Important in test interpretation is the awareness of research on cross cultural variation in the prevalence and presentation of psychopathology, behavioral risk factors, and disease rates.

To understand social system issues for an individual patient, the clinician needs knowledge of job-related information (e.g., a nursing home's policy about hiring an HIV+ nurse) and legislation pertaining to health care provisions for acutely or chronically ill and disabled employees. Such information promotes more feasible treatment planning, and can facilitate the patient coping with unexpected or abrupt lifestyle changes.

## Methods of assessment

There are a number of methods used by clinical health psychologists that can offer information about the various targets of assessment in our model. These include data obtained from archival sources, interview, observation, questionnaires and diaries, psychometric tests, and psychophysiological measures. Although we consider the interview and chart reviews to be cornerstone methods, we are not wedded to any other particular technique. Clinicians are encouraged to consider diverse sources of information and multiple types of data, using a convergent/divergent, hypothesis-testing approach. The purpose of the assessment, the target being assessed, the validity of the method, the skill of the clinician plus issues of feasibility and cost-effectiveness should all be considered in making choices among available methods.

In the hospital setting, interruptions and demands placed on patients can make data collection challenging. It is well known that medical and psychological states can influence test findings, thus assessment in health psychology requires a flexible, persistent, and thorough approach (Deshields et al., 1997). Although other chapters in this text critically evaluate specific methods for particular clinical problems, the following is a brief description of sources of data that should be considered in planning an assessment.

(1). *Archival data.* Medical record review and information from referral sources provide important information in assessment. A relevant literature search can also assist in the interpretation of test findings and formulation of treatment recommendations.

(2). *Interview.* The interview is a core clinical method in health psychology assessment; it provides both verbal and nonverbal information. Strengths include its potential to provide information in all blocks of the model. Unfortunately, unstructured interviews can be time consuming and sometimes diffuse in focus. Because of these limitations, structured or semi-structured interviews are often employed. Widely used structured interviews include the Type A Structured Interview (Rosenman, 1978), the Structured Clinical Interview for DSM-IV Axis I Disorders (SCID-I; First, 1997), and the Diagnostic Interview Schedule (DIS; Robins et al., 1981). Clinicians working with specific patient populations often design their own semi-structured interviews for particular problems. However, due to the potential reactive effects and bias with interview methods, it is recommended that interview data be supplemented with other assessment procedures such as those outlined below.

(3). *Observation.* Targets for observation include appearance, speech content, affect, cognitive status and style, and the whole range of interpersonal and health-related behaviors. Behavioral assessment may include observation of communication patterns and problem-solving techniques in patient-spouse, patient-family, patient-staff, and patient-peer relationships. The setting for observation can be highly structured (e.g., a laboratory) or natural (e.g., classroom, home, ward or treatment unit). Observations may be conducted by the clinician, family members or other health care providers, and may be accomplished *in vivo*, via one-way mirror, through video/audio recording, and even by utilizing advanced ambulatory monitoring technology.

The usefulness of observational data can be maximized through the development of coding systems and the use of trained observers. Rather than developing new coding systems, psychologists or trained observers may use previously developed observer rating scales such as the Measure of Overt Pain Behavior (Keefe & Block, 1982).

(4). *Questionnaires and Diaries.* Clinical health psychologists often develop problem-focused questionnaires that can be completed by patients prior to initial interview. For example, we have used such methods in the assessment of patients with headache, chronic back pain, facial pain, and those seeking penile prosthesis surgery, organ transplantation and *in vitro* fertilization. Questionnaires can be time-savers as well as provide for systematic recording of data for later program evaluation. Important features are clarity and ease of response.

Self monitoring through diary methods is a common method. Purposes include: (a) the acquisition of baseline information; (b) the facilitation of change; and (c) the evaluation of treatment interventions (Turk & Kerns, 1985). Self monitoring can be used to assess relationships among biological, psychological and social experiences. For example, tracking mood states, cognitions and external stressors associated with various symptoms (e.g., pain, binge eating, headache) can facilitate assessment of their interrelationships. Self monitoring complements treatment by enhancing patient awareness of the interplay among biological, psychological and social experiences.

(5). *Psychometric testing.* As noted by Nunnally (1978), standardized measures have many advantages over personal judgements or criterion-free ratings including improved objectivity, finer quantification, increased opportunities for replication, and improved communication.

According to a survey of health psychologists, psychological tests were used for diagnostic purposes by 88% of the 270 respondents, for direction of therapy (73%), for pre- and post-treatment measurement (50%), and for consultation involving litigation (33%) (Piotrowski & Lubin, 1990).

Within the past few decades, the number and nature of psychometric tests have steadily increased, providing clinicians with numerous alternatives for investigating issues pertinent to a variety of medical populations. Some have been more general in nature, e.g., Beck Depression Inventory (Beck, 1972), Sickness Impact Profile (Bergner et al., 1981), Psychosocial Adjustment to Illness Scale (Derogatis, 1986), Ways of Coping Inventory (Folkman & Lazarus, 1980), and the SF-36 Health Survey (Ware et al., 1993). Other measures are targeted to specific health problems, e.g., Arthritis Impact Measurement Scale (Meenan et al., 1982), McGill Pain Questionnaire (Melzack, 1975), Clinical Trauma Assessment (Ruch et al., 1991), Cardiac Depression Scale (Hare & Davis, 1996), and the Cancer Behavior Inventory (Merluzzi & Martinez Sanchez, 1997) just to name a few.

Measures have also been developed for staff to use. For example, in situations requiring complex medical and ethical decisions (e.g., the allocation of scarce resources for organ transplantation), it can be helpful for treatment team members to complete standardized rating scales for patient evaluation purposes (Olbrisch et al., 1989).

Prior to test selection it is important to define the behavior or attitudes of interest. Knowledge of a measure's reliability and validity for the specific usage intended is critical. Clinical practice guidelines and ethical principles for psychologists are violated when tests are misused in medical populations.

(6). *Physiological assessment.* The use of physiological measurement is common for patients presenting with problems of pain, hypertension, sexual dysfunction, sleep disruption and other stress-related disorders. Commonly measured variables include muscle tension, heart rate, skin conductance, blood pressure and respiration under both baseline and stress conditions. In many instances, psychophysiological techniques can facilitate understanding of the interplay among psychological and physiological factors, thus promoting "physiological insight" (Belar & Kibrick, 1986). Increasingly common in the assessment of chronic pain patients is the use of Quantitative Sensory Testing (QST) which provides information about how sensory stimuli are processed (Fillingim, 1997).

## Conceptualization and communication

Although for purposes of presentation we have described assessment as a building block process, the gathering and interpretation of data is not linear. As noted previously, blocks are integrally interrelated and information obtained in one will affect the nature or interpretation of data in another. For example, knowledge that a patient is from a Native American culture could affect interpretation of failure to maintain eye contact on interview. Age may mediate affective reaction to loss of childbearing capacity in women. High ammonia levels in liver disease will affect cognitive capacities on testing and interview. Religious beliefs will affect attitudes toward termination of pregnancy. A barrier-free home environment will facilitate mobility in the spinal cord patient. Negative staff attitudes regarding use of narcotics can result in undermedication of cancer pain. Legislative policies regarding disability can affect sick role behavior. Family knowledge and support can affect compliance with medical regimens. Diazepam can lower baseline EMG levels. And in one case we became aware that a foul-smelling discharge so pervaded a patient's hospital room that staff unwittingly avoided contact, which led to increased patient isolation and distress.

The demand characteristics associated with the assessment are also crucial to consider as they can differ substantially for the same problem (e.g., a patient with congestive heart failure making application for disability versus a waiting-list for transplantation). Furthermore, clinical settings may have different base rates of problems encountered (e.g., dementia in nursing homes, risk-takers in orthopedic wards, gunshot wounds in inner city emergency areas, child abuse in pediatric clinics, somatization disorders in pain clinics).

To practice competently in clinical health psychology, one must have a firm grounding in the theoretical and empirical bases of the specialty, including an ability to integrate knowledge about the biological, social, cognitive and affective bases of health and disease with biological, social, cognitive and affective bases of behavior. One must have an appreciation of the special ethical issues that can be encountered, and personal comfort in working with the physically ill and injured. In the United States, competency is recognized through board certification by the American Board of Professional Psychology. In addition, the American Psychological Association has formally recognized Clinical Health Psychology as a specialty in professional practice.

No matter how competent the professional, the most elegant and accurate conceptualization is of little value without the ability to effectively communicate with relevant stakeholders. "The rule of thumb is to be concrete, practical, brief and succinct" (Belar & Deardorff, 1995, p. 30). Psychological jargon, whether it be psychoanalytic or behavioral, is to be avoided, as is unnecessary revelation of personal information in the patient's medical chart. Recommendations should speak directly to the referral question and have clear implications for health care providers' behavior. To better capture their attention, we also recommend the development of report formats that speak directly to the kinds of referrals (e.g., using headings such as "Factors Impacting Pain Management", "Motivation for Oocyte Donation", "Readiness for Transplant Surgery"), and the avoidance of extensive summary sections.

Charting itself should be in accordance with the regulations of the particular facility; these rules can be as specific as identifying what color ink can be used and which abbreviations are authorized. Verbal communication with the referral source/health care providers is also encouraged, as it is through these communications that the psychologist is better able to ascertain whether there are misinterpretations of forwarded recommendations.

# Pitfalls in clinical health psychology assessment

This section highlights common pitfalls that clinical health psychologists may encounter during the assessment process. The examples offered are either ones we have experienced ourselves, or ones reported by colleagues. It is hoped that with increased awareness of potential problems, psychologists can develop their own prevention strategies.

## MISUNDERSTANDING THE REFERRAL QUESTION

Referrals are often too vague. For example, a post-cardiac transplant patient may be referred for "personality evaluation", a broad request that makes choice of assessment procedures difficult and can hinder practicality of recommendations for the referral source. It is also known that referrals are sometimes prompted more by staff-patient interaction or family issues than problems the patient is experiencing. Direct contact with the referring agent regarding the reason for assessment is always recommended. This also provides more opportunities for training consultees as to how to prepare patients for psychological consultation.

## INAPPROPRIATE REFERRALS

Sometimes requests are for services outside the scope of practice of clinical health psychologists (e.g., "please determine ability to drive", "are medications warranted for enuresis?"). Although psychologists can provide information very relevant to these decisions, consultees need to be educated regarding appropriate practice boundaries. Requests for individual tests (e.g., "give MMPI") are also inappropriate but not uncommon.

Some referrals are inappropriately timed. For example, we received a request for neuropsychological evaluation for attentional problems in a 17-year-old female who was suicidal and homicidal. Although testing was possible, emotional and motivational issues raised serious questions about the reliability and validity of the data. A recommendation for delay in testing until the patient was more stabilized was more judicious given the risk of future misapplication of the obtained test findings.

## FAILURE TO PROVIDE INFORMED CONSENT REGARDING ISSUES OF CONFIDENTIALITY

Clinical health psychologists often collaborate with other professions in the care of patients, thus patients must be informed of any limits to confidentiality in these arrangements. For example, psychologists performing pre-transplant evaluations must disclose to the patient that information obtained will be shared with transplant team members. Informing patients of psychologists' duties to protect and to safeguard the patient's welfare can also avert later misunderstanding and ill feelings by patients who might have assumed blanket confidentiality. Informed consent for psychological consultation includes a discussion of: (1) reasons for the referral; (2) the expected content (e.g., interview, questionnaires, psychological testing); (3) the expected participants (patient, spouse, interviewer); (4) the estimated length of the evaluation; and (5) the recipient(s) and use of the assessment information. In short, failure to discuss known limits to confidentiality is unethical.

## FAILURE TO CLARIFY THE MEANING OF PSYCHOLOGICAL CONSULTATION FOR THE PATIENT

Unlike mental health patients, medical patients often do not initiate their own psychological consultation. In fact they often hold health beliefs that significantly impede the establishment of rapport and the attainment of information. A common attitude is that referral to a psychologist means that their physician thinks their problem is "mental", an attitude that leads to considerable hostility and defensiveness on initial contact. It is critical to initially address potential misconceptions about the role of psychology in health. Patients usually respond well to such discussions since it can serve to demystify the evaluation. It also communicates respect for the patient, and can promote more active participation.

## FAILURE TO USE APPROPRIATE ASSESSMENT PROCEDURES

Assessments tools must be selected judiciously in health psychology assessment. For example, relying solely on interview information for chronic pain patients precludes the use of valuable information that could be obtained from psychometric instruments available for use in this population. In other cases, measures might be inappropriately applied. And in seriously ill patients, requesting extensive participation in energy consuming testing that provides little additional information is problematic; obtaining information from secondary sources (e.g., parents/caretakers) is often more helpful.

## USE OF INAPPROPRIATE NORMATIVE GROUPS

Clinicians sometimes select inappropriate norms for comparison of test results. For example, standard psychiatric interpretations of the Conversion V on MMPI are inappropriate for chronic pain patients, yet we have seen such statements in patients' charts. Although there is sometimes confusion over whether to use general or illness-specific norms, it is recommended that illness-specific norms be used when the question refers to a patient's psychological adjustment to illness (Rozensky et al., 1997). Clinicians should also consult up-to-date norms that are developed locally, or published in research journals (e.g., Putzke et al., 1997).

## FAILURE TO CONSIDER SETTING-RELATED ISSUES

Salient factors which can affect hospital-based evaluations include lack of privacy with a roommate present, sense of isolation due to confinement after a bone marrow transplant, lack of rest due to emergent activities with other patients in an intensive care unit, increased nervousness due to nicotine withdrawal in a nonsmoking environment and stress of treatment itself for claustrophobic individuals needing hyperbaric chamber treatment. We have seen over, under, and inappropriate interpretation of data from failure to consider the impact of setting-related issues.

## FAILURE TO CONSIDER THE PATIENT WITHIN THE DEVELOPMENTAL CONTINUUM

Life stage (e.g., child, adolescence, young adult, senior citizen) is a critical factor in determining attitudes and beliefs about health, disease, and traumatic events. For example, although the overall level of distress might be similar, the psychological components of reactions to a proposed hysterectomy may be substantially different for a 20-year-old than a 60-year-old female, with subsequent differing treatment implications.

## FAILURE TO CONSIDER ISSUES OF DIVERSITY

Eurocentric psychologists can inappropriately interpret poor eye contact as deceitfulness or sullenness in some ethnic groups (e.g., Native American, African American), or nodding and smiling as agreement in others (e.g., in Asians). Failure to inquire about indigenous health practices (e.g., coining) can lead to erroneous conclusions about child abuse. Young and Zane (1995) provide an excellent overview of ethnocultural influences in evaluation.

## FAILURE TO RECOGNIZE PSYCHOPATHOLOGY

Clinicians who overlook identifiable psychological problems risk inaccurate test interpretation and treatment recommendations. For example, if consulted to treat a patient with frequent vomiting post gastric bypass surgery, the clinician assuming only medical problems as precursors to the surgery might neglect important psychological problems that have significant implications for treatment (e.g., eating disorder, anxiety). And for a cancer patient beginning chemotherapy, the diagnosis and treatment of Bipolar Disorder may be crucial to ensure consistent adherence to treatment. Identification of psychopathology can also alert to the potential for self-destructive behavior (e.g., reckless driving, excessive drinking). Although psychopathology is not the major focus of practice in clinical health psychology, competence in its diagnosis and treatment is important in providing truly integrated care.

## FAILURE TO CONSIDER THEORY, OR OVERRELIANCE ON ONE THEORETICAL MODEL

In health psychology assessment, consideration of a variety of psychological models of health and disease is essential for case conceptualization and treatment planning (Di Scipio & Weigand, 1989). In fact, without theory, integration of seemingly divergent data can be a rather arduous, if not fruitless task. Consider a liver transplant recipient who shows a nonchalant attitude towards ongoing alcohol consumption. The use of the Health Belief Model can facilitate the development of an intervention program that targets relevant variables such as perceived susceptibility, severity, benefits and barriers of action (Becker, 1974). In the area of chronic pain, the design of contingency management aspects of a rehabilitation program relies heavily on an operant learning model, while affective components in pain (e.g., depression) might be best treated utilizing a cognitive-behavioral model. It is our belief that over-reliance on a single theoretical framework is not warranted given the variety of problems encountered in clinical health psychology. For example, it would be a mistake to be wedded to an operant learning model when attempting to deal with a classically conditioned response such as anticipatory nausea.

## FAILURE TO OBTAIN BACKGROUND INFORMATION

Valuable time and effort can be saved by reviewing previous medical records prior to evaluation. Clinicians can avoid the repetition of known facts, can check for consistency where important, and may more adeptly elaborate on ideas and issues related to the referral question. Psychologists who have the patient "start from scratch" are often seen as "outsiders" to the health care team. We are also aware of numerous incidents when lack of knowledge that had been available in the medical record led to serious misinterpretations of behavior during the initial interview (e.g., hearing deficits interpreted as confusion, medication effects interpreted as anxiety).

## FAILURE TO FOLLOW-UP
Consultees often complain about lack of follow-up after referral to psychologists. This is sometimes due to lack of communication as in large health care systems psychological records are often kept separately for reasons of confidentiality. However, integrated care requires that at least some information be communicated; all follow-up efforts should be documented.

Sometimes lack of follow-up is the result of unclear role expectations. For example, when a recommendation is made for a repeat evaluation, the consultee may assume the psychologist will take primary responsibility for scheduling, while the psychologist may be awaiting another consultation request. At the time of the initial consultation feedback it is wise to clarify (in writing) who will be responsible for which aspects of follow-up. It is also prudent to track such patients in one's own practice. When operating as a member of a health care team, the risk of diffusion of responsibility appears even greater.

## FAILURE TO RECOGNIZE BOUNDARIES OF COMPETENCE
Psychological assessment in the medical setting requires specialized knowledge and skills that are not always part of traditional education and training programs (Belar, 1980). Practitioners must have knowledge of biological, social, cognitive and affective bases of health and disease as well as behavior. They must have skills with health psychology assessment methods as detailed throughout this text, and understand the sociopolitical aspects of the health care system. In addition, they must be prepared for the special ethical, legal and professional issues encountered. The risks of incompetent practice are not only to the patient, but to the credibility of the profession as well.

## IGNORANCE OF THE ROLE OF OTHER HEALTH PROFESSIONALS
Significant contributions to health care are made by a variety of disciplines, sometimes with overlapping roles and functions. Although psychology has unique contributions to make, discipline pride must not be

confused with professional chauvinism. There is overlap in roles and functions between disciplines and psychologists may overlook the usefulness of other health care providers. One example is the provision of therapeutic services. In some cases, supportive care provided by a Social Worker or Chaplain may be sufficient. However, intervention decisions will depend on factors such as the patient's needs, health status, resources, and preferences.

## Future directions

The purpose of assessment in clinical health psychology is to understand interactions between the person, his or her health status, and the environment. It requires the integration of physiological, psychological, and sociological information, and its future is dependent upon the development of new knowledge about interrelationships in these areas. Historically, clinical health psychology has developed through the integration of research with practice. We foresee continued growth given the steady discovery of new knowledge and the failure of the biomedical model to adequately explain health and illness.

We predict that the trend to develop health-specific measures with appropriate normative data will continue and, in fact, expand. We will also witness the development of more ecologically valid methods of measurement of biopsychosocial components through the use of advanced technologies such as that used in ambulatory monitoring. And with the increased use of psychological assessment for tracking cognitive, affective and behavioral outcomes of medical treatments, we expect an increased focus on the development of measures concerning quality of life.

We also anticipate increased use of computer technology in the assessment process and do have some concerns that easy access to computerized assessments can bypass those professionals who are psychometrically trained and skilled in the integration of test information with clinical data. If inappropriate diagnostic labels or treatment decisions are made from the use of such methods, patients could suffer. There is a need for more research on the potential of untoward consequences of widespread psychological risk assessment, such as that found by Cummings (1985). Without sufficient attention to these issues, there may be a backlash in health care regarding clinical health psychology assessment similar to what we have witnessed regarding intelligence assessment in school systems. Psychologists may need to assume more professional and patient advocacy in these areas.

But we are more encouraged than discouraged. Clinical health psychology is a growing specialty that is rapidly becoming mainstream in the discipline and in health care.

# References

Andersen, B.T., & Haley, W.E. (1997). Clinical geropsychology: Implications for practice in medical settings. *Journal of Clinical Psychology in Medical Settings, 4,* 193–205.

Beck, A.T. (1972). *Depression: Causes and treatment.* Philadelphia: University of Pennsylvania Press.

Becker, M.H. (Ed.) (1974). *The health belief model and personal health behavior.* Thorofare, NJ: Charles B. Slack.

Belar, C.D. (1980). Training of clinical psychology students in behavioral medicine. *Professional Psychology, 11,* 620–627.

Belar, C.D. (1997). Clinical health psychology: A specialty for the 21st century. *Health Psychology, 16,* 1–6.

Belar, C.D., & Kibrick, S. (1986). Biofeedback in the treatment of chronic back pain. In: A. Holzman & D. Turk (Eds.), *Pain management: A handbook of psychological treatment approaches* (pp. 131–150). New York: Pergamon Press.

Belar, C.D., & Deardorff, W.W. (1995). *Clinical health psychology in medical settings: A practitioner's guidebook* (rev. ed.). Washington, DC: American Psychological Association.

Belar, C.D., Deardorff, W.W., & Kelly, K.E. (1987). *The practice of clinical health psychology.* New York: Pergamon Press.

Benton, A.L., Sivan, A.B., Hamsher, K. deS., Varney, N.R., & Spreen, O. (1983). *Contributions to neuropsychological assessment.* New York: Oxford University Press.

Bergner, M., Bobbitt, R.A., Carter, W.B., & Gilson, B.S. (1981). The Sickness Impact Profile: Development and final revision of a health status measure. *Medical Care, 19,* 787–806.

Bornstein, R.A. (1985). Normative data on selected neuropsychological measures from a nonclinical sample. *Journal of Clinical Psychology, 41,* 651–659.

Center for Disease Control and Prevention (CDC) (1997). Cigarette smoking among adults—United States, 1995. *Morbidity and Mortality Weekly Report (MMWR), 46,* 1217–1220.

Cummings, N.A. (1985). Assessing the computer's impact: Professional concerns. *Computers in Human Behavior, 1,* 291–300.

Deshields, T.L., Mannen, K., Tait, R.C., & Bajaj, V. (1997). Quality of life in heart transplant candidates. *Journal of Clinical Psychology in Medical Settings, 4,* 327–341.

Derogatis, L.R. (1986). The Psychosocial Adjustment to Illness Scale (PAIS). *Journal of Psychosomatic Research, 30,* 77–91.

Di Scipio, W.J., & Weigand, P.A. (1989). In: S. Wetzler & M.M. Katz (Eds.), *Contemporary approaches to psychological assessment* (pp. 325–334). New York: Brunner/Mazel.

Engel, G.L. (1977). The need for a new medical model: A challenge for biomedicine. *Science, 196,* 129–136.

Eriksson, B.S., & Rosenquist, U. (1993). Social support and glycemic control in non-insulin diabetes mellitus patients: Gender differences. *Women and Health, 20,* 59–70.

Fillingim, R.B. (1997). The future of psychology in pain management. *Journal of Clinical Psychology in Medical Settings, 4,* 207–218.

First, M.B. (1997). *Structured clinical interview for DSM-IV axis I disorders SCID-I: Clinical version, administration booklet.* Washington, DC: American Psychiatric Press.

Folkman, S., & Lazarus, R. (1980). An analysis of coping in a middle-aged community sample. *Journal of Health and Social Behavior, 21,* 219–239.

Hare, D.L., & Davis, C.R. (1996). Cardiac depression scale: Validation of a new depression scale for cardiac patients. *Journal of Psychosomatic Research, 40,* 379–386.

Jewell, D.A. (1989). Cultural and ethnic issues. In: S. Wetzler & M.M. Katz (Eds.), *Contemporary approaches to psychological assessment* (pp. 299–309). New York: Brunner/Mazel Publishers.

Keefe F., & Block, A. (1982). Development of an observational method for assessing pain behavior in chronic low back pain patients. *Behavior Therapy, 13,* 363–375.

Keh-Ming, L. (1996). Cultural influences on the diagnosis of psychotic and organic disorders. In: J.E. Mezzick, A. Kleinman, H. Falirega Jr., & D.L. Parron (Eds.), *Culture and psychiatric diagnosis: A DSM IV perspective* (pp. 49–62). Washington, DC: American Psychiatric Press.

La Greca, A.M., Swales, T., Klemp, S., Madigan, S., & Skyler, J. (1995). Adolescents with diabetes: Gender differences in psychosocial functioning and glycemic control. *Children's Health Care, 24,* 61–78.

Leigh, H., & Reiser, M.F. (1980). *Biological, psychological and social dimensions of medical practice.* New York: Plenum.

Melzack, R. (1975). The McGill Pain Questionnaire: Major properties and scoring methods. *Pain, 1,* 277–279.

Meenan, R., Gertman, P., & Mason, J. (1982). The Arthritis Impact Measurement Scales: Further investigation of a health status measure. *Arthritis and Rheumatology, 25,* 1048–1053.

Merluzzi, T.V., & Martinez Sanchez, M.A. (1997). Assessment of self-efficacy and coping with cancer: Development and validation of the cancer behavior inventory. *Health Psychology, 16,* 163–170.

Nunnally, J.C. (1978). *Psychometric theory* (second edition). New York: McGraw-Hill.

Olbrisch, M., Levenson, J., & Hamer, R. (1989). The PACT: A rating scale for the study of clinical decision-making in psychosocial screening of organ transplant candidates. *Clinical Transplantation, 3,* 1–6.

Piotrowski, C., & Lubin, B. (1990). Assessment practices of health psychologists: Survey of APA Division 38 clinicians. *Professional Psychology: Research and Practice, 21,* 99–106.

Putzke, J.D., Williams, M.A., Millsaps, C.L., Azrin, R.L., LaMarche, J.A., Bourge, R.C., Kirklin, J.K., McGiffin, D.C., & Boll, T.J. (1997). Heart transplantation candidates: A neuropsychological descriptive database. *Journal of Clinical Psychology in Medical Settings, 4,* 343–355.

Raczynski, J.M., & Lewis, C.E. (1992). Scientific needs. In: D.M. Becker, D.R. Hill, J.S. Jackson, D.M. Levine, F.A. Stillman, & S.M. Weiss (Eds.), *Health behavior research in minority populations: Access, design and implementation* (NIH Publication No. 92–2965, pp. 218–228). Washington, DC: U.S. Department of Health and Human Services.

Robins, L.N., Helzer, J.E., Croughton, J.L., & Ratcliff, K.S. (1981). National institute of mental health diagnostic interview schedule. *Archives of General Psychiatry, 38,* 381–389.

Robinson, L.A., & Klesges, R.C. (1997). Ethnic and gender differences in risk factors for smoking onset. *Health Psychology, 16,* 499–505.

Rodrigue, J.R. (1997). An examination of race differences in patients' psychological adjustment to cancer. *Journal of Clinical Psychology in Medical Settings, 4,* 271–280.

Rosenman, R. (1978). The interview method of assessment of the coronary-prone behavior pattern. In: T.M. Dembroski, S.M. Weiss, J.L. Shields, S.G. Haynes, & M. Feinleib (Eds.), *Coronary-prone behavior* (pp. 55–70). New York: Springer-Verlag.

Rozensky, R.H., Sweet, J.J., & Tovian, S.M. (1997). *Psychological assessment in medical settings.* New York: Plenum.

Ruch, L., Gartell, J., Ramelli, A., & Coyne, B. (1991). The Clinical Trauma Assessment: Evaluating sexual assault victims in the emergency room. *Psychological Assessment, 3,* 404–411.

Turk, D.C., & Kerns, R.D. (1985). Assessment in health psychology: A cognitive behavioral perspective. In: P. Karoly (Ed.), *Measurement strategies in health psychology* (pp. 335–372). New York: Wiley.

Ware, J.E., Jr., Snow, K.K., Kosinski, M., & Gandek, B. (1993). *SF-36 Health Survey: Manual and interpretation guide.* Boston: The Health Institute, New England Medical Center.

Weidner, G., Boughal, T., Connor, S.L., Pieper, C., & Mendell, N.R. (1997). Relationship of job strain to standard coronary risk factors and psychological characteristics in women and men of the Family Heart Study, *Health Psychology*, 16, 239–247.

Young, K., & Zane, N. (1995). Ethnocultural influences in evaluation and management. In: P.M. Nicassio & T.W. Smith (Eds.), *Managing chronic illness. A biopsychosocial perspective* (pp. 163–206). Washington DC: American Psychological Association.

# 2 SOME METHODOLOGICAL CONSIDERATIONS IN THE STUDY OF PSYCHOSOCIAL INFLUENCES ON HEALTH

Stanislav V. Kasl and Beth A. Jones

We begin by describing our orientation and the scope and aims of this chapter. Our perspective is that of *psychosocial epidemiology*, that is, the interdisciplinary domain of investigations dealing with social and psychological risk factors for health and disease outcomes in the population. These psychosocial risk factors can influence:

(1) *Incidence:* new cases of a disease in a defined population, initially free of the disease, within a specified period of time.
(2) *Recurrence:* development of additional episodes of a disease, among the incident cases, within a specified period of time.
(3) *Case Fatality:* the proportion of cases of a disease who die within a specified period of time.
(4) *Cause Specific or Total Mortality:* deaths over a specified period of time in a cohort not selected for presence or absence of disease at baseline.

The above are the major outcomes in population epidemiology. Within the framework of clinical epidemiology, psychosocial risk factors can also be examined as influences on the *recovery* process, the rate at which a person achieves functional recovery or becomes symptom free.

In psychosocial epidemiology, the frequently studied major risk factors include: position in social structure and characteristics of the social or interpersonal environment; stable personality traits or characteristics and indicators of psychological functioning and well-being; exposure to chronic stressors arising out of performance of major social roles; and exposure to changing life circumstances, often labeled "stressful life events."

The influence of social and psychological variables on health status indicators is typically examined in the context of a comprehensive set of biological variables, above all those which can be viewed as established risk factors for a particular disease outcome. The intent here is usually to demonstrate the independent contribution of the psychosocial risk factor above and beyond the contribution of the established biomedical risk factors and to explore the interplay of the psychosocial and the biomedical variables in contributing to disease etiology and disease progression.

The aim of this chapter is to discuss selected methodological issues which uniquely pertain to the study of psychosocial risk for physical illness. This discussion is organized around several broad topics: epidemiological guidelines for inferring causality, an idealized research paradigm from a disease development perspective, observational designs and their strengths and limitations, and potential biases in the measurement of psychosocial risk factors for disease.

These issues are selected because the overwhelming majority of studies use observational designs (a term from epidemiology) or quasi-experimental designs (a term from the social sciences). While excellent texts exist for epidemiology (e.g., Kelsey et al., 1996) and for the social sciences (e.g., Cook & Campbell, 1979), there is no methodological textbook for psychosocial epidemiology. Thus our organization of these topics cannot depend on precedents established in available textbooks. The overarching objective of this chapter is to help us determine *whether or not* a psychosocial risk factor is truly involved in the etiology of a particular adverse health outcome, and *how* it is involved in such etiology. We draw on our previous examinations of the issues (e.g., Kasl, 1985; Kasl & Cooper, 1987) for the organization of this material.

It should be appreciated that the apparently separate topics of study designs and measurement biases are usually intertwined in psychosocial epidemiology studies. For example, the possible influence of disease on the putative risk factor ("reverse causation") in case-control retrospective designs is generally absent in prospective designs using an initially healthy cohort (hopefully also free of subclinical disease). As another example, the concern over conceptual and methodological overlap in the operationalization of both the independent and dependent variables, such as reported exposure to stressors and symptoms of disease, is negligible when the measured outcome is instead a physiological variable.

## Epidemiological guidelines for inferring causality

In epidemiology, as in the social sciences, the fundamental assertion in causal relationships is that the manipulation of a cause will result in the manipulation (change) of an effect (e.g., Rothman, 1988; Susser, 1991). While epidemiologists prefer the term "risk factor" over "cause," there would be little interest in risk factors if they were not, at least indirectly, involved in the etiology of disease. Given that epidemiology uses mostly observational designs, guidelines or criteria have evolved for judging the likelihood of an association being causal without depending on direct demonstration of experimental change. We shall examine the major ones as they may be applicable to the study of psychosocial risk factors (Hill, 1965; Susser, 1991). It should be noted that the epidemiological tradition of examining the extent to which the evidence meets the criteria for causal inference needs to be supplemented by the social science tradition, so ably begun by Campbell and Stanley (1966), of posing rival hypotheses or rival causal processes and examining the extent to which the evidence allows the rejection of such rival explanations.

Below, we discuss five of the most important "criteria" for inferring a causal relationship. Our comments are selected to be particularly pertinent to psychosocial epidemiology.

## CORRECT TEMPORAL SEQUENCE OF CAUSE AND EFFECT

Given that the prospective follow-up of an initially healthy cohort for later development of incident episodes of disease is considered the best design in observational epidemiology (albeit expensive and almost infeasible for rare outcomes), the evidence of the proper temporal sequence is clearly important: it allows us to argue that the disease outcome did not influence the risk factor. But of course, many non-causal associations could be of the right temporal order and thus this evidence is far from sufficient. Furthermore, in psychosocial epidemiology, it is often very difficult to determine the correct temporal location of the risk factors or exposure variables. A few examples: (a) While retirement can be a temporally discrete event, planning for retirement and anticipating its consequences can have health consequences before the actual formal date of retiring. (b) Separation and divorce can be preceded by years of a changing marital relationship and determining the proper sequence between divorce and depression may be extremely difficult. (c) Health status changes after death of spouse may be difficult to establish if there was a long period of burdensome care giving which produced worsened health status in the surviving spouse well before the death of the spouse.

In cross-sectional and retrospective designs the temporal order is likely to be difficult to establish. One influence on the relative difficulty are the clinical features of the disease and the associated medical care seeking behavior. Conditions which have a sudden and memorable onset, such as the first attack of gout, are relatively easy to locate in time and individual differences in medical care seeking are relatively small. On the other hand, rheumatoid arthritis can be an episodic condition of gradual onset, may be fully remitting, and has considerable variation in medical care seeking. Here onset may be difficult to pin down and its temporal relation to psychosocial risk factors will be unclear.

## CONSISTENCY OF EVIDENCE

This guideline suggests that consistent evidence of an association is needed before it becomes a candidate for causal interpretation. It needs to be noted that consistent findings are not impressive if studies share the same design weaknesses and we are thus unable to reduce the number of plausible rival hypotheses. However, consistency of results based on designs that use different methods and have different limitations to them is much more valuable. The difficulty with this criterion, as with the previous one, is that many non-causal associations can be quite consistent as well and thus this requirement is again not sufficient.

Another dilemma is how to distinguish between inconsistent evidence and high specificity of etiological dynamics. The latter may be due to the presence of strong moderators which define the specific circumstances under which the (causal) association will be observed. Such specificity puts limits on the generalizability of the observed effects but need not force us to doubt its causal nature. For example, the influence of social networks on mortality can be truly different depending on whether it is an urban or a rural setting (Seeman et al., 1993). It is tempting to argue that in classical epidemiology, the underlying biological processes are less likely to vary according to time and place than are psychosocial etiologic processes involved in studies in psychosocial epidemiology.

Non-replication can also come from inadequate operational specificity of a particular construct. For example, hostility appears to play an etiological role in coronary heart disease but many measures of anger-hostility do not zero in on what appears to be the crucial behavioral component (Siegman & Smith, 1994) and thus will not show the association. This kind of a situation, again arguably more common in psychosocial than classical epidemiology, need not undermine our interpretation that causal dynamics are involved in such an association.

## STRENGTH OF THE ASSOCIATION

It is generally suggested that stronger associations are more likely to be causal than weaker associations. Immediately, however, one has to spell out some qualifiers and explanations in order to prevent thoughtless application of this simple guideline. The basic assumption here seems to be that biases and confounders can produce weak associations but are unlikely to produce a strong one. A related assumption is that biases producing weak associations can be subtle and hard to detect, but biases producing strong associations are likely to be obvious and easily detected, thus reducing the likelihood that we would even propose a causal interpretation until that bias was controlled.

Those assumptions about biases may be correct in specific instances but seem unconvincing across the board. Powerful biases can be present under some circumstances: (a) If one relies on a single method and a single occasion to collect both exposure and outcome data, then strong influences on self-report (recall, social desirability, "negative affectivity") are shared by both sets of measurements (e.g., Watson & Clark, 1984; Watson & Pennebaker, 1989). (b) If there is an inadequate conceptual separation of exposure and outcome, such as treating "vital exhaustion" as a risk factor for a heart attack when it could reflect the prodromal period preceding overt clinical disease (Appels & Mulder, 1988); however, the issue is not clear cut since vital exhaustion can predict new cardiac events even after controlling for severity of coronary atherosclerosis (Kop et al., 1994). (c) If there exists a popular lay notion of etiology, such as stress and heart disease (Marmot, 1982; Shekelle & Lin, 1978), then the search for explanation among cases of heart disease in a case-control design may produce strong retrospection biases.

The guideline regarding strength of association is particularly inappropriate when one is comparing risk factor data across diseases. For example, when the sufficient cause for a multifactorial disease consists of several component causes (which must all be present), then the low prevalence of one of the components in a particular population lowers the estimate of the impact of another component cause, one with greater prevalence. But a comparison unifactorial disease may have a sufficient cause which consists of a single variable and this may produce a strong association.

There are also technical reasons for mistrusting the guideline regarding strength of association. For example, when a continuous risk factor is dichotomized at an extreme cut point, it will produce higher risk estimates for a disease than when it is dichotomized at a more moderate level. Another example is that individual matching of cases and controls leads to higher estimated risk than is obtained in unmatched designs because of the way the data are analyzed.

## DOSE-RESPONSE EFFECT (BIOLOGICAL GRADIENT)

The basic idea here is that an association which shows a dose-response relationship is more likely to be causal than one which doesn't. The fact that this is also referred to as the "biological gradient" suggests that biological theory (about underlying biological mechanisms) usually leads to the expectation of such a gradient. Therefore its absence points to the influence of non-biological (non-causal) variables, such as biases and confounders. The value of this guideline seems to hinge pretty much on the assumption that dose-response gradients are less common for the rival hypotheses involving alternate explanations of the obtained association. Several comments are in order here. First, dose-response effects are exceedingly common for biases and confounders as well; e.g., the uncontrolled effects of age or education are very likely to be linear as well. Thus one needs additional evidence to suggest that a particular confounder would not produce a dose-response effect. For example, the association between body mass and mortality in adults (but not the elderly) shows a U-shaped curve with higher mortality at both ends of the body mass distribution. However, controlling for smoking status and pre-existing illnesses does produce the expected gradient. Second, non-linear effects can still reflect a causal relationship. For example, the evidence for an association between social isolation and adverse health outcomes (e.g., Berkman, 1995; Kaplan, 1992) suggests that there may be a threshold effect rather than that the benefits of social relations continue to increase as size of networks or quantity of interaction goes up. Similarly, the research literature on the effects of residential crowding on mental health (Kasl, 1977) suggests that there is a non-linear but (suggestively) causal association: increasing levels of crowding do not have an adverse impact until very high levels of crowding are examined.

## BIOLOGICAL PLAUSIBILITY

The idea here is that the proposed causal relationship should be biologically plausible and not violate any firm principles about known biological pathways or mechanisms. The applicability to psychosocial epidemiology is somewhat limited, particularly in designs and analyses where the risk factor of interest is shown to act independently of the known biological risk factors. Here the biological plausibility cannot be appraised since the statistical model building intentionally controls for the plausible (known) biological risks.

The value of this guideline is limited by two considerations: (a) Given the great complexity of human biology and the many possible pathways of influence, coming up with a plausible biological mechanism may not be a very discriminating requirement. For example, almost any psychosocial variable can be linked, theoretically, to stress hormone dynamics (Baum & Grunberg, 1995) or to immune system functioning (Kiecolt-Glaser & Glaser, 1995). (b) What is plausible is tied to the state of contemporary evidence. For example, the relatively recent information about the role of helicobacter pylori in the etiology of peptic ulcer disease (Dunn et al., 1997) changes the meaning of biological plausibility drastically from the period during which much of the psychosomatic research on ulcers was conducted (Weiner, 1977) but the role of this bacterium was unrecognized. Similarly, before Ader's pioneering work in psychoneuroimmunology (Ader et al., 1991), the notion of a conditioned immunological response was considered biologically implausible.

## OTHER GUIDELINES

Among the original criteria proposed for inferring causality, Hill (1965) listed also specificity, coherence, and experimental manipulation. Specificity refers to the situation where a single putative cause produces a specific health effect. This appears to be a criterion of limited applicability. In classical epidemiology, the fact that a risk factor such as cigarette smoking has multiple disease consequences does not increase our suspicion that the associations are non-causal. In psychosocial epidemiology, it is even more common to deal with multiplicity of health consequences when dealing with broad constructs such as poverty or social support. However, it should be recognized that should we decompose highly complex exposures such as smoking or poverty into constituent elements, we might observe more specificity of effects. The criterion of coherence refers to the notion that the association should be compatible with existing theory and knowledge; however, this appears to be no more than a more general restatement of the biological plausibility criterion. And the criterion of experimental manipulation is more or less a restatement of the fundamental notion of what is a causal relationship.

As indicated already, studies in psychosocial epidemiology generally seek to demonstrate that the psychosocial risk factor affects the health outcome independently of known biological risk factors. This is typically done in multivariate modeling rather than through original study design, such as matching subjects. It is thus tempting to conclude that, for psychosocial epidemiology, another criterion for causal inference is that the relationship of the putative psychosocial risk factor be maintained after controlling for biological risk factors. However, this is incorrect whenever the variable for which we are controlling is not a confounder but a mediator. Thus vigorous exercise influences cardiovascular health through raising High-Density Lipoprotein (HDL) cholesterol. Adjusting for HDL levels may wipe out the association of vigorous exercise with cardiovascular health but this in no way demonstrates that the original association was not causal.

## Formulating an idealized research paradigm

Thus far we have discussed guidelines or criteria for causal inference. Clearly, whether or not the findings allow such inference is closely linked to types of research designs, our next topic. We approach this in two steps: formulating an idealized research paradigm and then evaluating specific research designs common to observational epidemiology.

Since evaluating an association between a psychosocial variable and a health outcome in relation to possible underlying etiological processes is based both on the use of the guidelines for causation and the strategy of ruling out rival hypotheses, it is useful to have a formulation of an "ideal" study which can then facilitate the systematic evaluation of data from actual studies. We will consider such an ideal design from two perspectives: the *disease development paradigm* and *the natural experiment paradigm*. While the two perspectives complement each other, the former is more useful when one is studying stable psychosocial characteristics as influences on the disease process, while the latter is more useful when we are looking at psychosocial exposures (experiences) affecting the disease process.

*The disease development paradigm* starts with a formulation of the natural history of progression of a particular disease from the biomedical viewpoint. For coronary heart disease (CHD), the important stages in the development can be characterized as follows:

(a) asymptomatic status, risk factor(s) absent;
(b) asymptomatic status, risk factor(s) present;
(c) subclinical disease susceptible to detection;
(d) intial symptom experience;

(e)  initial episode of disease, with diagnostic criteria being met;
(f)  course of disease (repeat episodes, residual disability, etc.);
(g)  mortality (case fatality).

Admittedly, this paradigm could be made more complicated by grafting onto it a medical care perspective. That is, each of the above transitions can be preceded or followed by medical care contacts which can affect the transitions to later stages.

One purpose of the above paradigm is to guide our evaluation of existing evidence. When we have informative designs, the paradigm enables us to pinpoint the role of the psychosocial variable. More often, unfortunately, we will be using the paradigm to acknowledge uncertainties in the evidence and to catalogue the possible ways in which an association could be interpreted. For example, when a community sample of adults is followed for CHD mortality (e.g., Berkman & Breslow, 1983) and we only have the baseline data and the outcome, it becomes very difficult to determine the specific way a psychosocial variable acts to influence mortality. On the other hand, a study of the impact of marital status on in-hospital survival after acute myocardial infarction (Chandra et al., 1983), was a design which enabled the investigators to pin down the influence precisely. Thus in looking at in-hospital case fatality, they adjusted for 12 potential confounders (e.g., sociodemographics, clinical history, treatment received, etc.) so that marital status was an independent effect on short term survival. Of course, while the design allows one form of precision (locating the influence of the variable of interest), on the other hand the measure of the psychosocial variable, marital status, is quite imprecise in terms of telling us which of many possible underlying processes could be producing the result: marital status could be linked to level of social and emotional support, frequency of visits at the hospital, sense of responsibility for dependents, will to live, lower depression, and so on.

Another purpose of the paradigm is for planning one's study. For example, it can guide us to the segment of disease development which is in the greatest need of clarification or new information. Similarly, if we wish to study several stages (transitions) of development, it reminds us of the need to be thoughtful about the monitoring and scheduling of repeat data collections before final outcome is assessed. It needs to be noted that the usefulness of the disease development schema changes as new technologies emerge. For example, with our recent ability to measure progression of carotid atherosclerosis noninvasively with ultrasonography, we can now study effects of psychosocial variables, such as hostility, on subclinical progression (Julkunen et al., 1994).

Different diseases obviously have different developmental schemata, while those with unknown etiology may not allow any guiding schema at all. For infectious mononucleosis (IM), the role of psychosocial variables can be seen as follows: (a) those which influence immunity status (presence vs. absence of antibody to Epstein-Barr virus) at the beginning of prospective follow-up: those immune (antibody present) at the start need not be followed; (b) those which influence seroconversion of the susceptibles during follow-up: those who do not become infected cannot develop IM; (c) those which influence the development of overt clinical disease: only about 1/4 of infected have more than a subclinical infection. In our study of IM in West Point cadets (Kasl et al., 1979), these distinctions among psychosocial influences were crucial: high commitment to a military career measured at baseline was protective of becoming infected among susceptibles, but increased the risk of overt disease among those who did become infected. If the design had not included monitoring for seroconversion and military commitment were treated as only a baseline predictor of the ultimate clinical outcome (development of IM during the four years), we would not have been able to detect an association.

*The natural experiment paradigm* highlights the occasional opportunities to conduct an observational field study that has the appearance of an "experiment." In research on the health effects of job loss, we have studies of unexpected factory closures where all the workers lose their jobs (Morris & Cook, 1991). In research on the effects of job insecurity, we have studies of downsizing and planned mergers (Ferrie et al., 1995). In occupational stress research, we have studies of unexpected changes in job demands and work environment (Kittel et al., 1980). In bereavement research, we have prescheduled longitudinal monitoring of cohorts of elderly, some of whom become widowed during follow-up (Mendes de Leon et al., 1994).

These natural experiments, at their best, tend to have the following characteristics: (a) the total cohort of subjects is picked up before anyone is exposed; (b) proximate preexposure (for those who become exposed) status is nonreactive, i.e. no anticipatory effects or selective preexposure attrition; (c) the environmental condition (exposure) is objectively defined and measured; (d) self-selection factors, which influence exposure status, are minimal or negligible; (e) surveillance for target outcomes is complete (no attrition) and of sufficient duration for health outcomes to manifest themselves; (f) health outcomes are measured objectively.

The salient features of these natural experiments are that self-selection is minimized and that the cohort is picked up before exposure. This is different from the classical epidemiological prospective study which follows an initially healthy cohort; in this approach, the follow-up starts with the cohort already separated at baseline into exposed and unexposed, and the transition from all unexposed to some exposed is not, or cannot be, studied. This makes sense for exposures that are early acquired life-style habits, such as smoking, or for more-or-less stable traits, such as Type A behavior. But for exposures that are adult-onset life circumstances, such as job loss, picking up the cohort before anyone is exposed is valuable.

The notion that the exposure should be measured objectively does not preclude assessing subjective perceptions of, and reactions to, the exposure. However, the subjective measures need to be anchored to some objective operationalization of exposure, even if the latter is rather limited and the former are rich and detailed. We recognize that this point is controversial with those with a strong psychological formulation of exposures as risk factors and we return to an additional discussion of this issue below.

# Methodological concerns linked to specific research design characteristics

Having discussed criteria for causal inference and idealized research paradigms that are optimally informative, we turn to a discussion of the major types of designs utilized in psychosocial epidemiology. We will proceed from strong designs to progressively weaker ones.

### RANDOM ASSIGNMENT TO EXPOSURE OR BENEFICIAL INTERVENTION

It has already been noted that most epidemiologic evidence is observational, not experimental. Thus the rather rare true experimental design is likely to involve randomization to beneficial or ameliorative exposures rather than the unethical strategy of randomly exposing individuals to disease risk. For example, the literature on health effects of job loss does contain social experiments designed to improve the unemployed workers' job seeking skills (Price, 1992).

In principle, the superiority of a randomized design is based on ensuring the comparability of two (or more) groups of subjects on all characteristics except the one(s) under experimental manipulation. In addition, it imposes a temporal ordering on the exposure and outcome variables. Even so, a number of problems can arise which can compromise this design. And if they can arise in this setting, then they are certainly applicable in weaker designs as well. A few illustrative points: (a) The length of follow-up is inadequate for detecting the expected outcome. (b) The intervention fails to show the expected benefit because irreversible subclinical disease development is already under way. (c) The intervention is an incomplete operationalization of the totality of the sufficient cause. (d) The intervention contains more components than intended and identifying the underlying specific relevant causal process becomes difficult. (e) Non-compliance among study subjects is considerable and analysis by compliance status destroys randomization. (f) When investigators are not blinded to exposure or treatment status, the potential for additional problems arises, such as communicating expectations about efficacy of treatment to treated subjects, and biasing assessment of outcome. (g) When subjects are not blinded to treatment status, additional problems (not listed in (f), above) may arise, such as untreated subjects initiating some treatment (crossover) or influences on self-reports (e.g., social desirability, denial) become differential by treatment condition.

## PROSPECTIVE DESIGNS IN WHICH SOME COHORT MEMBERS CHANGE EXPOSURE STATUS

Probably the strongest observational design is one in which the cohort is picked up prospectively with respect both to the development of disease as well as the onset of exposure. Pre-exposure baseline data are thus available and are not influenced by either disease or exposure status. If the design mimics a natural experiment, self-selection is not a major concern (as discussed above). Otherwise, self-selection may be the chief weakness; prior variables which influence both the move into exposure status and disease development could confound the observed association. A limited collection of information regarding potential confounders and a limited understanding of the dynamics of exposure status changes increase the potential problem due to self-selection. For example, in the literature on health effects of unemployment (Kasl & Jones, 2000), unless the whole plant or company closes down, those becoming unemployed could be workers in poorer health, with substance abuse problems, more interpersonal difficulties, and so on. Baseline data on the cohort may be inadequate to adjust for all these variables.

A somewhat weaker design is one in which a cohort consisting of already exposed and unexposed individuals is not only followed for outcomes but is also monitored for change in exposure status among those who have not yet developed the outcome of interest. In the unemployment and health literature, there are studies of employed and unemployed subjects followed over time, with benefits of re-employment examined among the unemployed with new jobs. Better health or lower depression after re-employment could mean the benefits of a new job, but only close and frequent monitoring of the cohort could rule out the alternative scenario, e.g., that they recovered from depression first and then found work. Another weakness is that when we start out with an already unemployed cohort, and they have been unemployed for some time, they are really a subset of a larger group of unemployed, some of whom have self-selected out of eligibility for the study by becoming successfully re-employed.

## TRADITIONAL PROSPECTIVE COHORT DESIGNS

The classical design here is one in which a representative sample of individuals, who are free of a target disease, are assessed at baseline for exposure status and then monitored for the development of the target disease. As noted already, this is considered the premier strong design in observational epidemiology. However, as we discuss below, there will be specific instances where plausible rival hypotheses cannot be easily ruled out and where causal inferences may seem less appropriate.

Strictly speaking, this design only ensures the temporal ordering of exposure and outcome, and even then, subclinical disease may influence exposure status or its measurement, thus rendering this design rather weak. Another possible weakness is that the cohort may not be periodically re-assessed after baseline for changes in exposure status, a particularly important shortcoming with psychosocial risk factors, many of which could be somewhat labile (e.g., conflict with boss, marital difficulties). The need for frequent monitoring was noted above.

At its best, this design can be a very strong one if: (a) the cohort is widely representative of persons who are in the life cycle stage during which typical cases of the disease develop; (b) there is a clear-cut and clinically meaningful separation between being free of disease and having positive history of disease, and presence of subclinical disease can be detected; (c) follow-up for outcome is without serious attrition and without bias in assessing the disease; (d) the exposure variable is relatively non-reactive ("silent"), such as HDL cholesterol levels, rather than, say, deadline pressures at work, to which the respondent has been accommodating over some period of time; (e) a plausible biological mechanism or hypothesis links the exposure variable to the disease outcome; (f) possible self-selection characteristics linked to differential exposure are relatively stable, can be assessed retrospectively at baseline, and can be statistically controlled in analysis.

The historical cohort design (prospective study in retrospect) is an effective variation on the usual prospective design to the extent that data are complete and available so as to permit the full reconstruction of a particular definable cohort, as it existed at some point in the past, and the complete and unbiased determination of outcomes from that point on. The two areas in which the historical cohort design tend to fall short, compared to the usual prospective design, are: (a) limited information about the cohort at baseline (including exposure status), thus precluding extensive statistical adjustments for potential confounders; (b) incomplete tracing of respondents and of disease outcomes to the present.

While the traditional prospective cohort design has served classical epidemiology well, it is less serviceable in psychosocial epidemiology. Consider the following scenario: We are conducting a study of work stress and CHD incidence. At baseline workers free of CHD are assessed for established CHD risk factors, work stress, sociodemographics, life style habits, and so on. At 10 year follow-up, high work stress is found associated with higher incidence of CHD. Adjustments for blood pressure and cholesterol and lipid fractions do not alter this conclusion, but adjustments for smoking status wipe out this effect: workers on high stress jobs have more current smokers while low stress jobs have more former smokers. Is smoking a confounder or an explanatory variable? Do we conclude that "proper" adjustments reveal no effect of work stress or do we argue that work stress affects CHD and the effect is mediated by smoking status? The latter is speculative since we do not have the prospective design for answering the relationship between work stress and smoking status, i.e., rule out self-selection of smokers into high stress jobs. This is a common dilemma in psychosocial epidemiology: the classical prospective design doesn't allow us to disentangle the causal priorities among and between the psychosocial and the biological risk factors measured at baseline, even though this is often crucial for a full understanding of the combined role of biological and psychosocial risk factors. This dilemma is less common in classical epidemiology, but it does occur. In cardiovascular epidemiology, obesity usually has no independent effect, once we account for the contribution of blood pressure, cholesterol and lipid fractions. Yet, obesity is likely to be causally antecedent to these risk factors.

## CROSS-SECTIONAL POPULATION SURVEYS

At its strongest, this design involves a broadly representative sample (not selected because of exposure or disease status), who are assessed for: (a) past and current history of exposure or level of risk factors; (b) presence-absence of a particular disease (and perhaps some retrospective information such as date of onset); and (c) a wide variety of other characteristics for which statistical adjustments can be made.

This design is vulnerable to the limitations already mentioned for the stronger designs discussed above. In addition, there are other limitations not specifically applicable to the earlier designs. The salient ones are: (a) Cases of disease identified in the survey may be a biased portion of all relevant cases of disease in the population, notably also those who didn't survive and, to a lesser extent, those who are in remission at time of survey (and history of disease is inaccurate). (b) Risk factor information may become biased when obtained after disease has developed; this would be both because (i) risk factors are truly altered after initial episode of disease (e.g., blood pressure after MI), and (ii) measurement becomes biased (e.g., presence of disease influences recall). (c) Temporal sequence among many variables may be difficult to determine. (d) Self-selection factors which influence both the exposure variable and the disease outcome may be difficult to identify and may remain uncontrolled.

## CASE-CONTROL RETROSPECTIVE DESIGNS

This is a common design in epidemiology, particularly useful for very rare disease outcomes; in cancer epidemiology it is still the standard design and it has yielded many trustworthy leads on potential risk factors. Still, the specifics of execution of this design may make this an extremely weak and biased research strategy and this danger is particularly great in psychosocial epidemiology. In addition to the limitations which have already been mentioned above in connection with the stronger designs, the following are some salient additional limitations which may apply: (a) Cases of disease which are enrolled in the study are a biased subset of all cases of the disease in the population (e.g., they are only cases in specific treatment, the cases have more severe disease or some additional comorbidity); (b) Selection of controls may be inappropriate in at least two ways: (i) they may be unrepresentative of persons free of that disease in known and unknown ways; (ii) they may be insufficiently comparable to cases on those variables which the investigator wishes to rule out as alternative explanations of the difference in prevalence of a risk factor between cases and controls.

A variation on a case-control retrospective design is the purposive selection of a group of subjects known to be exposed and a comparison group of unexposed individuals is then also assembled. The two groups are then compared on prevalence of a particular disease. The two major concerns listed above apply here as well, with small change in terminology (e.g., "cases" are the exposed, not those with disease). In addition, there is a new concern labeled "detection (ascertainment) bias": if there is a more complete ascertainment of disease among those known to be exposed, then their disease rates are higher than the rates for controls which are thus underestimated. Similarly, if measurement of outcome is not objective, then knowledge of exposure may bias determination of outcome.

## Biases and limitations in the measurement of psychosocial risk factors

In the introduction we referred to our broad aim of discussing study design and methodological issues that undermine our ability to establish *whether or not* a psychosocial risk factor is involved in the etiology of a disease, and *how* it is involved. So far we have discussed primarily study design issues and only secondarily measurement issues. In this section we wish to focus more exclusively on measurement. By biases (a more precise term would be "potential biases") we mean those conditions of measurement which prevent us from ruling out other explanations of the association between a psychosocial risk factor and a health outcome than the etiological one of interest. By limitations we mean those conditions of measurement which prevent us from learning more about how the psychosocial risk factor influences the etiology.

As we noted already, a particular operationalization of a psychosocial risk factor does not produce the same set of biases and limitations, irrespective of other methodological issues. Rather, a changing subset of these may be applicable, depending upon the study design utilized, the procedures for measuring the health outcome, and the availability of additional variables for statistical control of rival hypotheses.

Clearly, one of the major concerns is *the possible influence of the presence of disease on the measurement process*. (Equally clearly, this applies to cross-sectional and retrospective designs but should not normally be a concern in prospective designs where baseline data are collected on a cohort free of the disease.) The concerns are that the disease has altered the presumptively antecedent risk factor or has influenced its assessment, or both. The impact of the "presence of disease" could refer to somewhat different processes: (a) the effects of the distress and pain of having the condition; (b) the effects associated with the process of detection (diagnosis) and treatment, and (c) the effects of knowledge and beliefs about the condition (e.g., about its etiology and its prognosis). The effects could impact on different domains: (a) primarily affective, such as anxiety and depression, or (b) cognitive such as causal reattribution as one looks back at the period before diagnosis, or (c) functional, such as social interaction with friends and relatives.

Of course, the degree of actual bias present is difficult to assess since we don't have the necessary longitudinal methodological studies which examined how various measures change when prospective assessments are compared to post-disease assessments. One might speculate that relatively neutral data, such as occupational history, would be reasonably unaffected, while sensitive variables, such as health locus of control after cancer diagnosis, would seem pretty much useless. Adverse life style habits could be underreported if the respondent is trying to avoid "blame" for the disease, or could be overreported if they are trying to "explain" why the disease occurred. Accounts of marital closeness could also be distorted in either direction, depending on individual differences or the particular disease, e.g., cancer vs. coronary heart disease. And in spite of labels put on scales that imply stable characteristics, such as trait anxiety (Spielberger et al., 1970), it would be unwise to assume that such trait measures are insensitive to disease events.

Finding remedies for the possible biasing effect of presence of disease is equally hampered by the absence of empirical data from studies that have explicitly demonstrated such biases. If, for example, the effect on a particular measure is due to the painful symptoms, then assessing cases at the time they are in remission would seem to remove the bias. But that assumes that previous painful episodes have a reversible rather than enduring impact. Or, as another example, we could use proxy respondents who know the case well and who themselves are free of the disease. But such proxies tend to be close family members and the disease of the case could have a strong impact on them as well.

Assessing patients while they are awaiting diagnostic results, such as biopsy findings, seems, at first blush, like an attractive strategy (Schmale & Iker, 1971). Some patients find out they are free of disease, while others are diagnosed with it, but both groups are presumably equally affected, at time of assessment, by the fear of the results. This strategy, too, has its limitations: (a) it controls for the *knowledge* of diagnosis results, but not for any possible physiological effects of the disease itself; (b) it assumes that results cannot be anticipated more than chance by either the patient or the physician, or if the physician can anticipate results, that s/he will not communicate them to the patient; (c) certain risk factors cannot be examined, such as stressful life events during the previous months, since such a variable is at best contemporaneous with the disease rather than truly preceding it; (d) certain diseases cannot be studied if being free of the disease means that the person has a benign precursor, such as polyps in the case of colorectal cancer, and if the risk factors for the precursor are the same as for the disease itself.

In addition to the potentially biasing influence of the presence of disease on the measurement process, the other major concern in psychosocial epidemiology focuses on the measurement of exposures. We shall discuss some of the issues in the language of a dilemma between "objective" vs. "subjective" strategies of measurement, even though these terms are quite imprecise and unnecessarily polarizing. But in the stress and disease health research domain, particularly occupational stress, this distinction represents a major ongoing debate (Frese & Zapf, 1988; Hurrell et al., 1998). Incidentally, because of the crucial importance of self-reports in epidemiologic surveys, we are quite unwilling to view self-reports as synonymous with subjective. Rather, "subjective" means measures that *intentionally* involve the respondent's cognitive and emotional processing (Frese & Zapf, 1988); the term is not linked to source of information.

In the research on the job strain model (Karasek & Theorell, 1990; Theorell & Karasek, 1996), the two primary dimensions are *decision latitude* and (psychological) *job demands*. Differences between occupations explain about 35% of the variance in latitude but only about 4% in demands. What is the meaning of this difference in explained variance and what are the implications for measurement of work stress dimensions? There would seem to be a number of issues here: (a) Are occupational titles too crude a classification to pick up variation in job demands, or are job demands a subjective reaction almost uncorrelated with objective work conditions, so that a more refined grouping of jobs would not increase the explained variance? (b) Do job demands measure psychological reactions to objective work conditions, albeit with enormous individual differences, or do they measure mostly pre-existing personal characteristics which would manifest themselves in a similar way on different jobs? And what data do we need to decide which it is? (c) Is the health impact of the work setting most appropriately understood as a link to the objective work conditions, to the subjective measures, or to some unique combination of the setting and the reactions? (d) How does one know how to develop ameliorative intervention strategies; does one try to change the work conditions, the reactions of the workers, or some specific reactions of workers in specific settings? (e) And if one is measuring psychological outcomes (mental health, well-being, job satisfaction), how does one eliminate the potential for shared biases in the measurement of the subjective exposure and the outcome?

The above questions are quite generic: they can be repeated for many other measures in the occupational health sphere, as well as exposures (experiences) in other life domains. Admittedly, for some domains, such as the work setting and the residential environment, we need to be more determined to capture some of the objective dimensions than for other domains, such as the marital relationship, where presumably the subjective dimensions are paramount.

We also need to recognize that the theories surrounding our psychosocial risk factors are psychological or social-psychological theories designed to understand psychological and behavioral outcomes. Thus for these outcomes, the emphasis on subjective measurement of exposures makes sense. But when the outcomes are biomedical variables, we cannot be equally wedded to these subjective exposures. We need to give ourselves an adequate opportunity to find out what the role of the objective aspects of the exposure is and how this may be altered by the cognitive and emotional processing.

The considerations in the "subjective" vs. "objective" dilemma may be summarized as follows:

(1) The arguments in favor of objective measurement strategies are: (a) We will have a clearer linkage to the "actual" environmental conditions and will know better what aspects of the environment needs changing; (b) We will have a clearer picture of the etiological process, since it is less clear what are all the influences on the subjective measures; (c) There will be less measurement confounding when outcomes are psychological and behavioral; (d) There will be

a clearer separation of where the independent variable ends and the dependent variable begins, while with subjective measures we are already somewhere along the trajectory of reactions and impact.

(2) The arguments in favor of subjective measurement strategies are: (a) They are needed when the "meaning" of exposure varies substantially across individuals; (b) Cognitive and emotional processing moderates the overall etiological process and the subjective exposure clarifies the etiological mechanism; (c) Environmental manipulation is not possible, only differential reactivity of subjects can be addressed; (d) Objective measures are irrelevant or are outside of any possible causal chain (in Lewin's (1951) terminology, not part of the life space but in the foreign hull).

Pragmatic considerations have also been part of this debate. Fundamentally, self-report measures tend to be more easily available, cheaper, and more convenient. Objective measures, such as for the work environment, can be expensive, clumsy, difficult to obtain (e.g., Hacker, 1993). Given the greater convenience of self-reports on the one hand, and our reluctance to rely exclusively on subjective strategies, on the other hand, we need to find strategies for collecting information from respondents while minimizing cognitive and emotional processing. For example, many of our scales ask not only about whether some environmental conditions exist but also if they were bothersome or distressing, all in the same item. Similarly, we can get at the meaning of an event, such as job loss, by asking what it meant and how the person reacted. Or we can formulate ideas about differential vulnerability, such as stage of life cycle, dependents at home, other wage earners, and create the "meaning" of the event out of a combination of relatively objective characteristics.

## Concluding comments

Epidemiologic methods evolved as a strategy for the study of risk factors for various diseases at the level of the population. They are generally not suitable for the additional study of the various mechanisms which could be involved as links between the risk factor and the disease outcome. Thus typical epidemiologic data leave a fairly large "black box" unopened. The recent and growing prominence of the role of molecular biomarkers in epidemiology (e.g., McMichael, 1994) holds considerable promise of letting us peer inside the black box. For example, for occupational cancers, the molecular biomarkers can assist with the following: (a) the measurement of internal exposure; (b) the measurement of early biologic response; (c) the measurement of effect-modifying host characteristics; (d) elaboration of biologic mechanisms in disease induction; (e) the refinement of risk quantification; and (f) differentiation of disease outcomes.

The inclusion of psychosocial variables in classical epidemiology holds the promise of similarly expanding the reach of epidemiologic methods, albeit in a different way. The primary difference is that it adds to the scope of the risk factors outside of the "black box", and attempts to demonstrate the psychosocial antecedents of the biological risk factors. Psychosocial dynamics however could also illuminate the processes inside the "black box". The possible contributions from psychosocial epidemiology are the measurement of: internal exposures, early stages of reacting, and effect-modifying host characteristics. However, as this chapter demonstrates, the challenges are considerable.

# References

Ader, R., Felten, D.L., & Cohen, N. (Eds.) (1991). *Psychoneuroimmunology.* New York: Academic Press.

Appels, A., & Mulder, P. (1988). Excessive fatigue as a precursor of myocardial infarction. *European Heart Journal, 9,* 758–764.

Baum, A., & Grunberg, N. (1995). Measurement of stress hormones. In: S. Cohen, R.C. Kessler, & L.U. Gordon (Eds.), *Measuring stress* (pp. 175–192). New York: Oxford University Press.

Berkman, L.F. (1995). The role of social relations in health promotion. *Psychosomatic Medicine, 57,* 245–254.

Berkman, L.F., & Breslow, L. (1983). *Health and ways of living.* New York: Oxford University Press.

Campbell, D.T., & Stanley, J.C. (1966). *Experimental and quasi-experimental designs for research.* Chicago: Rand McNally.

Chandra, V., Szklo, M., Goldberg, R., & Tonascia, J. (1983). The impact of marital status on survival after an acute myocardial infarction: A population-based study. *American Journal of Epidemiology, 117,* 320–325.

Cook, T.D., & Campbell, D.T. (1979). *Quasi-experimentation: Design & analysis issues for field settings.* Chicago: Rand McNally.

Dunn, B.E., Cohen, H., & Blaser, M.J. (1997). Helicobacter pylori. *Clinical Microbiology Review, 10,* 720–741.

Ferrie, J.E., Shipley, M.J., Marmot, M.G., Stansfeld, S., & Smith, G.D. (1995). Health effects of anticipation of job change and non-employment: Longitudinal data from the Whitehall II study. *British Medical Journal, 311*, 1264–1269.

Frese, M., & Zapf, D. (1988). Methodological issues in the study of work stress: Objective vs. subjective measurement of work stress and questions of longitudinal studies. In: C.L. Cooper & R. Payne (Eds.), *Causes, coping, and consequences of stress at work* (pp. 375–411). New York: Wiley.

Hacker, W. (1993). Objective work environment: Analysis and evaluation of objective work characteristics. In: *A healthier work environment: Basic concepts and methods of measurement* (pp. 42–57). Copenhagen: WHO Regional Office for Europe.

Hill, A.B. (1965). Environment and disease: Association or causation? *Proceedings of the Royal Society of Medicine, 58*, 295–300.

Hurrell, J.J., Jr., Nelson, D.L., & Simmons, B.L. (1998). Measuring job stressors and strains: Where we have been, where we are, and where we need to go. *Journal of Occupational Health Psychology, 3*, 368–389.

Julkunen, J., Salonen, R., Kaplan, G.A., Chesney, M.A., & Salonen, J.T. (1994). Hostility and the progression of carotid atherosclerosis. *Psychosomatic Medicine, 56*, 519–525.

Kaplan, G. (1992). Health and aging in the Alameda County Study. In: K.W. Schaie, D. Blazer, & J.S. House (Eds.), *Aging, health behaviors and health outcomes* (pp. 69–88). Hillsdale, NJ: Lawrence Erlbaum.

Karasek, R., & Theorell, T. (1990). *Healthy work.* New York: Basic Books.

Kasl, S.V. (1977). The effects of the residential environment on health and behavior: A review. In: L.E. Hinkle, Jr. & W.C. Loring (Eds.), *The effect of the man-made environment on health and behavior* (pp. 65–127). Washington, DC: DHEW Publication No. (CDC) 77–8318.

Kasl, S.V. (1985). Environmental exposure and disease: An epidemiological perspective on some methodological issues in health psychology and behavioral medicine. In: J.E. Singer & A. Baum (Eds.), *Advances in environmental psychology, Vol. 5: Methods and environmental psychology* (pp. 119–146). Hillsdale, NJ: Lawrence Erlbaum.

Kasl, S.V., & Cooper, C.L. (Eds.) (1987). *Stress and health: Issues in research methodology.* Chichester: Wiley.

Kasl, S.V., & Jones, B.A. (2000). The impact of job loss and retirement on health. In: L. Berkman & I. Kawachi (Eds.), *Social epidemiology.* Oxford: Oxford University Press.

Kasl, S.V., Evans, A.S., & Niederman, J.C. (1979). Psychosocial risk factors in the development of infectious mononucleosis. *Psychosomatic Medicine, 41*, 445–466.

Kelsey, J.L., Whittemore, A.S., Evans, A.S., & Thompson, W.D. (1996). *Methods in observational epidemiology.* New York: Oxford University Press.

Kiecolt-Glaser, J.K., & Glaser, R. (1995). Measurement of immune response. In: S. Cohen, R.C. Kessler, & L.U. Gordon (Eds.), *Measuring stress* (pp. 193–212). New York: Oxford University Press.

Kittel, F., Kornitzer, M., & Dramaix, M. (1980). Coronary heart disease and job stress in two cohorts of bank clerks. *Psychotherapy and Psychosomatics, 34*, 110–123.

Kop, W.J., Appels, A.P.W.M., Mendes de Leon, C.F., Swart, de H.B., & Bar, F.W. (1994). Vital exhaustion predicts new cardiac events after successful coronary angioplasty. *Psychosomatic Medicine, 56*, 281–287.

Lewin, K. (1951). *Field theory in social science.* New York: Harper & Rowe.

McMichael, A.J. (1994). Invited commentary—"Molecular epidemiology:" New pathway or new traveling companion. *American Journal of Epidemiology, 140*, 1–11.

Marmot, M.G. (1982). Hypothesis-testing and the study of psychosocial factors. *Advances in Cardiology, 29*, 3–9.

Mendes de Leon, C.F., Kasl, S.V., & Jacobs, S. (1994). A prospective study of widowhood and changes in symptoms of depression in a community sample of the elderly. *Psychological Medicine, 56*, 557–563.

Morris, J.K., & Cook, D.G. (1991). A critical review of the effect of factory closures on health. *British Journal of Industrial Medicine, 48*, 1–8.

Price, R.H. (1992). Impact of preventive job search intervention on likelihood of depression among unemployed. *Journal of Health and Social Behavior, 33*, 158–167.

Rothman, K.J. (Ed.) (1988). *Causal inference.* Chestnut Hill, MA: Epidemiology Resources.

Schmale, A.H., & Iker, H.P. (1971). Hopelessness as a predictor of cervical cancer. *Social Science and Medicine, 5*, 95–100.

Seeman, T.E., Berkman, L.F., Kohout, F., LaCroix, A., Glynn, R., & Blazer, D. (1993). Intercommunity variation in the association between social ties and mortality in the elderly. *Annals of Epidemiology, 3*, 325–335.

Shekelle, R.B., & Lin, S.C. (1978). Public beliefs about causes and prevention of heart attacks. *Journal of the American Medical Association, 240*, 756–758.

Siegman, A.W., & Smith, T.W. (1994). *Anger, hostility, and the heart.* Hillsdale, NJ: Lawrence Erlbaum.

Spielberger, C.D., Gorsuch, R.L., & Lushene, R.E. (1970). *Manual for the State-Trait Anxiety Inventory (STAI).* Palo Alto, CA: Consulting Psychologists Press.

Susser, M.W. (1991). What is a cause and how do we know one? *American Journal of Epidemiology, 133*, 635–648.

Theorell, T., & Karasek, R.A. (1996). Current issues relating to psychosocial job strain and cardiovascular disease research. *Journal of Occupational Health Psychology, 1*, 9–26.

Watson, D., & Clark, L.A. (1984). Negative affectivity: The disposition to experience aversive emotional states. *Psychological Bulletin, 96*, 465–490.

Watson, D., & Pennebaker, J.W. (1989). Health complaints, stress, and distress: Exploring the central role of negative affectivity. *Psychological Review, 96*, 234–254.

Weiner, H. (1977). *Psychobiology and human disease*. New York: Elsevier.

# 3 METHODOLOGICAL CONSIDERATIONS FOR PSYCHOSOCIAL INTERVENTION STUDIES

Carolyn E. Schwartz, Sally Brotman, and Evguenia Jilinskaia

As the field of behavioral medicine has matured, the empirical issues which require attention have changed focus. Pioneer behavioral medicine researchers were faced with simply demonstrating that behavior can influence health, and that modifying behavior can affect health outcomes. In the current climate, such precepts are accepted and an increasing number of behavioral intervention options are available to patients. With the rapid and recent explosion of interest in alternative and complementary therapies, the number of available patient-initiated, behavioral, and non-allopathic intervention options are ever increasing. This dynamic situation presents current behavioral medicine specialists with a context in which the assumptions and methods of our work must be reconsidered as we face the task of demonstrating which of several behavioral interventions is most effective for a given problem and for a specific patient population. The purpose of this chapter is to discuss conceptual, implementation, and measurement issues of particular methodological relevance in current psychosocial intervention research.

## Conceptual issues

### THE CONTROL GROUP DILEMMA

Given the availability of numerous psychosocial, behavioral, and complementary intervention options, the no-treatment control group is no longer a feasible arm in a psychosocial randomized trial. Even if one were to attempt to do such a study, it would likely suffer from confounding due to unmeasured or unmentioned treatments which have become standard cultural fare; a problem which speaks to the successful first two decades of behavioral medicine research. Consequently, the astute researcher is forced to derive a control condition which shares a number of non-specific factors with the psychosocial intervention of interest (e.g., attention, frequency of contact, credibility), but not the operant factor(s) which the investigator believes to be most important. The ethical, theoretical, scientific, and statistical challenges involved in deriving the appropriate control condition(s) are described in depth by Schwartz et al. (1997a). The culmination of all of these factors is that current behavioral intervention research will require a greater number of participants to have adequate statistical power. Detecting treatment effects is largely a function of the comparison group. Accordingly, the more active the comparison condition is, the less likely one is to detect large differences between groups. Consequently, studies comparing two active interventions should be designed to detect a moderate to small effect size and thus will require a greater number of subjects than past research (e.g., 64 to 375 as compared to 15 patients per treatment arm). Indeed, the majority of recent studies of psychotherapy and behavioral medicine interventions did not have sufficient sample sizes to yield adequate statistical power (Kazdin & Bass, 1989; Rossi, 1990). Results of meta-analyses suggest that most psychosocial interventions for cancer patients, for example, yield an effect size of 0.17–0.28 (Meyer & Mark, 1995), requiring at least 64 to 393 participants per treatment arm to yield adequate power (assuming an inactive control condition) (see Lipsey & Wilson, 1993 for broader review).

As mental health professionals are forced to compete for third-party reimbursement in an increasingly restrictive health care market, demonstrating short-term effects is not sufficient to justify expenditures. Consequently, it may not be feasible to do standard cross-over designs (i.e., waiting-list controls serving as the comparison group) because they do not allow an investigation of long-term effects. Studies which aim to focus on long-term outcomes will require at least two distinct study groups, one of which receives the intervention of interest and the other of which receives some non-specific treatment control condition.

## THE PROBLEM OF CAUSAL INFERENCE

Given the difficulties in selecting a feasible and appropriate control condition, the behavioral researcher might prefer to examine the effectiveness of an intervention using a case-control design. In this design, patients who receive a particular treatment might be followed over time and compared to patients who do not receive the exposure. This design has the advantage of avoiding the ethical and other difficulties of randomization. However, it has a fundamental difficulty which can make results difficult to interpret. That is, one is unable to make unequivocal causal inference using a case-control design. An empirical example of such a problem was a retrospective follow-up study of 102 participants in a psychosocial support program for women with breast cancer (Morgenstern et al., 1984). Participants in the program were matched for several prognostic factors and both groups were tracked using hospital registry data. Preliminary findings suggested a strong beneficial effect of the program on survival. Further investigation revealed, however, that this effect was due to the failure to match on the duration of the lag period between cancer diagnosis and program entry. This example illustrates how a case-control design does not get around the third factor problem which plagues much of behavioral science research. Although there is some evidence that appropriate covariate adjustment can mitigate this problem to some extent (Shadish & Ragsdale, 1996),[1] it is not always possible to know what third factor is playing a critical role in treatment outcomes. For these reasons, investigators continue to rely upon the randomized controlled trial for evaluating treatments which are expected or hoped to have a long-term impact on patients' well-being. We will thus address variations and modifications to this preeminent study design.

One of the strongest proponents of the randomized controlled trial and of meta-analysis, Thomas Chalmers, M.D., was often cited for saying "randomize the first patient". His experience as a physician revealed numerous "medical miracles" which failed to maintain their stature when subjected to the neutrality imposed by random allocation of patients to treatments. Thus, the randomized controlled trial provides a neutral slate for investigating the true benefit of treatments. Since all patients have an equal chance of being assigned to any treatment arm, it is assumed that patients in all treatment arms will be comparable on the innumerable unmeasured factors. This assumption is not always true, especially when the study sample size is small (Hsu, 1989). There are specific steps, however, which can be implemented to maximize the probability of such a situation.

## Implementation issues

### ISSUES IN RANDOMIZATION
The importance of random allocation cannot be overstated. There are several issues which arise in working within a randomized design, and which suggest specific steps that should be taken before randomization

occurs. First, important prognostic variables should be considered as stratification factors for the randomization. This stratified randomized design (Pocock, 1983) helps to ensure that patients are comparable in terms of disease severity or prognosis. It is best to select a small number of stratification factors to create blocks for randomization, since more than three or four will approximate a random distribution and thus will not accomplish the goal of a stratified randomized design. An example of relevant stratification variables for a trial of breast cancer patients would be age at diagnosis (pre- versus post-menopausal) and stage of disease (I, II versus III, IV). These two factors have important prognostic value, as pre-menopausal and later-stage patients have significantly worse prognoses (Fisher et al., 1997).

A second important issue in randomization is to identify a neutral party to assign treatments based on a process like a coin-toss. Given the strong degree of commitment to the precepts of behavioral medicine which must be prevalent in our clinicians, it is preferable to have someone other than the clinician who is implementing the intervention assign the treatment. Our experience has been that asking clinicians who have a vested interest in demonstrating the efficacy and effectiveness of their favorite intervention(s) is not straightforward. For example, a clinician may believe that her approach to cognitive behavioral therapy is eminently helpful for chronically ill patients suffering from depression. Allowing this clinician to implement the randomization would be problematic, since she may feel impelled to treat the most afflicted patients with her cognitive behavioral treatment. She may thus not randomize such patients. Alternatively, she might peek to ensure that they would get the treatment she wished. Ironically, if the above clinician were allowed to randomize participants, it is likely in this case that her treatment trial would suggest no benefit of her cognitive behavioral intervention. That is to say, the biased clinician is handicapping her own study. If she only randomizes the more afflicted patients conditional on their being assigned to her treatment arm of choice, she is likely to randomize this subgroup only 50% of the time (assuming a two-arm design). Thus, 50% of the patients who would be most likely to be helped, would not be enrolled in the clinical trial and thus would not contribute valuable information about the treatment's effectiveness. For this reason, it is recommended that treatment assignment be done by a neutral party, and not by the clinician who is implementing the intervention.

A third issue is related to the fact that an intention-to-treat analysis is the most rigorous and thus the recommended approach. This approach refers to the idea that participants' data are analyzed according to the treatment arm to which they were assigned, irrespective of their adherence to the treatment protocol (Armitage, 1983). Thus, the patient who attended one of eight group meetings and dropped out would be analyzed as belonging to the same treatment arm as the patient who attended all eight sessions. Such an approach may yield estimates of treatment gain which are substantially different from an analysis which drops all participants who did not receive the full treatment dose (Nich & Carroll, 1997), although this is not always the case (Schwartz, 1999).

The successful implementation of an intention-to-treat analysis may be facilitated if potential participants are required to prove that they can be good study subjects prior to randomization. That is, the behavioral medicine researcher might consider the accrual process as similar to a job interview: the participant must prove to the investigator that he is committed to the study, intends to attend all treatment sessions, and will provide data for as long as is defined in the study protocol. Although the informed consent process requires that potential participants be aware that they are free to withdraw from the study at any time, it behooves the clinical investigator to screen them adequately prior to randomization in order to minimize patient attrition. This screening can be done by asking potential participants to think about the commitment required and contact the investigator some number of days later, and perhaps even to complete the baseline questionnaire so that the full implications of study participation are understood. The more steps required for participant enrollment in a trial, the higher the likelihood that the response rate of the long-term follow-up will be high. Each step introduces potential selection biases, but these biases can be quantified (Schwartz & Fox, 1995). Our experience is that such screening steps can help to yield a very high (e.g., 96%) follow-up rate over two years.

## THE SCIENTIFIC IMPORTANCE OF PERSEVERENCE

Perseverence is critical for ensuring not only the careful implementation of randomization, but perhaps most importantly for guaranteeing a high follow-up rate. A recent study which was completed by our group illustrates the biases that can be introduced if a high response rate were not ensured. In this study, a survey-by-mail was sent to investigate sexual functioning and quality of life among a group of men who had undergone radical prostactectomy for prostate cancer. It should be noted that this surgery results in erectile dysfunction for 42–89% of patients at 12 months after surgery (Talcott et al., 1998). Approximately 50% of the participants returned the completed surveys without further ado. The remaining 50%, however, found the questionnaire bothersome to answer because the issues addressed were perceived to be too personal in nature. After some modification of the questionnaire in which the more sensitive items were deleted, the patients were asked to reconsider their participation in the study. After a series of persistent phone calls implemented by a clinical psychologist, we were able to achieve a 72% response rate, which is closer to an

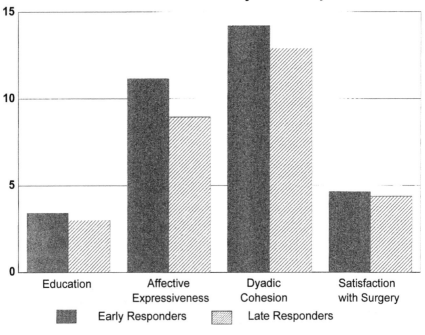

Figure 3.1. *Selection biases introduced by low response rate*: Approximately 50% of the participants in a study-by-mail returned the completed surveys without further ado (Early Responders). The remaining 50% (Late Responders) required persistent follow-up efforts to ensure compliance. The Early Responders were found to be better educated ($t = 2.7$, $p < 0.01$), to be more affectively expressive ($t = 4.8$, $p < 0.0001$), tended to report higher levels of dyadic cohesion ($t = 1.8$, $p < 0.10$), and tended to report higher levels of satisfaction with their surgery ($t = 1.7$, $p < 0.10$). Thus, pushing the data collection phase of the study to ensure an adequate response rate yielded a more representative sample in terms of some key sociodemographic and quality-of-life factors.

acceptable level (Dillman, 1978). Of particular interest, we found that those men who had provided the completed questionnaires initially were significantly more likely to be better educated, to be more affectively expressive, tended to report higher levels of dyadic cohesion, and tended to report higher levels of satisfaction with their surgery. Thus, pushing the data collection phase of the study to ensure an adequate response rate yielded a more representative sample in terms of some key sociodemographic and quality-of-life factors (see Figure 3.1).

## ENSURING EQUIVALENT TREATMENT PREFERENCES ACROSS STUDY ARMS

An additional relevant issue to the successful implementation of a randomized trial is to track that all treatment arms are equally attractive. This can be done very simply at the intake interview by asking potential participants to which study arm they would prefer to be assigned. Treatment arms of equal valence would yield similar proportions of patient preference endorsement. If there are significant differences in treatment assignment, one can do subgroup analyses to determine how different the effect size is for patients who receive their preferred treatment as compared to those who do not. For example, Schwartz et al., (1997a) illustrated the impact of pre-randomization preference by showing that patients who were randomized to the treatment they preferred were more likely to report improvement in psychosocial role limitations after two months, whereas those who were not randomized to their preferred intervention reported no change. Ensuring that the treatments being evaluated have similar appeal will thus facilitate an evaluation of the true impact of treatment, independent of patient expectations or a placebo effect.

## STANDARDIZATION OF TREATMENT

An important consideration in an intervention trial involves ensuring that the treatment being delivered has some standardized parameters. Since clinical work needs to be responsive to the individual's or group's needs, some tailoring of the intervention will be necessary. Having some codification will thus be an important step toward ensuring that one is evaluating a relatively homogenous phenomenon, and perhaps more importantly, that the intervention can be reliably replicated. This treatment manual could be published as a peer-reviewed journal article (e.g., Fawzy & Fawzy, 1994; Schwartz & Rogers, 1994) or can be copyrighted and distributed by the primary investigator (e.g., Spira, 1997).

If an intervention is tailored to each individual in such a way that all recipients actually receive very distinct treatments, then the clinical investigator may have some difficulty because a given intervention is far from codified. For such treatments, an extended phase of pilot testing might be useful so that the relevant parameters can be identified. This phase can be critical for determining whether an overarching schema can be defined that contains quite a bit of variation. For example, the assigned topic of a particular session within a behavioral medicine intervention might be coping with stress at home. Although the specific issues which participants choose to discuss may vary, the suggested strategies may be quite similar. In contrast, other clinical interventions may entail extensive tailoring in the dosage (e.g., number of sessions), topics covered, or complexity. For example, if the intervention involves implementing a varying number of neuropsychological and personality tests to improve diagnostic sensitivity and subsequent pharmacotherapeutic management and cognitive remediation for a particular condition, then the protocol may be quite variable. Accordingly, it might be necessary to keep close track of exactly what tests were done, how feedback was provided to the patient as well as to the pharmacotherapy provider, and what steps were taken to manage the subsequent care of the patients who received the neuropsychological testing. Characterizing these relevant parameters would facilitate a decision as to whether all patients who received the neuropsychological testing and cognitive remediation received similar enough management to be analyzed as one group or would be more appropriately analyzed as more than one group.

## DETERMINING AN APPROPRIATE SOURCE FOR TREATMENT INFORMATION

Behavioral medicine research which seeks to address the complementary or synergistic relationship between behavioral and psychopharmacotherapeutic interventions will need to consider a further issue, that of determining an appropriate source for dosage information. Imagine a trial which seeks to determine whether a behavioral intervention given in conjunction with pharmacotherapy is more effective for reducing anxiolytic responses to medical treatment than either one alone. It might be hypothesized, for example, that the behavioral intervention will reduce the required dosage level of potentially toxic pharmacotherapy regimens. Although the medical record may be a reasonable place to determine the prescribed dosage for the pharmacotherapeutic regiment, this information is not equivalent to what patients actually take.

Relying strictly on patient report may present problems of recall bias. The careful investigator would thus be well-advised to consider the various methods for evaluating treatment adherence (cf. Dunbar-Jacob et al., 1998) which can complement medical record abstraction.

## ACCRUING A REPRESENTATIVE SAMPLE

An increasingly relevant concern within behavioral medicine research concerns the racial, gender, and generational representativeness of the study sample. The National Institutes of Health (USA) now have strict guidelines for ensuring the representativeness of proposed research, such that the study sample reflects the true patient population in terms of race, gender and age. If a study excludes some subgroup, then this exclusion must be justified.

The well-meaning investigator may, however, end up with an unrepresentative sample due to the same societal barriers that prevent people of minority groups from adequate access to health care. These barriers include an interplay of individual, societal, and institutional factors. An illustration of these factors is provided by work done by our group to examine the barriers which prevented African Americans from participating in health services research. Through a series of interviews and focus groups with African Americans, it was revealed that lack of trust was the primary barrier to their involvement. They expressed a lack of trust in both the motives and impartiality of the institution and investigators. They expressed a fear of being used as a guinea pig to demonstrate harmful outcomes or side-effects. Further, there was a prevalent belief that study results would not be applied to help African Americans. Finally, there was a strong cultural barrier which saw medical treatment as a crutch that could result in dependency.

Each of these barriers may be expressed on an individual, institutional, or societal level. For example, lack of trust on an individual level may be expressed as, "… they only tell you so much". At the institutional level, lack of trust derives through experience with perceived discrimination. For example, a focus group member recalled that her treatment protocol was different when directed by a Caucasian doctor than by an African American doctor. The former examined her and was prepared to send her home. In contrast, "… then a black doctor checked me out and said, 'she needs surgery'". On the societal level, lack of trust is expressed as, "… they come to the African American community to study drug abuse, [but] you never hear about prostate cancer." In addition to these barriers, minority groups are disproportionately affected by the factors that make it more difficult for individuals of lower socio-economic status to obtain and follow through with meeting their health care needs. By becoming more aware of these barriers, behavioral medicine investigators may be able to design studies so that the impact of the barriers is reduced. For example, employing study staff who are of similar ethnic background may reduce the perceived barriers. Rigorous studies which address the effectiveness of various strategies for reducing barriers to ethnic minorities will be an important area for future behavioral medicine research.

## THE DOUBLE-EDGED SWORD OF STRICT ELIGIBILITY CRITERIA

In addition to concerns about the ethnic representativeness of a study sample, there are other concerns which are relevant to defining appropriate eligibility criteria for a study. The goal of eligibility criteria is to define a patient sample that is relatively homogenous. However, it is possible that the actual situation is more complicated than one initially imagines. For example, research on chronically ill patients may seek not only to confirm the diagnosis but also to ensure that there are no other co-morbid conditions. A number of medical illnesses have psychiatric co-morbidities that are quite prevalent and may indeed be a normal aspect of the disease. For example, affective disorders are quite prevalent among people with multiple sclerosis (Minden & Schiffer, 1990). The same may be true for psychiatric populations where the proportion of patients with a singular diagnosis is quite low. An example of this situation is adults with Attention Deficit Hyperactivity Disorder, where such patients are quite likely to suffer from personality and affective disorders in addition to their primary diagnosis (Kane et al., 1990). Thus a study which aims to exclude patients with other co-morbid conditions may be seeking a patient sample of exceptions and may lead to study results which cannot be generalized to the general population of patients with such a diagnosis.

One way to determine whether the eligibility criteria are inappropriately restrictive would be to track reasons for ineligibility as well as for why eligible individuals decline to participate. This information can provide insight into possible confounders or biases, as well as into possible avenues for recourse to reduce such attrition. For example, if transportation difficulties play a significant role in eligible patients' refusal to participate, then it would be worthwhile to consider budgetary appropriations to mitigate transportation difficulties (e.g., providing cab vouchers or reimbursement for handicapped-accessible car service).

## SITE-SPECIFIC CONFOUNDERS

In addition to explicit decisions of the investigator, other more implicit factors may influence study accrual. Studies which are implemented in teaching hospitals are likely to accrue a different segment of the population than studies which have community-based clinical sites. Similarly, accruing patients who participate in a managed care health service delivery system will yield patients from a different socioeconomic stratum than those which are aimed at the uninsured or the privately insured. This selection has already taken place before one has even started the study. Accordingly, it would behove the clinical investigator to consider the implications of recruiting patients from only one site and, if multiple sites are selected, to ensure that large enough samples are accrued at each site to enable subgroup analysis by site. This type of analysis can help to highlight the types of biases introduced by each site, even though the whole study sample may be relatively unbiased.

# Measurement issues

The field of outcomes measurement has developed in theoretical as well as methodological ways in the past two decades. Anyone who peruses academic journals in psychology and the health sciences will acknowledge a greatly expanded repertoire of ways of operationalizing impact as compared to the first generation of empirical intervention research. Developments in psychometrics and related advances in the ease of complex statistical computing have contributed to this increasing sophistication, and promise to yield more sensitive outcomes assessment. Finally, recent developments over the past decade in biostatistical methods have yielded longitudinal analytic techniques which can accommodate individual growth over time and model relationships among a system of constructs (see below). All of these developments represent great promise for future psychosocial intervention research, and have important implications for planning appropriate measurement strategies. The purpose of this section is to introduce some relevant considerations to planning psychosocial intervention research which reflect recent developments in analytic and measurement methodology.

## TIMING OF MEASUREMENT: WHEN AND HOW OFTEN IS ENOUGH?

Baseline measurement might take place before or after randomization, depending on the specific randomization protocol. For study populations where attrition is a concern, the investigator might minimize patient drop-out by using the baseline data collection time point as one of the proofs which demonstrates that the potential participant is likely to be a good study subject (see Issues in Randomization above). Having patients complete the baseline questionnaire prior to randomization might also be desirable if a stratification variable will be measured by self-report (e.g., depression). Alternatively, the baseline questionnaire might be collected after randomization if attrition is unlikely to be a problem and/or if the investigator is using a randomized consent design (Zelen, 1979), in which patients are randomized to a treatment prior to informed consent being obtained (see Schwartz [1998] for a discussion of the advantages and disadvantages of this design). In all cases, informed consent should be obtained before patients are asked to provide self-report data, whether this is before or after randomization.

The issue of how often one should collect self-report data will depend on the patient population being studied. It is important to remember that the goal of outcomes assessment is to elucidate the impact of an intervention by quantifying variations from the underlying disease process. For patient populations with linearly progressive diseases, less frequent outcome assessment may be required than for patient populations with relapsing-remitting illness (e.g., multiple sclerosis, chronic fatigue syndrome, systemic lupus erythematosus). Figure 3.2 illustrates this idea by showing three possible trajectories over a given period of follow-up (time interval $t$) for one multiple sclerosis patient. Trajectory A reflects a decreasing linear function. Trajectory B reflects a quadratic function, characterized by a temporary increase in functional problems followed by remission to the original (baseline) state. Trajectory C reflects a cubic function, characterized by an asymptotically increasing and then decreasing function. These trajectories can be mathematically described as first-order, second-order, and third-order polynomials, respectively. That is to say, they can be modeled as an additive model with linear, quadratic and cubic components to estimate the mean and variance of the trajectory. The data collection implications are that for a first-order model, a minimum of two time points within the time interval $t$ are required. In contrast, a second-order polynomial requires a minimum of three time points, and a third-order polynomial requires a minimum of four time points.

Our group examined monthly data on self-reported symptoms for a group of 80 multiple sclerosis patients and found that over a year approximately 43% had a first-order trajectory, 30% had a second-

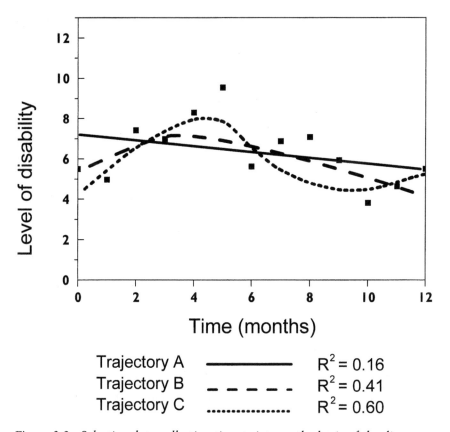

Figure 3.2. *Selecting data collection time points on the basis of the disease or treatment trajectory:* By characterizing patients accurately about their disease trajectory, one might be better positioned to measure outcomes as frequently as would be necessary to reveal changes in the underlying disease trajectory. This idea is illustrated using data from one multiple sclerosis patient followed monthly for a year. We found that a first-order (i.e., linear) polynomial model explained approximately 16% of the variance in the patient's scores (Trajectory A), a second-order (i.e., quadratic) polynomial model explained 41%, and a third order (i.e., cubic) polynomial model explained 60%. By explicitly considering the underlying disease (or treatment) trajectory, the appropriate number of data collection time points can be determined, and a more sensitive trial protocol will result. Alternative ways of conceptualizing desirable treatment outcomes and/or methods of working with the data are suggested as a consequence of acknowledging the non-linearity of patients' trajectories.

order trajectory, and 28% had a third-order trajectory. These results suggest that the data collection time points need to be selected based on the anticipated trajectory of the disease and/or of the treatment. Not doing so may result in a lack of precision, which could account for some of the unexplained variation in outcomes of patient populations characterized by variability and uncertainty.

Conceptualizing trajectories as first-, second-, and third-order polynomials led us to consider concomitantly more than one parameter in investigating treatment outcomes. That is, rather than being solely concerned with reducing reported mean levels of symptoms, one might consider an additional relevant outcome to be reducing the variability (i.e., variance) of the patients' experience. An example of such a statistic might be the coefficient of variation (i.e., SD/mean) or a variant of it, the range of the patient's scores divided by the individual's mean level. Accordingly, if an intervention might help patients to reduce the fluctuations of their symptom experience as well as the perceived level, this might be significantly more useful than simply reducing the perceived level.

A notable finding of the above-mentioned work was that the patients characterized by trajectories with higher-order polynomials were not distinguished by clinical variables such as overall neurological functioning or frequency of relapses. Rather they were more likely to report having emotional problems not including depression, suggesting that a psychosocial intervention might have an impact in helping patients to develop strategies for reducing the variability of their symptom experience by learning alternative coping strategies. By characterizing patients accurately on the basis of their disease trajectory, one might be better positioned to measure outcomes as frequently as would be necessary to reveal changes in the underlying disease trajectory or illness experience.

## HOW MANY PATIENTS IS ENOUGH?

An important consideration before beginning a randomized trial is what statistical analyses will be most appropriate for answering the primary research questions. For behavioral medicine specialists who took the minimum required number of statistics courses to complete their doctoral degree, the ordinary least squares analysis of variance may be the only analytic technique with which they are familiar or comfortable. It should be noted, however, that analysis of variance is a relatively inefficient way to analyze data, especially in cases where there are missing data (Nich & Carroll, 1997). Recent advances in longitudinal methods have yielded promising, statistically efficient methods which should replace analysis of variance as the analytic method of choice. For example, growth curve analysis (Bryk & Raudenbush, 1987; Francis et al., 1992; Willett et al., 1991) assumes that each individual has his/her own growth trajectory and which utilizes slopes generated for each individual as the new dependent variable of interest. A more complex variation of growth curve includes mixed effect models (Laird & Ware, 1982), which include fixed (group) and random (individual) parameters to model growth, thereby allowing for group effects and individual variation about the group mean trajectory. Finally, an even more complex variation includes Markhov simplex and unconditional latent trajectory models which are outgrowths of structural equation modeling (cf. Muthén & Curran, 1997), and can even examine dynamic, non-linear models of change (e.g., Boker & McArdle, 1995). This family of models involves a multi-step analytic process in which the measurement model (i.e., that constructs are measured invariantly) is tested before the structural (theoretical relationships among constructs) model.

As the statistical method increases in complexity, the sample size requirements for estimating its models increase. For example, an analysis of variance for a balanced design (i.e., equal numbers of subjects per treatment arm) with no covariates, a time factor, and two intervention groups would require 34, 76, or 547 patients per treatment arm, depending on whether one expects a large, medium, or small effect size, respectively (Cohen, 1992). If any data point were missing for a given subject, then listwise deletion would remove that subject from the analysis, necessitating larger accrual or higher follow-up rate to maintain the intended statistical power. A growth curve analysis would require similar numbers of subjects per group, but listwise deletion would not take place since a slope can be estimated as long as there are at least two data points. It is thus a more efficient method than analysis of variance. Mixed effect models might require more subjects since both fixed and random effects are being estimated, and models may have difficulty converging (i.e., estimating a reliable solution) if there are too few subjects included in the computation. Structural equation modeling, however, will require at least 200 subjects in order for standard errors and goodness of fit indices to be correct. Sample size should be rather large if multivariate normality does not hold and also if any model diagnostics (e.g., Lagrange tests, modification indices based on partial derivatives) are to be used (Tanaka, 1987). Thus the more complex methods in longitudinal analysis present a trade-off of additional subtlety in the research questions that can be asked at the cost of a larger requisite sample size.

## LONGITUDINAL FOLLOW-UP: HOW LONG IS ENOUGH?

Longer follow-up also increases the statistical power of a study (Kraemer & Thiemann, 1989), due to the reduced variance that results from having multiple, reliable measurements on each subject. Having considerable follow-up (e.g., two years or longer) facilitates asking a substantive question of increasing relevance, that is the cost-effectiveness of the intervention(s) in question. The literature which addresses the efficacy of various psychosocial interventions can be difficult to synthesize because studies differ widely in length of follow-up. A number of studies report the impact of an intervention immediately (i.e., two months) after the intervention or perhaps six months later (e.g., Kaplan & Calfas, 1991). However, longer-term follow-up (e.g., one year follow-up) of these same studies might suggest no apparent benefit (e.g., Calfas et al., 1992; Kaplan & Calfas, 1991). Although it is possible that psychosocial interventions have a relatively short shelf life, it is also possible that the impact is subtle but grows over time. It may thus only be detectable with long-term follow-up. One example of this subtle effect is the work of Spiegel and colleagues (1989) who found that a support group for metastatic breast cancer patients yielded a significant survival benefit which only began to be apparent 20 months after study entry (i.e., eight months after the intervention ended). Schwartz (1999) reported a significant enhancement in quality-of-life outcomes after two years of follow-up among multiple sclerosis patients who received one of two psychosocial interventions. These differences were less dramatic than those revealed six months after completing the intervention (Schwartz, 1994). These studies suggest that psychosocial intervention studies with longer follow-up intervals may yield more clinically relevant information.

# Other factors which can mitigate the detectable treatment effect

The detectable impact of a psychosocial intervention may also be obscured by other unmeasured but systematic factors. An emerging construct in behavioral medicine research, response shift, has particular relevance to this discussion. Response shift refers to the idea that as a result of health state changes, an individual may undergo changes in: (a) internal standards; (b) values; or (c) conceptualization of quality of life (cf. Sprangers & Schwartz, 1999). Research has documented that medically ill patients indeed undergo response shift over the course of their illness (e.g., Breetvelt & Van Dam, 1991), and that these changes can obscure medical treatment effects if appropriate designs and measures are not utilized (Sprangers, 1996). In work done by our group, response shift was found to have a different effect depending on stage of follow-up (Schwartz et al., 2000). Whereas the immediate effects suggested that response shift may heighten the apparent benefit of a psychosocial intervention, the longer-term effects may actually be in the opposite direction as standard analyses would suggest. Indeed, response shift may serve as a buffer for participants as they cope with the post-intervention void. In another study done by our group, a lack of differences between treatment groups could be explained by a different underlying structure to quality of life (Schwartz et al., 2000), suggesting that differences in the conceptualization of quality of life may obscure the true impact of an intervention.

Although the response shift phenomenon has a historical foundation in management sciences research, the reported work is plagued with difficulties. The primary problem in the management science work is that the methods used to evaluate response shift do not consistently point in similar directions even when the same data are analyzed (cf. Armenakis, 1988). Recent work by Sprangers and Schwartz (1999) has proposed a theoretical model which can help to guide the research questions for future response shift investigations. A range of methods for evaluating response shift are proposed by Schwartz and Sprangers (1999), including design, statistical, individualized, preference-based, successive comparison, and qualitative methods.

Regardless of the approach selected for measuring response shift and quality of life outcomes, the behavioral medicine investigator would be well-advised to ensure that at least one objective, clinical measure, be included in the battery of outcomes assessed. Clinical assessments can help to distinguish objective change from changes in internal standards, values, and conceptualization. Further, objective and subjective data can complement each other and increase the amount of explained variance in psychosocial outcomes (Schwartz et al., 1996).

# Integrating cost-effectiveness analysis into behavioral medicine trials

For behavioral medicine interventions to compete for resources in a market increasingly dominated by cost concerns, their impact must be conveyed in language that is meaningful to medical economists, health care providers, and patients (Schipper et al., 1996). Thus a further consideration for current intervention research must be to link the intervention with lower medical costs, while demonstrating a synchrony between primary care and behavioral medicine interventions. In addition to measuring relevant quality of life outcomes, this synchrony can be revealed by integrating analytic methods from cost-effectiveness and cost-offset studies, which balance cost and quality concerns by integrating subjective and objective treatment outcomes. Friedman et al. (1995) describe several theoretical models which can be invoked to explain how behavioral medicine interventions might be cost-effective, including accurately diagnosing psychiatric problems and providing services directly appropriate to the emotional problems at the root of the patient's complaint. In general, however, most cost-effectiveness and cost-offset studies have not demonstrated a significant impact. Rather they have suggested only a small cost-offset as mental health services transiently reduce medical service utilization, and replace it with lower cost care delivered by mental health professionals (Strain et al., 1991). Kashner and Rush (1999) have proposed a number of explanations of how mental health interventions could actually cause an increase in utilization. It may also be the case, however, that heretofore unacknowledged cost-savings would be documented if cost-effectiveness were one of the standard metrics for reporting study results. This benefit might be easy to detect if conclusions about cost-effectiveness were based on a more representative sample of studies.

The interested reader is referred to Sieber and Kaplan (chapter 17 in the current volume) for an explanation of the Quality-Adjusted Life Year (QALY), a metric which summarizes the benefits of health care in terms of years of healthy time gained. This metric can be very useful for behavioral medicine studies, since physical and mental health symptoms covary across patient groups (Schwartz et al., 1999), supporting the behavioral medicine tenet of addressing both aspects of the illness experience. The Sieber and Kaplan chapter also summarizes a family of QALY-based approaches. One specific method, The Extended Q-TWiST

(Schwartz et al., 1995), was designed for evaluating interventions which have an impact on multidimensional quality of life domains and social cost (e.g., work productivity). Further, this method integrates response shift into a treatment evaluation in that it considers individual patient preferences at each point in time, and integrates changes in patient values into the estimate of treatment gain. Preliminary analyses inspired by the Extended Q-TWiST method suggest that it is useful in understanding the trade-off between treatment costs and improved clinical response (Schwartz et al., 1997b). This approach facilitates treatment decisions which can be tailored to patient values.

## Conclusion

The present chapter discussed conceptual, implementation, and measurement issues of particular methodological relevance to current psychosocial intervention research. It is clear from the data and literature discussed that behavioral medicine researchers are faced with significant challenges, due to the increased acceptance of their methods into the current *zeitgeist*, as well as to the requisite attention that must be paid to the economic consequences of their interventions. The advances in analytic methodologies and in measurement subtlety and sophistication provide useful tools to the keen investigator. It is hoped that the theoretical and empirical work discussed herein will facilitate the growth of this dynamic field.

**Acknowledgments:** The author gratefully acknowledges the assistance of Rebecca Feinberg and Amy Carey for their assistance with data management for studies discussed in this chapter, and Marvin Zelen, Ph.D., Herman Chernoff, Ph.D., Mikhail Malioutov, Ph.D., and Yen-Pin Chiang, Ph.D., for helpful discussions. This work was funded by a grant from the Agency for Health Care Policy and Research (1RO1 HSO 8585–03) to Dr Schwartz.

## Notes

1.  It is interesting to note that a subsequent randomized trial published by Spiegel et al. (1989) supported the survival effect of support groups for metastatic breast cancer. This study is discussed above.

# References

Armenakis, A.A. (1988). A review of research on the change typology. In: W.A. Pasmore & R.W. Woodman (Eds.), *Research in organizational change and development: An annual series featuring advances in theory, methodology, and research, Vol. 2* (pp. 163–194). Stamford, CT: JAI Press.

Armitage, P. (1983). Exclusions, losses to follow-up, and withdrawals in clinical trials. In: S.A. Shapiro & T.A. Louis (Eds.), *Clinical trials: Issues and approaches* (pp. 99–113). New York: Marcel Dekker.

Boker, S., & McArdle, J.J. (1995). Statistical vector field analysis applied to mixed cross-sectional and longitudinal data. *Experimental Aging Research, 21*, 77–93.

Breetvelt, I.S., & Van Dam, F.S.A.M. (1991). Underreporting by cancer patients: The case of response shift. *Social Science and Medicine, 32*, 981–987.

Bryk, A.S., & Raudenbush, S.W. (1987). Application of hierarchical linear models to assessing change. *Psychological Bulletin, 101*, 147–158.

Calfas, K.J., Kaplan, R.M., & Ingram, R.E. (1992). One-year evaluation of cognitive-behavioral intervention in osteoarthritis. *Arthritis Care and Research, 5*, 202–209.

Cohen, J. (1992). A power primer. *Psychological Bulletin, 112*, 155–159.

Dillman, D.A. (1978). *Mail and telephone surveys: The total design method.* New York: Wiley.

Dunbar-Jacob, J., Sereika, S., Rohay, J., & Burke, L. (1998). Electronic methods in assessing adherence to medical regimens. In: E.S. Krantz, A. Baum et al. (Eds.), *Technology and methods in behavioral medicine* (pp. 95–113). Mahway, NJ: Erlbaum.

Fawzy, F.I., & Fawzy, N.W. (1994). A structured psychoeducational intervention for cancer patients. *General Hospital Psychiatry, 16*, 149–192.

Fisher, B., Osborne, C.K., Margolese, R.G., & Bloomer, W.D. (1997). Neoplasms of the breast. In: J.F. Holland, R.C. Bast, D.L. Morton, E. Frei, D.W. Kufe, & R.R. Weichselbaum (Eds.), *Cancer medicine, fourth edition* (Chapter 136, pp. 2349–2429). Baltimore: Williams and Wilkins.

Francis, D.J., Fletcher, J.M., Stuebing, K.K., Davidson, K.C., & Thompson, N.M. (1992). Analysis of change: Modeling individual growth. In: A.E. Kazdin (Ed.), *Methodological issues and strategies in clinical research* (pp. 607–630). Washington, DC: American Psychological Association.

Friedman, R., Sobel, D., Myers, P., Caudill, M., & Benson, H. (1995). Behavioral medicine, clinical health psychology, and cost offset. *Health Psychology, 14*, 509–518.

Hsu, L.M. (1989). Random sampling, randomization, and equivalence of contrasted groups in psychotherapy outcome research. *Journal of Consulting and Clinical Psychology, 57*, 131–137.

Kane, R., Mikalac, C., Benjamin, S., & Barkley, R.A. (1990). Assessment and treatment of ADHD. In: R.A. Barkley (Ed.), *Attention-deficit hyperactivity disorder: A handbook for diagnosis and treatment* (pp. 613–638). New York: Guilford Press.

Kaplan, R.M., & Calfas, K. (1991). Evaluation of a behavioral intervention in osteoarthritis. [Abstract.] *Proceedings of the Fellows 40th Anniversary Conference*, arthritis clinical research conference, June 21–23, Snowbird Resort, Utah.

Kashner, T.M., & Rush, A.J. (1999). Measuring cost offsets of psychotherapy. In: N.E. Miller & K.M. Magruder (Eds.), *The cost-effectiveness of psychotherapy: A guide for practitioners, researchers and policymakers* (pp. 109–121). New York: Wiley.

Kazdin, A.E., & Bass, D. (1989). Power to detect differences between alternative treatments in comparative psychotherapy outcome research. *Journal of Consulting and Clinical Psychology, 57*, 138–147.

Kraemer, H.C., & Thiemann, S. (1989). A strategy to use soft data effectively in randomized controlled clinical trials. *Journal of Consulting and Clinical Psychology, 57*, 148–154.

Laird, N.M., & Ware, J.H. (1982). Random-effects models for longitudinal data. *Biometrics, 38*, 963–974.

Lipsey, M.W., & Wilson, D.B. (1993). The efficacy of psychological, educational, and behavioral treatment: Confirmation from meta-analysis. *American Psychologist, 48*, 1181–1209.

Meyer, T.J., & Mark, M.M. (1995). Effects of psychosocial interventions with adult cancer patients: A meta-analysis of randomized experiments. *Health Psychology, 14*, 101–108.

Minden, S.L., & Schiffer, R.B. (1990). Affective disorders in multiple sclerosis: Review and recommendations for clinical research. *Archives of Neurology, 47*, 98–104.

Morgenstern, H., Gellert, G.A., Walter, S.D., Ostfeld, A.M., & Siegel, B.S. (1984). The impact of a psychosocial support program on survival with breast cancer: The importance of selection bias in program evaluation. *Journal of Chronic Disease, 37*, 273–282.

Muthén, B., & Curran, P. (1997). General longitudinal modeling of individual differences in experimental designs: A latent variable framework for analysis and power estimation. *Psychological Methods, 2*, 371–402.

Nich, C., & Carroll, K. (1997). Now you see it, now you don't: A comparison of traditional versus random-effects regression models in the analysis of longitudinal follow-up data from a clinical trial. *Journal of Consulting and Clinical Psychology, 645*, 252–261.

Pocock, S.J. (1983). *Clinical trials: A practical approach*. New York: Wiley.

Rossi, J.S. (1990). Statistical power of psychological research: What have we gained in 20 years? *Journal of Consulting and Clinical Psychology, 58*, 646–656.

Schwartz, C.E. (1994). How do psychosocial interventions influence functional status in multiple sclerosis? Result of a randomized trial. *Psychosomatic Medicine, 56,* 147–180.

Schwartz, C.E. (1998). Design issues for clinical research in health psychology. In: M. Johnston & D. Johnston (Eds.), *Comprehensive clinical psychology: Health psychology* (Vol. 8, pp. 137–151). Oxford: Elsevier Science.

Schwartz, C.E. (1999). Teaching coping skills enhances quality of life more than peer support: Results of a randomized trial with multiple sclerosis patients. *Health Psychology, 18,* 211–220.

Schwartz, C.E., & Fox, B. (1995). Who says yes? Identifying selection biases in a psychosocial intervention study of multiple sclerosis. *Social Science and Medicine, 40,* 359–370.

Schwartz, C.E., & Rogers, M. (1994). Designing a psychosocial intervention to teach coping flexibility. *Rehabilitation Psychology, 39,* 61–76.

Schwartz, C.E., & Sprangers, M.A.G. (1999). Methodological approaches for assessing response shift in longitudinal quality of life research. *Social Science and Medicine, 48,* 1531–1548.

Schwartz, C.E., Cole, B.F., & Gelber, R.D. (1995). Measuring patient-centered outcomes in neurologic disease: Extending the Q-TWiST methodology. *Archives of Neurology, 52,* 754–762.

Schwartz, C.E., Kozora, E., & Zeng, Q. (1996). Towards patient collaboration in cognitive assessment: Specificity, sensitivity, and incremental validity of self-report. *Annals of Behavioral Medicine, 18,* 177–184.

Schwartz, C.E., Chesney, M.A., Irvine, M.J., & Keefe, F.J. (1997a). The control group dilemma in clinical research: Applications for psychosocial and behavioral medicine trials. *Psychosomatic Medicine, 59,* 362–371.

Schwartz, C.E., Coulthard-Morris, L., Cole, B., & Vollmer, T. (1997b). The quality-of-life effects of Interferon-Beta-1b in multiple sclerosis: An extended Q-TWiST analysis. *Archives of Neurology, 54,* 1475–1480.

Schwartz, C.E., Feinberg, R., Jilinskaia, E., & Applegate, J. (1999). An evaluation of a psychosocial intervention for survivors of childhood cancer: Paradoxical effects of response shift over time.

Schwartz, C.E., Sprangers, M.A.G., Carey, A., & Reed, G. (Under review). Exploring response shift in longitudinal data. *Psycho-oncology, 8,* 344–354.

Schwartz, C.E., Covino, N., Morgantaler, A., & DeWolf, W. (2000). Quality-of-life after penile prosthesis placed at radical prostatectomy. *Psychology & Health, 15,* 651–661.

Schwartz, C.E., Kaplan, R.M., Anderson, J.P., Holbrook, T., & Genderson, M.W. (1999). Covariation of physical and mental symptoms across illnesses: Results of a factor analytic study. *Annals of Behavioral Medicine, 21,* 122–127.

Schipper, H., Clinch, J.J., & Olweny, C.L.M. (1996). Quality of life studies: Definitions and conceptual issues. In: B. Spilker (Ed.), *Quality of life assess-*

*ments in clinical trials* (second edition, pp. 11–23). Philadelphia: Lippincott-Raven Press.

Shadish, W.R., & Ragsdale, K. (1996). Random versus nonrandom assignment in controlled experiments: Do you get the same answer? *Journal of Consulting and Clinical Psychology, 64,* 1290–1305.

Spira, J. (1997). Existential group psychotherapy for women with advanced breast cancer and other life-threatening illnesses. In: J. Spira (Ed.), *Group therapy for medically ill patients* (pp. 165–222). New York: Guilford Publications.

Spiegel, D., Bloom, J.R., Kraemer, H.C., & Gottheil, E. (1989). Effect of psychosocial treatment on survival of patients with metastatic breast cancer. *The Lancet, October 14,* 888–891.

Sprangers, M.A.G. (1996). Response shift bias: A challenge to the assessment of patients' quality of life in cancer clinical trials. *Cancer Treatment Reviews, 22SA,* 55–62.

Sprangers, M.A.G., & Schwartz, C.E. (1999). Integrating response shift into health-related quality-of-life research: A theoretical model. *Social Science and Medicine, 48,* 1507–1515.

Strain, J.J., Lyons, D.S., Hammer, J.S., Fahs, M., Lebovits, A., Paddison, P.L., Snyder, S., Strauss, E., Burton, R., Nuber, G., Abernathy, T., Sacks, H., Noralie, J., & Sacks, C. (1991). Cost offset from a psychiatric consultation-liaison intervention with elderly hip fracture patients. *American Journal of Psychiatry, 148,* 1044–1049.

Tanaka, J.S. (1987). "How big is enough?" Sample size and goodness of fit in structural equation models with latent variables. *Child Development, 58,* 134–146.

Talcott, J.A., Rieker, P., Clark, J., Propert, K.J., Weeks, J.C., Beard, C.J., Wiskow, K.I., Kaplan, I., Loughlin, K.R., Richie, J.P., & Kantoff, P.W. (1998). Patient-reported symptoms after primary therapy for early prostate cancer: Results of a prospective cohort study. *Journal of Clinical Oncology, 16,* 275–283.

Willett, J.B., Ayoub, C.C., & Robinson, D. (1991). Using growth modeling to examine systematic differences in growth: An example of change in the functioning of families at risk of maladaptive parenting, child abuse, or neglect. *Journal of Consulting and Clinical Psychology, 59,* 38–47.

Zelen, M. (1979). A new design for randomized clinical trials. *New England Journal of Medicine, 300,* 1242–1245.

# 4 THEORY AND MEASUREMENT: CONCEPTUALIZATION, OPERATIONALIZATION AND THE EXAMPLE OF HEALTH STATUS

Jane Ogden

The relationship between theory and measurement takes many forms (see Figure 4.1). Firstly, a theoretical perspective is implicit within any discipline. In line with this, this chapter will primarily examine the relationship between theory and measurement in terms of matching a theoretical perspective with whatever is being measured. Secondly, a theory needs to be translated into a measurement tool. This itself involves a theory of measurement concerned with how best this can be done. Therefore, this chapter will examine the processes of conceptualization and operationalization, and the strategies of reliability and validity as these are described by the theory of measurement as essential to this translation process. Finally, the belief that theories can be measured is itself a theoretical position. To conclude, the chapter will explore the origins of this belief and the role of the relationships between theory and measurement in supporting and perpetuating the perspective inherent within any attempts at measurement.

## Matching a theoretical perspective to what is measured

Researchers working within the field of health measure a range of variables. Those interested in laboratory science may measure cell replication or decay and the impact of a new drug upon this process. For those interested in clinical medicine, blood pressure, weight, and glucose metabolism may form their focus of attention and for the epidemiologists illness prevalence and incidence are important. Such research involves questions such as "how many cells are there?", "what is their rate of decay?", "what is an individual's level of insulin production?" or "how many new cases of cancer are there each year?".

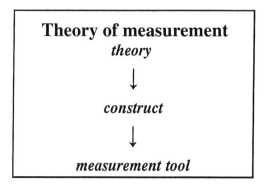

Figure 4.1. Relationships between theory and measurement

These questions require a simple process of measurement. The cells and cases are counted, and the numbers shown on weighing scales or blood pressure machines are recorded. The machines may need to be calibrated but that is all. No one asks the questions "how do you know?", "are you sure?" or "says who?". What it is, is what is measured. Measurement is simple. However, for social scientists the story is completely different. Although our historical roots lie in the science of an observable variable, namely behavior, the increasing emphasis on the complexity of human beings has brought with it an interest in cognitions and emotions. Such constructs cannot simply be counted or read from a meter. They are complex. For social scientists, measurement is a complicated process. This shift from simplicity to complexity is particularly apparent in the range of attempts at measuring health status.

# From simple to complex measures of health status

## THE MORTALITY RATE

The bottom line measurement of health status is the mortality rate. At its most basic it takes the form of a very crude mortality rate which can be calculated by simply counting the number of deaths in one year compared to either previous or subsequent years. The question being asked is "has the number of people who have died this year gone up, down or stayed the same?". An increase could be seen as a decrease in health status and a decrease in mortality rate as an increase in health status. This approach, however, requires a denominator, a measure of who is at risk. The next most basic form of mortality rate therefore includes a denominator reflecting the size of the population being studied. Such a measure allows for comparisons to be made between different populations: more people may die in a given year in London when compared to Bournemouth, but London is simply bigger. However, does this measure really now tell us about health status? To provide any meaningful measure of health status mortality rates are corrected for age (Bournemouth has an older population and therefore we would predict that more people would die each year) and gender (men generally die younger than women and this needs to be taken into account). Furthermore, mortality rates can be produced to be either age specific such as infant mortality rates, or illness specific such as sudden death rates. As long as the population being studied is accurately specified, corrected and specific mortality rates provide an easily available and simple measure: death is a good reliable outcome.

## THE MORBIDITY RATE

Laboratory and clinical researchers and epidemiologists may accept mortality rates as the perfect measure of health status. However, the juxtaposition of social scientists to the medical world over the past few decades has managed to challenge this dichotomous model of health to raise the now obvious question "is health really only the absence of death?". In response to this there has been an increasing focus upon morbidity. However, in line with the emphasis upon simplicity inherent within the focus on mortality rates, many morbidity measures still use methods of counting and recording. For example, the expensive and time consuming production of morbidity prevalence rates involves large surveys of "caseness" to simply count how many people within a given population suffer from a particular problem. Likewise, sickness absence rates and caseload assessments simply count days lost due to illness and the numbers of people who visit their General Practitioner or hospital respectively within a given time frame. Such morbidity measures are still relatively simple. In contrast, other measures of morbidity have embraced the more complex nature of health status and are often called measures of subjective health status.

## SUBJECTIVE HEALTH STATUS

In line with this approach, measures of functioning such as activity of daily living scales (Katz et al., 1970) and self report measures ranging from single items such as "How would you rate your own health?" (Idler & Kasl, 1995) to composite scales such as the Nottingham Health Profile (Hunt et al., 1986) and the SF-36 (Ware & Sherbourne, 1992) ask for the individuals' own assessment of their health status. Quality of life scales also largely focus on the individual's own assessment of how their own quality of life has been impaired (e.g., Fallowfield, 1990). In fact more recent quality of life scales ask the subject not only to rate their own assessment of their health status but also to define the dimensions along which it should be rated (McGee et al., 1991; O'Boyle et al., 1992). From a pure science perspective such measures can be seen as problematically unobjective and far removed from simply counting the number of deaths. Social scientists are, however, concerned with cognitions and emotions, not the absence or presence of death. Therefore, from a social science perspective the measures are complex because health status is itself regarded as a complex construct.

## A SHIFT IN PERSPECTIVE

The shift from an emphasis on mortality to one on quality of life reflects a shift from simplicity to complexity. However, it also reflects a shift along a series of other dimensions. Firstly, it represents a shift from implicit value to attempts to make this value explicit. For example, mortality and morbidity measures assume that what they are measuring is an absolute index of health. The value of the events is assumed to be inherent within the constructs themselves. However, the areas being measured are value laden but this value is implicit; it is assumed that not being able to walk up stairs and death are negative events. Accordingly, the subjects being studied are not asked "Is it a bad thing that you cannot walk upstairs?". However, it could be argued that mortality and aspects of morbidity are not always negative. The more complex measures attempt to make the value within the constructs being studied explicit. In line with this, subjective measures of health may ask "to what extent are you prevented from doing the things you would like to do?" or "is your present state of health causing problems with your. ..." (e.g., Hunt et al., 1986). Furthermore, some measures ask the subjects to describe "what are the five most important aspects of your life at the moment" (O'Boyle et al., 1992). Both these approaches make explicit the value that is implicit within simplistic measures of health. The next dimension which varies between the simple and complex measures of health is the subjectivity of the individual being studied. Mortality and morbidity measures are assumed to be objective scientific measures which access a reality which is uncontaminated by bias. In contrast, the complex measures make this bias the essence of what they are interested in. For example, whereas mortality data are taken from hospital records or death certificates, and morbidity ratings are often made by the health professional not the individual being studied, subjective health measures ask the individual for their own experiences and beliefs in terms of "How do you rate?" or "How do you feel?". They make no pretence to be objective and, rather than attempting to exclude the individuals beliefs, they make them their focus. The final shift in perspective concerns the subjectivity of the researcher. It could be assumed that mortality rates would be the same regardless of who collected them or that morbidity would be consistent for the same individual across different raters. Studies of caseness, however, require definitions of diagnoses and evaluations of sickness absence rates require a decision to be made about what constitutes an absence due to illness (having a sick note? not taking annual leave?). Perhaps individual researchers differ in their choice of population and vary in the way they rate levels of functioning. Olsson et al. (1986) suggested that morbidity should be rated by the health professional on a scale "dead" (1) to "alive" (4). There is obvious room for researcher bias in this approach. However, choice of data for mortality rates may also be open to bias (in addition, the definition of death may vary across both researchers and time – when does a miscarriage become a stillbirth which is registered as a death?). The more complex measures of health attempt to address the issue of researcher subjectivity. However, whereas explicit value and the beliefs of the individual being studied have become accepted foci, the subjectivity of the researcher remains unresolved and still provokes debate. Methods such as using self report questionnaires or asking only closed questions attempt to address this issue. However, the questions being asked and the response frames given are still chosen by the researcher. An alternative approach can be found within qualitative methods with the use of in depth open ended interviews to elicit the beliefs of the interviewee with minimal input from the interviewer. Further, the quality of life scale developed recently (O'Boyle et al., 1992) also offers a method for dealing with the researchers' subjectivity by in effect presenting the subject with a blank sheet and asking them to devise their own scale. However, both the interview transcript and the individual's own scales still require coding and analysis by the researcher.

Accordingly, the shift from mortality rates to quality of life scales reflects a change from a simple to a complex approach to health status. It also reflects a shift from implicit to explicit value and from attempts at objectivity to an emphasis on the subjectivity of both the individual and the researcher. Further, such shifts epitomise the different biomedicine and social science perspectives. Therefore, if health status is regarded as the presence or absence of death, then mortality rates provide a suitable assessment tool. Death is a reliable outcome variable and mortality is appropriately simple. If, however, health status is regarded as more complex than this, more complex measures are needed. Morbidity rates account for a continuum model of health and illness and facilitate the assessment of the more gray areas and some morbidity measures accept the subjective nature of health. However, only measures which ask the individual themselves to rate their own health are fully in line with a social science model of what health means. Such subjective measures not only accept but highlight and emphasize health as a complex construct. They provide a measure of health status which is in accordance with the perspective of the discipline.

Therefore, complex measures of health status solve the problem of matching the measure to the theoretical perspective. But are such measures really a solution? Rather than simply providing an answer to the question of how to measure social science constructs, such a perspective opens up a whole set of other measurement problems for researchers as adult theories of measurement have been developed.

## Theories of measurement

### THE PROBLEMS OF MEASURING COMPLEX CONSTRUCTS

In the 1920s scientists began to suspect a link between asbestos and inflammation of the lining of the lung and subsequent lung cancer. In the 1950s clinicians had a theory that smoking caused lung cancer. In the early 1980s competing research groups hypothesized that a lentivirus which they called HIV1 was responsible for the sudden increase in deaths from previously rare forms of cancers and pneumonia. To test these theories the researchers needed to confirm significant links between the different pairs of variables involved. Primarily, this involved translating theory into a set of constructs which could be measured. This was easy as the theories themselves were made up of constructs: asbestos, lung cancer, smoking and so on. However, for social scientists this process is more complex and highlights the first problem encountered by attempts at measurement. Social science researchers theorize that beliefs influence behavior and that behavior influences health. Such theories need to be refined. Translating theory into constructs highlights the problem of conceptualization. The second stage involves developing a suitable and accurate measurement tool for each of the relevant constructs. For example, the existence of asbestos would have been established, the number of cigarettes smoked counted and the presence of the HIV virus confirmed. Likewise diagnoses of the appropriate diseases would have been made. However, if, as social scientists, we have a theory that a particular medical intervention may impact upon an individual's quality of life, how do we know that our measurement tool for quality of life is actually measuring what we want it to do (perhaps it measures depression, or anxiety or learned helplessness?). This illustrates the second problem associated with measuring complex constructs: that of operationalization. These two problems are not independent of each other and often the process of measurement involves a return to the conceptualization stage when operationalization does not appear to have been satisfactory. However, the problems of conceptualization and operationalization are central to any attempts at measurement within social science. Aspects of validity and reliability are strategies which have developed as their solution. These aspects of the theory of measurement are illustrated in Figure 4.2.

## THE PROBLEM OF CONCEPTUALIZATION

Conceptualization describes the stage involved with the clarification of ideas and concepts which enable the resulting theoretical construct to be distinguished from any other. It therefore involves the translation of a vague notion into a clearly bounded construct and is essential to any attempts at measurement. It is also essential for communication both within and between academic disciplines. Poorly conceptualized constructs can lead to confusion between research groups and an appearance of contradictory findings. Accordingly, happiness could be conceptualized as "the absence of depression", or "the absence of

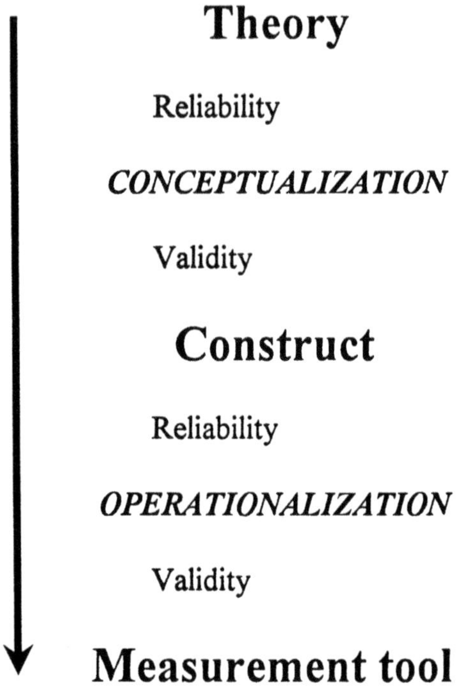

# Theory

Reliability

*CONCEPTUALIZATION*

Validity

# Construct

Reliability

*OPERATIONALIZATION*

Validity

# Measurement tool

Figure 4.2.  Theories of measurement

negative thoughts" or "the presence of positive thoughts". Suppose a group of researchers were interested in the impact of cervical screening on health. The two variables being studied, "cervical screening" and "health", first need to be conceptualized before they can be assessed. A biomedical paper describing this relationship may conclude that cervical screening improved health status whereas a psychology paper may conclude the reverse. Poor conceptualization could account for this apparent contradiction. The role of conceptualization is particularly apparent in the area of quality of life. Reports of a Medline search for the term "quality of life" indicate a surge in its use from 40 citations between 1966 and 1974, to 1,907 citations from 1981 to 1985, to 5,078 citations from 1986 to 1990 (Albrecht, 1994). Quality of life is obviously in vogue. Researchers have differentiated between quality of life in the last year of life (Lawton et al., 1990), quality of life in individuals with specific illnesses (e.g., Meenan et al., 1980), quality of life from a health economics perspective (Rosser & Kind, 1978) or with an emphasis on survival (Bush, 1983). Measures of quality of life have ranged in complexity from single item scales (Idler & Kasl, 1995) through to multifactorial scales (e.g., Hunt et al., 1986) and have used either a unidimensional approach which focuses on a single aspect of health such as mood (e.g., Goldberg, 1978) or pain (e.g., Melzack, 1975) or a multidimensional perspective (e.g., Fallowfield, 1990). Further, it has been defined in a multitude of ways including "the value assigned to duration of life as modified by the impairments, functional states, perceptions and social opportunities that are influenced by disease, injury, treatment or policy" (Patrick & Ericson, 1993), "a personal statement of the positivity or negativity of attributes that characterize one's life" (Grant et al., 1990) and more recently by the World Health Organization as "a broad ranging concept affected in a complex way by the person's physical health, psychological state, level of independence, social relationships and their relationship to the salient features in their environment" (WHOQOL Group, 1993). However, it remains unclear whether quality of life is different to health status, whether it is to be defined as separate to health related quality of life; as a construct, quality of life remains poorly conceptualized. In fact, Annas (1990) argued that we should stop using the term altogether. However, given that at present its use continues, how can good conceptualization be achieved? Blood pressure, body temperature, cell replication have been clearly conceptualized. Can the same be done for social science constructs?

## USING RELIABILITY AND VALIDITY

Aspects of reliability and validity have been developed and used within social science as strategies to assess and promote the degree of conceptualization. In particular, although face validity is often described within the context of the actual measurement process, it is particularly relevant to the conceptualization process. Face validity requires researchers to agree that a concept makes sense and that its definition reflects the construct itself. Over recent years the WHO have set up a working group to define quality of life (WHOQOL Group, 1993). Similar meetings were also held to develop the EORTC QLQ-C30 (e.g., Aaronson et al., 1993). This has involved experts meeting to develop a definition; quality of life work tends to be collaborative. In order to be satisfactory, the resulting definition must have face validity and the belief that the definition has face validity must be shared. Conceptualization is also facilitated through interrater reliability. Again, although this term is usually used within the descriptions of actual measurement, the fact that several researchers agree about a given definition creates consensus which in turn aids conceptualization. In addition, methods such as focus groups and, in particular, the Delphi method of asking individuals to generate new ideas and then comment on each idea until they can agree upon a definition are also approaches to facilitate conceptualization. A clearly conceptualized construct is therefore one which has been clearly defined and can be easily differentiated from other constructs; quality of life will have been clearly conceptualized when we know what it is and what it is not. The gap between idea and construct involves the process of conceptualization and is bridged by face validity and interrater reliability.

## THE PROBLEM OF OPERATIONALIZATION

Once the objects of study have been conceptualized, the measurement process involves operationalization. This stage requires the development of an indicator which is an acceptable measurement of the construct in question. For constructs such as patient, health professional, child and so on, this involves a process not dissimilar to conceptualization. For example, on a simple level, if a study required on the assessment of the health of patients, the concept "patient" needs to be operationalized. It could be operationalized in many ways including "person requiring treatment", "person registered on a General Practice list", "person attending a general practice within a one year period" or, more specifically, "person over the age of 16 attending a general practice in order to see the GP for their own health problem (not accompanying a child or other adult) within a year". For most social scientists, however, their measurement tools are either interviews involving semistructured questions or selfreport questionnaires using statements or questions which are rated by the individual being studied. In line with this, definitions of more complex terms such as depression and anxiety can also be turned into suitable indicators in the form of a mood scale and the definition of quality of life can be translated into a quality of life scale. For example, following the discussions around an acceptable definition of quality of life, the European Organisation for Research on Treatment of Cancer operationalized quality of life in terms of "functional status, cancer and treatment specific symptoms, psychological distress, social interaction, financial/economic impact, perceived health status, and overall quality of life" (Aaronson et al., 1993). In line with this, their measure consisted of items which reflected these different dimensions. Likewise, the researchers who worked on the Rand Corporation health batteries operationalized quality of life in terms of "physical functioning, social functioning, role limitations due to physical problems, role limitations due to emotional problems, mental health, energy/vitality, pain and general health perception" which formed the basic dimensions of their scale (e.g., Stewart & Ware, 1992). Such tools are usually developed from items elicited from the literature, the researchers, the subjects of the research or all three. The items are then constructed into a questionnaire which is piloted and finalized. The operationalized construct and subsequent scale is assumed to measure the construct under scrutiny. However, the development of a measurement tool raises the question "does the tool really measure the construct in question?". We know that weighing scales measure weight, height charts measure height and sphygmomanometers measure blood pressure. How do we know that our constructs are being measured by our measurement tools; that the construct has been accurately operationalized?

## THE ROLE OF RELIABILITY AND VALIDITY

Social scientists have developed indices of reliability and validity as strategies for facilitating accurate operationalization; to know that the results from the measurement tool are not simply an artefact of the tool itself (Box 4.1). Firstly, if the construct is conceptualized as being constant, can the tool detect this constancy or does it produce different results at different times. Test-retest reliability deals with the problem of change over time by illustrating that the measurement tool can produce consistent results. Secondly, does the tool produce results which are comparable to those produced by other similar tools? Construct validity in the forms of both convergent and discriminant validity deals with this problem of variability by illustrating consistent results when compared to other measures. Finally, do all items used in the scale reflect different aspects of the same complex construct? This problem is dealt with by testing the scale for internal consistency using statistical procedures such as factor analysis and reliability coefficients. By determining a level of agreement between measures, over time and within measures, social scientists create a sense that the tool accurately measures the construct. The gaps between idea and construct, and between construct and measurement tool have been bridged and the conceptualization and operationalization process is complete.

## WHY DO THESE PROBLEMS ARISE WITHIN SOCIAL SCIENCE?

Biologists agree what cells are, epidemiologists agree what death is and biochemists agree what changes in cell structure look like. There is a consensus between the researchers working within these disciplines. Furthermore, sphygmomanometers clearly measure blood pressure,

**Box 4.1**    Reliability and validity

Contrary to the biomedical sciences, where a concept like validity is not known (because there is no reason to question the validity of heart rate, leukocyte counts, or noradrenaline plasma concentrations), for psychological measures reliability and validity are considered to be of crucial importance (e.g. Peck & Shapiro, 1990).

*Reliability* refers to the question of consistency. The crucial question is whether the measure as a whole, and the individual items, yield roughly similar results, when being applied under more or less the same conditions. Reliability estimates are generally given in the form of a correlation coefficient. It should be noted that for a test to be really considered reliable a minimum value of .80 has to be reached; measures with reliabilities of less than .70 should be applied with great caution. Unreliable measures include a great deal of random variability, which implies that both for clinical work and for research purposes the use of unreliable measures should be avoided. The most common forms of reliability are the following:

- Test-retest reliability: refers to consistency of the measure. The measure is applied to the same respondents under similar conditions at two different times. Applying this measure, of course, only makes sense for the measurement of more stable characteristics
- Alternative form reliability: indicates to what extent similar results are obtained with alternative forms of the instrument The same respondents complete an alternative form of the measure under similar circumstances
- Split-half reliability: provides information about the correlation between the scores on two halves of the measure The measure is divided into two halves which are completed by the same respondents under the same conditions. Assuming that the items in the two halves assess the same feature, a high correlation might be expected.
- Inter-rater reliability: provides insight into the degree of agreement among observers in their judgement of the same materials or persons.
- Intra-rater reliability: focuses on the consistency in the judgements of the same observers over time of the same materials.

In addition to these traditional methods of reliability assessment, there are a number of important new developments and extensions for the determination of the reliability, e.g., generalizability theory and item-response theory. Designers of new measures should consider the application of this new methodology when developing or refining assessment tools.

*Validity* is the second criterion to evaluate measures. Validity refers to the question whether the device indeed measures what it intends to measure. Some kinds of validity are reported in the form of a correlation, whereas in other cases authors report descriptive statistics for different groups or any other information. Also for validity it is recommended that coefficients, if appropriate, have a value of at least .70. Whereas this criterion generally suffices to warrant the use of a specific measure, occasionally measuring tools may be evaluated with more sophisticated methods to assess their utility for specific research questions. The most frequently reported forms of validity are:

- Face validity: refers to the extent to which a measure appears to be measuring the feature of interest. Note that there is no standard criterion and that there exists no summary statistic.
- Sampling or content validity: indicates to what extent the measures tap all relevant aspects of the characteristic in question. This important aspect of validity also lacks a statistic and there are neither standard ways nor guidelines to determine it objectively.
- Concurrent validity: refers to the patterns of association of the measure with a pre-existing criterion or already existing measurement methods with proven validity and reliability. Strongly positive (or negative) correlations indicate concurrent validity.
- Predictive validity: this type of validity is especially relevant if one aims to predict future (clinical) state. It is less important if one wishes to monitor changes in clinical state. The statistic employed is typically a correlation between a measure and some future criterion.
- Incremental validity: indicates not only whether a new tool "works" adequately, but rather whether it also is a better instrument than existing measures. According to Mischel (1972), subjects' own simple direct self-ratings and self-reports often are not inferior to more costly and sophisticated assessment instruments including combined batteries, interviews, and expert clinical judgements.

weight scales measure weight and height charts clearly measure height because although the value of these variables may vary from individual to individual their essence does not. Likewise, it is believed that cells are the same wherever they are and death is death regardless of who has died. Biologists, biochemists and epidemiologists have consensus among themselves. In addition, their objects of study are also consistent. Accordingly, their constructs do not need to be conceptualized because there are no dissenting voices; the researchers already have a consensus. Further, their constructs do not need to be operationalized because the object they are measuring is the same wherever it is and whoever it belongs to. In contrast, the social scientists need to reach a consensus in order for their concepts to be clearly conceptualized. Quality of life cannot be clearly conceptualized because researchers will not and do not agree what it is. Further, it is not only a lack of consensus between researchers which makes the process of measurement problematic. The constructs studied by social scientists also vary. In fact, central to the social science perspective is the belief that these constructs do vary both between individuals and within individuals over time; it is the variation that is studied. Social science lacks consensus both among the researchers and among the objects of study. Reliability and validity can be used by social scientists to generate a sense of good conceptualization by creating consensus between the researchers as to the appropriate definition. Further they can be used to provide confidence that a concept has been effectively operationalized by asserting a sense of consensus among the object being measured. If all the researchers agree, then a concept has been clearly conceptualized and if the concept can be shown to have consistency across time and between individuals then the measure can be seen as an accurate indicator of this concept.

## Why is there a problem of consensus?

Whether it be biology research examining cell function, epidemiology research examining mortality or psychology research assessing the predictors of smoking, there is a biologist, an epidemiologist and a psychologist examining a cell, death certificates, or selfreports of smoking. Any research process involves two components: the researcher and the researched. However, different disciplines regard these two elements very differently. Within the natural sciences both the researcher and the researched are homogenous. It doesn't matter where the researcher is located, what their age, gender or culture is or what they think. Researchers are homogenous, undifferentiated entities; it is as if they are headless. Accordingly, it is no wonder that conceptualization within the natural sciences is so simple because its researchers are automatically a consensual group. In addition, French cells are believed to be the same as those in the US. Death is regarded as the same in the UK as in Africa. Their objects of study are uniform. Accordingly, operationalization is simple because the thing "out there" being measured is also homogenous. Social science, however is the study of individuals. Furthermore, it is the study of individuals who vary. Therefore, these individuals are a heterogenous group. Whether it be along the dimensions defined by demographic variables such as age, gender, class, geographical location or whether it be according to beliefs and behaviors, individuals differ from each other. Accordingly, operationalization is problematic because of variation in the object being operationalized. Furthermore, if the individuals being studied are heterogenous, then the researchers, who are also individuals, must also be heterogenous. They must also vary; social science studies individuals but is also studied by individuals. The social science researcher has a head. Accordingly, conceptualization is also problematic. The attempt to diversify from the natural sciences has both problematized the object of study and by default has problematized the objects doing the studying. In doing so it has lost the consensus inherent within the natural sciences. Reliability and validity are attempts at regaining this status.

## Measurement as a theoretical position

Central to empiricism is the belief that the objects of study can be measured and that things "out there" can be accessed by measurement tools. Empiricism depends upon the faith that the results produced by these measurement tools are not simply artefacts of the tools themselves; depression exists in individuals not in depression scales and quality of life exists even when it is not being measured. Therefore, if the researcher is regarded as a disembodied being who passively records what is happening in the world, then the gap between themselves and the "out there" is straightforward; the "out there" is all there is. Accordingly, reliability and validity are central to the process of bridging this gap between the idea and the construct (conceptualization) and ensuring that the assessment results are accurate reflections of things in the world (operationalization). If, however, we accept that the researcher is an individual who has cognitions and emotions comparable to the individuals being studied then this gap is more problematic. Can we ever measure what is "out there"? Perhaps reliability and validity do not bridge the gaps between idea and construct and between construct and measurement tool but create them. Without such strategies to give credibility to the process of operationalization, the measurement tool would be the construct, nothing else. Furthermore, without such strategies to substantiate the process of conceptualization, the construct would simply be the creation of the researcher. The researcher would be studying what was inside his/her own head – it would bear no relation to the outside world. We need conceptualization, operationalization and strategies of reliability and validity, not to create accurate measurement tools which reflect the outside world but to prevent us from simply reporting our fictional stories as we see them.

## Conclusion

Social science represents the study of complex individuals and their cognitions and emotions. In terms of health related research, it has elaborated upon the simple constructs of mortality and morbidity to develop more complex constructs which match its theoretical perspective. However, this shift has brought with it the problems inherent with measuring diverse factors such as quality of life. Such measurement involves the processes of conceptualization to clarify the concept being studied and operationalization to develop the appropriate indicator. Further, it utilizes the strategies of reliability and validity to check that these processes have been effectively executed. Such processes are required due to the absence of consensus both between researchers and within the objects being researched. Social science emphasizes heterogeneity. However, if social science studies individuals who are deemed to be heterogenous, they must therefore be studied by individuals who are equally varied. If it is not only the researched that is seen to be heterogenous but also the researcher, how can we know that the measurement tool is not simply the construct itself or that the construct is not simply in the mind of the researcher? Perhaps, rather than being strategies to bridge the gaps between idea and construct and tool, reliability and validity have been developed to serve an important function; to construct these gaps. Without them we would only have our scientific faith that empiricism was possible. Theories can be matched to their objects to be measured and translated into suitable measurement tools. However, the very belief that all this is possible is itself a theoretical position and the processes involved in both matching and translating theory are themselves essential to sustaining and perpetuating the credibility of this position.

# References

Aaronson, N.K., Ahmedzai, S., Bergman, B., Bullinger, M., Cull, A., Duez, N.J., Filiberti, A., Flechtner, H., Fleishman, S.B., & de Haes, J.C. (1993). The European Organisation for Research and Treatment of Cancer QLQ-C30: A quality of life instrument for use in international clinical trials in oncology. *Journal for the National Cancer Institute, 85*, 365–76.

Albrecht, G.L. (1994). Subjective health status. In: C. Jenkinson (Ed.), *Measuring health and medical outcomes* (pp. 7–26). London: UCL Press.

Annas, G.J. (1990). Quality of life in the courts: Early spring in fantasyland. In: J.J. Walter & T.A. Shannon (Eds.), *Quality of life: The new medical dilemma* (pp. 319–322). New York: Paulist Press.

Bush, J.W. (1983). *Quality of well being scale: Function status profile and symptom/problem complex questionnaire.* San Diego, CA: University of California Health Policy Project.

Fallowfield, L. (1990). *The quality of life: The missing measurement in health care.* London: Souvenir Press

Goldberg, D.P. (1978). *Manual of the General Health Questionnaire.* Windsor: NFER-Nelson.

Grant, M., Padilla, G.V., Ferrell, B.R., & Rhiner, M. (1990). Assessment of quality of life with a single instrument. *Seminars in Oncology Nursing, 6*, 260–270.

Hunt, S.M., McEwen, J., & McKenna, S.P. (1986). *Measuring health status.* Beckenham: Croom Helm.

Idler, E.L., & Kasl, S.V. (1995). Self ratings of health: Do they predict change in function as ability. *Journals of Gerontology, Series B-Psychological Sciences and Social Sciences. 50B*, S344-S353.

Katz, S., Downs, T.D., Cash, H.R., & Grotz, R.C. (1970). Progress in development of the index of ADL. *Gerontology, 10*, 20–30.

Lawton, M.P., Moss, M., & Glicksman, A. (1990). The quality of life in the last year of life of older persons. *The Millbank Quarterly, 68*, 1–28.

McGee, H.M., O'Boyle, C.A., Hickey, A., O'Malley, K., & Joyce, C.R. (1991). Assessing the quality of life of the individual: The SEIQoL with a healthy and a gastroenterology unit population. *Psychological Medicine, 21*, 749–759.

Meenan, R.F., Gertman, P.M., & Mason, J.H. (1980). Measuring health status in arthritis: The arthritis impact measurement scales. *Arthritis and Rheumatism 23*, 146–152.

Melzack, R. (1975). The McGill pain questionnaire: Major properties and scoring methods. *Pain, 1*, 277–299.

Mischel, W. (1972). Direct versus indirect personality aseesment: Evidence and implications. *Journal of Consulting and Clinical Psychology, 38*, 319–324.

O'Boyle, C.A., McGee, H., Hickey, A., O'Malley, K., & Joyce, C.R. (1992). Individual quality of life in patients undergoing hip replacement. *The Lancet, 339*, 1088–1091.

Olsson, G., Lubsen, J., & Van Es, G.A. (1986). Quality of life after myocardial infarction: Effect of long term metroprolol on mortality and morbidity. *British Medical Journal, 292*, 1491–1493.

Patrick, D.L., & Ericson, P.E. (1993). *Health status and health policy: Allocating resources to health care.* Oxford: Oxford University Press.

Peck, D.F., & Shapiro, C.M. (1990). Guidelines for the construction, selection, and interpretation of measurement devices. In: D.F. Peck & C.M. Shapiro (Eds.), *Measuring human problems. A practical guide.* (pp. 1–12). Chichester: Wiley

Rosser, R.M., & Kind, P. (1978). A scale of evaluations of states of illness: Is there a social consensus? *International Journal of Epidemiology, 7*, 347–358.

Stewart, A.L., & Ware, J.E. (Eds.) (1992). *Measuring functioning and well being: The Medical Outcomes Study Approach.* Durham, NC: Duke University Press.

Ware, J.E., & Sherbourne, C.D. (1992). The MOS 36 item short form health survey (SF-36). Conceptual framework and item selection. *Medical Care, 30*, 473–483.

WHOQOL Group (1993). *Measuring quality of life: The development of a World Health Organisation quality of life instrument (WHOQOL).* Geneva: WHO.

# 5 DEVELOPING SELF-REPORT MEASURES IN HEALTH CARE

Fred Tudiver

The purpose of this chapter is to give the reader an understanding of the principles and various approaches that health care researchers have used for developing and utilizing measures of self report. In particular, I will describe several uses of these types of measures by reporting on actual examples of self report measures that have been used by investigators in recent years. These examples will illustrate the principles, approaches and uses.

## Self-report measures in health care research: what are they?

Measures of self-report are used in virtually every corner of health care research. One would have to eliminate a significant part of modern health research if we did not have these measures, whether they be face-to-face or telephone interviews, "paper-and-pencil" questionnaires or surveys. Self-report measures have many uses in data collection, but today they are used most widely in the survey. Self-report measures are now accepted as scientific tools for use in health research—tools that are as appropriate and suitable for research as any other. The main proviso is that investigators using these tools apply as much scientific rigor to their data collection and analyses as with any other data collection. There are excellent tried and proven means for doing this with a survey, and we will explore these later in this chapter.

### DEFINITION
Perhaps it is the definition of the survey that best describes what we will be discussing in this chapter: "A survey is a research technique where informational requirements are specified, a population is identified, a sample selected and systematically questioned, and the results analyzed, generalized to the population, and reported to meet

the informational needs" (Albreck & Settle, 1985). The self-report measure is essentially an organized set of questions, directly asked of a population to answer a specified research question.

## THEORETICAL UNDERPINNINGS

With any good quality research, there needs to be a recognized, substantial theory that holds the various components of the research together. Without the theory, the research question and hypothesis, the methodology, the data collection, and the analyses will not comprise a uniform whole. The same goes for any measures we use for collecting our data (Henry, 1992, p. 111). If investigators use a measure of self-report without a theoretical underpinning they are attempting to do research without the guide or beacon that is essential to drive the research, and provide the platform that is critical, yet this is still not carried out as frequently as required.

To illustrate, we can look at a common example. A lot of health promotion studies in recent years have focused on the process of change, in particular, the process of getting people to adapt to healthier lifestyles that are associated with lower morbidity and mortality. Many of the studies in the past decade have used the transtheoretical model of behavior change of Prochaska and DiClimente (1986) to link their questions with this theory. Without the theory, it would hardly make sense to design a survey that purports to measure the process an individual may go through in order to quit smoking, or to discover how physicians adopt clinical practice guidelines into everyday clinical decisions.

## STRENGTHS, WEAKNESSES, AND LIMITATIONS

Self-report measures are among the most commonly used instruments in health care research, yet they are not a panacea. They will not always be the appropriate tool for answering research questions. A major advantage of using these measures is that they are very efficient for collecting personal and sensitive health related data. The cost of training and hiring personnel for interviews is usually spared, and it often takes little time to collect data. Further, they can be administered to large numbers of subjects by hand or through a postal system quickly and with relatively low cost. More than one measure can be administered at a time, and there are no geographical limitations. Personal and sensitive questions can be asked with relative ease, and there are many efficient methods for ensuring confidentiality. A major disadvantage, however, is that these instruments may be insensitive to what the investigator is trying to measure. Much of the time this happens when an existing measure, which was initially designed for an older study with a different population, is used in a new study. Another problem is that when one tries to avoid this first problem by designing new measures, they often incur large costs, are time consuming, and psychometric expertise is required. We will look at these issues again in more detail later in this chapter. Finally, the response rate on many self-report measures can be low, often lower than the unofficial standard of a minimum 60% response rate. This is a particular problem with surveys handed out by third parties or with those that are sent directly in the mail.

## Self-report measures: standards and applications

This section will offer details on what a health care researcher should look for in a high quality self-report measure. There is a lot more rigor and effort required in developing these types of measures than many realize. Many young clinical investigators resort to surveys early in their careers often because they believe they are simple and quick to produce and utilize. However, much science (and work) has to go into the development of a high quality instrument.

## Choosing and using existing self-report measures: what should you expect from a good measure?

Many researchers will opt for using an existing self-report measure, rather than face the daunting task of creating a new one to answer their question. The research disciplines are replete with measures for almost any question in the health, or for that matter, any other field. There are now many texts that focus on measures, books that provide anthologies of self-report measures. They often include detailed descriptions of the measure, they report on uses of the measure with descriptions of populations and settings. Most include psychometric properties; some even attach a copy of the measure in their appendix. Two excellent examples are McDowell and Newell (1996) and Grotevant and Carlson (1989).

## HOW CAN YOU EVALUATE WHETHER EXISTING MEASURES MEET THE REQUIREMENTS OF A CERTAIN PROJECT?

One of the first questions to ask when searching for existing measures is, does it meet the requirements of your project? If not, it is often necessary to adapt existing measures or create a new one altogether. What follows are some general guidelines for choosing an existing measure. These come under the headings: purpose of the measure; the type and how it was developed; its psychometric properties; its responsiveness; how it has been administered; types of populations and settings; and brevity.

It is important to know your question and the purpose for using a measure. Further, this all hinges on the theoretical underpinnings in which you are operating—assuming you know what they are. For example, if you were studying a symptom like pain, it would be critical to know whether your theoretical basis was neurophysiologic, psychologic, or social, because pain measures exist for all three domains (Culpepper, 1992).

The type of measure, and how it was developed and tested are critical for evaluation. This is discussed in some detail under new measure construction later in this chapter (e.g., see the seven steps, p. 100); it is important to know and understand these essential elements. These steps not only include the development of individual items for a measure, but the formats for the possible answers, the use of overall scores or indices, and types of scales for responses. In addition, the psychometric properties should be known. This is one of the most neglected areas when choosing existing measures. Statements that simply say, "the instrument has good reliability and validity" are inadequate. The investigator should take the effort and time to find out what they are. This is especially valuable if you can determine these properties for settings and populations similar to your study.

Responsiveness refers to the sensitivity of a measure to detect change. Often referred to as discriminant validity, responsiveness is crucial to self-report measures that are used to assess change, whether they are assessing interventions (e.g., psychiatric drug trials, education research) or to detect differences in longitudinal studies (e.g., memory changes over time, quality of life with a chronic disease). We will say more of responsiveness later in this chapter.

Researchers also need to heed logistical issues like how a measure has been administered in prior studies. We are often caught between rigor and carrying out the "perfect study" on the one hand, with down to earth issues such as time, cost, and the effort to run a survey and analyze the data on the other.

New investigators often underestimate these practical issues that are necessary to carry out their study, in particular the resources for conducting something like a survey. Unquestionably the one major advantage of most self-administered measures is that the subject does the data collection. For example, there is no need to hire, pay, and train interviewers. Further, they are frequently mailed to subjects or handed out face-to-face in clinical settings.

The next two questions to ask when choosing an existing measure are: "what sorts of populations and settings has it been tested and used in previous studies? and are these populations and settings similar to the ones for your planned study?" An example or two will illustrate. Suppose your study question is: what is the relationship between life stresses and health care utilization in a family practice population? You intend to measure and quantify life stresses in a randomly selected but representative population of the patients in your large group practice of six family physicians using a cross-section design. You chose, however, a self-administered measure that was developed, tested, and used exclusively on a typical North American, community-based sample of 10–12% elderly. However, most of the patients in your group practice come from a retirement community nearby, and the practice is a teaching, academic, university-based one with a population consisting of 75% elderly. The problem is that the intended sample and setting are not representative of those for whom the measure was created and tested. The language and issues used in the text of many of the items may not be relevant; for example, many may ask questions about work related stress.

## THE CASE FOR BRIEF AND "USER FRIENDLY" MEASURES FOR USE IN CLINICAL SETTINGS

Many of us have had the experience of being asked to complete very long and tedious surveys. Often the measure is complex, containing confusing or vague questions and distracters, with complicated directions for going elsewhere in the survey if certain conditions are met, etc. These sorts of surveys have usually been inadequately tested on representative populations—the investigators have simply not asked for feedback from subjects in pilot situations. They often contain too many items, and the language may not be suitable for the population being surveyed. We will have more on this topic later in the chapter.

Perhaps the best way to illustrate several of these guidelines for choosing and using good quality, existing self report measures is to describe an example from my own experience: the Widowers Surviving Project (see Box 5.1).

---

**Box 5.1    Using existing self-report measures: The "Widowers Surviving Project"**

The "Widowers Surviving Project" was a community-based study that used existing measures of self-report. The purpose of the study was to assess the effectiveness of a mutual-help group intervention that was designed to assist new widowers in their grieving (Tudiver et al., 1991; Tudiver et al., 1992).

*Methods*

The methodology was a randomized controlled non-blinded trial using waiting-list controls. Recently widowed men (conjugally bereaved for the previous 3–12 months) were recruited from a large urban Canadian center. They were asked to participate in a peer-group intervention that focused on working through their grief, and on learning about various aspects of health promotion. The 113 subjects that matched the selection criteria were randomly allocated to one of nine treatment groups (N = 61) or a waiting-list control group (N = 52). The intervention consisted of nine weekly semi-structured sessions which focused on issues such as the grief process, family, diet, new relationships, and physical exercise. Each group was led by two trained facilitators, most of whom were themselves widowed and had experience in bereavement counseling. Much of the time spent in the nine intervention sessions was on sharing and venting feelings, and on facilitating mutual support. We wanted to assess the effect of this intervention on psychological and social well-being through asking participants to complete self-administered measures. We used existing measures for the following reasons: first, the investigators had limited resources and expertise with the development of new measures; second, there were several high quality existing instruments with theoretical grounding similar to our needs; and third, these measures had already been used to assess interventions for the bereaved in prior studies. The one significant drawback was that none had been used specifically to assess interventions for the population of interest—elderly widowers.

The following self-report instruments were chosen: (1) the 28-item Goldberg General Health Questionnaire (GHQ; Goldberg, 1978), which rates psycho-emotional distress in terms of everyday functioning. It had previously been used to evaluate the benefits of mutual-help interventions for widows (Vachon et al., 1980) but not for widowers; (2) the 13-item short form of the Beck Depression Inventory (BDI; Beck & Beck, 1972; Beck et al., 1961) is a measure of depression that had been used previously for evaluating the benefits of mutual-help for widows (Marmar et al., 1988); (3) the 42-item Social Adjustment Scale (SAQ; Weissman & Bothwess, 1976; Weissman et al., 1978) which was designed to evaluate treatment for psychotherapy, by assessing social areas such as work outside and in the home, spare time, family, and children. It had also been used for evaluating the benefits of mutual-help for widows (Marmar et al., 1988); (4) the 27-item Social Support Questionnaire (SSQ; Sarason et al., 1983), which was designed to quantify the availability of, and satisfaction with, social support. This measure had, unfortunately, only been tested on young college coeds; and (5) the 20-item State-Anxiety Inventory (STAI; Spielberger, 1983), which rates anxiety levels at the time of administration.

The five measures were administered at baseline (before randomization), at the end of the nine-week intervention period, and six months post-intervention (eight months post-recruitment). Subjects reported several difficulties with the measures. The most common complaints were that the "battery" took too long to complete (at least one hour), and that the instructions were difficult to follow, in particular, those with multiple-choice responses. Many of the subjects were elderly—average age was 62.9 years—and most had had little or no prior experience with this type of measure. In addition, many complained that items and even entire scales were not relevant to their situation; and that they disliked "completing different questionnaires that kept asking me the same questions" (e.g., the BDI and the GHQ).

*Results*

There were no significant differences between treatment subjects and controls at baseline. Group-by-time analyses of variance over the three observations showed no improvements due to the intervention; in fact, the trend was in the opposite direction, with all psychological scores for the waiting-list control subjects showing greater improvement over time. The scores on the STAI were statistically significantly higher (a higher score means more anxiety) over the time period in the treatment groups.

*Discussion*

This study suffered from the fact that many of the five measures had been developed and validated on diverse populations, several of which did not resemble the study population. The instruments were burdened with unrelated or inappropriate items, and sometimes different measures asked the same questions. In two post-study focus groups, we discovered that a number of drop-outs had occurred because of resistance to these two frequently complained-about problems. In addition, many of the men complained about having to complete the same measures on three occasions in a short span of time.

An important issue that had not been considered in this study at the time of selecting the measures was whether they had been sensitive enough to detect the differences we were looking for—responsiveness. In the same focus group sessions the men in the treatment groups were assessed by four independent raters as being less depressed and anxious than their control group counterparts; however, the quantitative measures indicated the opposite trend (although not to a significant degree).

This study had chosen existing self-administered measures as the most acceptable and affordable method for collecting the required data. The investigators had decided that creating original measures would have required much more time, energy, and money to construct, test, and refine, and was only possible because of generous federal government resources. This sort of undertaking was beyond the scope and available resources of the researchers. Perhaps the most appropriate "compromise" would have been to adapt a single new measure from the five existing ones. This could have eliminated many of the problems of the study. A cut-and-pasted measure would have been developed, modified, and tested in a representative population—middle aged and elderly Canadian men. Further, we would have eliminated unrelated, inappropriate, and duplicate or similar items that asked the same questions. However, all these efforts may not have been enough to ensure the measure was sensitive enough to detect the differences we were looking for. Perhaps an original measure would have been the only type to satisfy this last requirement.

## Creating an original self-report measure

Despite the availability of many self-report measures it often seems necessary to tailor an instrument to the specific research question. Walking through the steps in the investigative process—developing a question and hypothesis, reading the literature, refining the question to fit the theory and former research, developing a design—will bring the investigator around to consider the requisites for the measure. After a careful evaluation of existing measures, the investigator may surmise that they do not meet these conditions. The next step, considering adapting existing measures in a cut-and-paste approach, may not have any appeal for the study as well. This leaves the sole option of creating an original measure. This process, however, is time consuming and requires expertise to do it properly. This is particularly relevant if the author wishes other investigators to regard it as useful, valid, and reliable, and to try it in their own studies. The time involved in creating a new measure of approximately 50 items from scratch along with the initial testing, rewriting, and evaluations is about 1–2 years. Pilot testing can add on another 3–6 months. The decision to create a new measure is therefore a serious one. A more detailed description of the topic of creating a new measure is in Tudiver and Ferris (1992).

The advantages of creating a new measure are obvious: the instrument will be "custom made" for a particular study, and an intended population and setting. It will focus exclusively on the study question rather than on some other, and it will be directly related to the theoretical underpinnings upon which the study is based. Further, it will be created with the study population in mind, and be tested on a representative sample of that population. All this will ensure a much easier time of obtaining good psychometric properties on the measure, in particular, content and construct validity (more of that later).

There are disadvantages. Perhaps the most substantial is the cost in terms of effort, time, and money. And related to these is the frequent need for consultants. Most primary care researchers will need some specialist in the field for this sort of task. It is clearly beyond the scope of creating a "quick-and-dirty" measure for a simple study in say a clinical setting. Too many of these measures are created without the rigor so necessary for creating a good measure.

A very detailed account of how to create and fully test a new measure is beyond the scope of this chapter. For a good overview of the subject, I suggest a series of papers by Del Greco and colleagues (Del Greco & Walop, 1987a; 1987b; Del Greco et al., 1987a; 1987b; 1987c). For much more detail, Goddard and Villanova (1996) offer a good recent text on the subject. However, we can give the reader a fairly detailed summary of the steps in this process. There are seven critical steps necessary to create and test a new self-report measure, particularly if one wishes to do it rigorously. We will assume the investigator already has a clear question, and knows the literature, including the theory underpinning the question.

## THE SEVEN STEPS IN DEVELOPING ORIGINAL MEASURES
### (1) Identifying and prioritizing content areas
This first step should be driven by the theory behind the study. For example, let us say the study question is: "why do family doctors request so many prostate specific antigen (PSA) screening tests on young male patients when the clinical practice guidelines are not clear and often conflicting?" The planned methodology would be to create a brief paper and pencil survey to administer to a group of physicians at a continuing medical education event. One way to go about creating the measure would be to develop the content areas and items (see step two below) from your impressions and notions, as well as from those of colleagues. This process is done quite often, it can be done quickly, but it ignores the theory. A search in MEDLINE would have found that a recent theory had been developed in this area (Pathman et al., 1996; Tudiver et al., 1998), and that this theory could provide many of the relevant content areas and items. Other sources of content could be the published proceedings of a symposium or expert panel, or the report of a focus group the investigator could conduct on experts in the field (this could include consumers such as patients). A description of the use of focus groups for survey research can be found in O'Brien (1993) and Wolff et al. (1993).

### (2) Generating items for each content area
The next step is to write the individual questions. There are many ways to do this. For example, you can use open-ended versus forced response questions. Open-ended questions ask for written statements

from the respondents, while forced responses could be YES-NO or scaled choices as in Likert scale choices (see more details below). The challenge is to be acutely aware of what you want to learn. It is important to place questions under the content area headings, such as demographics, or knowledge and attitudes about a particular area. This may sound straightforward, but it is easy to drop in items of casual or last minute interest, only to find out later that it is not clear where they fit, or that they may not be relevant for the study question. Further, it is important to consider how each item relates to others in the same content area, to the domain of the area itself, and to the question in the project itself. Two useful references for tips on generating items are Dillman (1978) and Sudman and Bradburn (1983).

*(3) Quantifying selected items*
After creating the individual items, it is necessary to quantify the closed ended questions. There is a science to this—it is a lot more than just arbitrarily choosing YES-NO, or Likert choice responses. The type of possible answers will dictate the type and degree of measurement utilized in the analysis part of the study; for example, nominal versus ordinal data. I suggest a chapter by David Wilkin (1992) for a detailed discussion of this topic. Other useful references for instrument construction include Woodward and Chambers (1986) and Goddard and Villanova (1996). For instrument design I suggest looking again at Dillman (1978), the Del Greco et al. series described above, and Goddard and Villanova (1996).

The three common types of answers for use in surveys are the forced choice YES-NO response, scales, and multiple-choice. YES-NO responses are most appropriate for detecting the presence or absence of details like patient symptoms or simple attitudes: for example, "Do you have pain in a joint every day?"; or "Do you believe in capital punishment?". Scales are mostly used for measuring behaviors or attitudes: for example, "How often do you use the internet to answer your health questions, rather than ask your doctor?" (1-never; 2-sometimes; 3-neutral; 4-often; 5-very often); or "I agree everyone should have an annual checkup." (strongly agree, agree, disagree, strongly disagree). One common decision at this point is whether to use neutral distractors versus forcing the respondents to a positive or negative choice.

*(4) Establishing the content and face validity*
The next step is to determine two very basic properties of the new measure: the content and face validity. Testing for the more detailed

psychometric properties, for example, internal consistency, test-retest reliability, criterion and construct validity, etc., is for after the development phase during testing on populations. Content and face validity are crucial to test at this early stage in order to ensure the instrument and the resulting analyses are measuring what they intend to measure.

Content validity refers to an organized method that tests if the items adequately investigate the domains in the measure, and whether they are constructed in the most suitable form. Content validity is often omitted and often confused with face validity; both should be performed. The usual way to test content validity is to ask a group of experts in the field of study to examine the measure and make quantitative and qualitative remarks on relevance (to the domain and the entire measure), and on the clarity of each item. They are also asked to suggest alternate positions in the measure of items, to consider alternate wordings for individual items, or to even delete items. For a more detailed discussion on this, see Tudiver and Ferris (1992; pp. 91–93).

Face validity simply refers to a superficial means of testing whether the instrument appears to measure what it claims to. Although this seems cursory, it is an important step in the development of a measure in terms of its meaning for the study population. The usual way this is done is to ask representative members of the target population to give feedback about the appearance of the measure. Common questions to ask are: "does the measure look valid?" and "are different questions asking for the same information?" Open-ended questions are also included: for example, "comment on the length of the survey" and "what do you think about order of the questions?" Most experts suggest that once changes are made, the instrument should be retested for face and content validity on a different group of experts and representative study population.

*(5) Final review of items*
For this step the investigator needs to first check the measure for its readability. This is done with the target population in mind. The Fog Index is a method of analyzing written material to see how easy it is to read and understand. It is roughly equivalent to a grade level of reading. The "ideal" Fog Index level is 7 or 8. Several versions of computer software, often bundled with word processors, can calculate the index in a survey in seconds. A final step is to have 5–10 people from the target population complete the measure, in order to determine whether they complete it, how long it takes, whether they answer the appropriate questions, and if they follow the directions correctly. Also,

the investigator should ask them about their overall experience and if they had any difficulties completing it.

## (6) Formatting the new measure

Many researchers pay little attention to this step despite the fact that it is critical for a successfully completed project that utilizes a self admin-istered measure. A poorly formatted measure will often result in incor-rect and unreliable responses, incomplete surveys with missed items, and confusion among the participants. All this will result in threats to the validity and reliability of the measure. My favorite two references for formatting the measure are Dillman (1978) which also includes a lot of detail on mailing surveys, and Sudman and Bradburn (1983). These sources provide aspects on what I consider the most important components of the physical aspect of a self report measure: (1) overall appearance; (2) layout of the questions and response choices; (3) size and format of the actual text including fonts; (4) layout choices for multiple choice questions, including "skip" instructions; and (5) place-ment of demographic questions. For example, although many surveys locate the demographic questions at the beginning, Dillman (1978) suggests placing them at the end of the measure as most respondents find them tedious to complete. See also Tudiver and Ferris (1992) for a brief overview on these particular components.

## (7) Preliminary or "pilot" testing

The final step is to test the measure on a representative sample of the target population. This is often referred to as pilot testing. The purpose here is twofold: (1) to test the feasibility of administering the newly completed measure on a sample of subjects that will respond similarly to the ultimate study population; and (2) to determine the psychomet-ric properties of the measure. Unfortunately the testing of self-report measures for psychometric properties is beyond the scope of this chapter. Further, it usually requires the help of an expert, often a bio-statistician. For in-depth discussions on psychometric theory, I suggest Nunnally and Bernstein (1994).

The common validity tests an investigator would include are: crite-rion validity and construct validity. Criterion validity involves the testing of a measure for its predictive ability with respect to a standard outcome which is measured by a criterion or standard. There are two types of these criteria: concurrent and predictive. With concurrent cri-terion validity, the investigator would be checking the new measure against a standard at the same time: for example, comparing a new depression scale against a recognized "gold standard" like the Beck Depression Inventory. An example of predictive criterion validity would be to check for the presence of depression with clinical evaluations several months after the administration of the new measure.

The need for various tests for reliability will depend on the eventual uses of the measure. For example, if it will be used for multiple observations, particularly to assess an intervention, then knowledge of the measure's test-retest reliability or stability will be required. If the measure contains summative rating scales composed of specified items in the measure, then the internal consistency will need to be determined using the statistic, the Cronbach's alpha coefficient, or a split-half measure, like the Spearman-Brown correlation coefficient. Last, the inter-rater reliability will need to be tested if the score of the measure will be subject to scorer judgement. Most self-report measures, however, incur little if any scorer judgement.

Again, I will provide an example from my experience to illustrate the guidelines for creating original measures, this time related to physicians' awareness of spousal abuse (see Box 5.2).

---

**Box 5.2    Creating an original self-report measure: The "physicians' awareness of spousal abuse" project**

In this example we were interested in family physicians' awareness of the problem of spousal abuse, as well as their perceptions and approaches to this problem. In particular, we wished to examine whether postgraduate training in this specialty had an impact on family physicians' awareness, detection, and management of spousal abuse in their practices.

A major search of the literature found no existing self-report measures on this topic, although one study had examined family physicians' attitudes towards prevalence rates, detection of, and physician response to spousal abuse (Trute et al., 1988). The measure used in that study, however, did not contain the desired items for rigorous testing and assessment. In fact, it had never been pilot tested. We decided that an original measure was required.

*Development of the original measure*

A spousal abuse questionnaire was developed and tested over a two-year period. This development is described in detail elsewhere in a previous publication (Ferris & Tudiver, 1992). First, content areas were established and prioritized; then items were generated and quantified as described earlier in this chapter. Next, the establishment of face and content validity, clarity, and relevance were evaluated independently by 25 health care professionals with an interest in spousal abuse. A final review of items was completed and the questionnaire was formatted using many suggestions from Dillman (1978).

The questionnaire was then pilot tested on a sample of 650 Ontario, Canada-based family physicians (FPs) who were randomly selected from three targeted regions using the membership listing of College of Family Physicians of Canada. A computerized modified Dillman technique was used to administer the surveys (Dillman, 1978; Tudiver & McQuaig, 1990). This pilot study is described in detail elsewhere (Tudiver & Ferris, 1992). No items were altered or eliminated after the pilot study.

## Methods

The basic design was cross-sectional. A randomly selected, but representative sample of FPs was used in this study. It was derived from a national physician data base maintained by a private Canadian company. The inclusion criteria were English speaking FPs and general practitioners who were active in practice in a Canadian province, and not part of the original pilot study sample. The final version of the questionnaire was mailed to participants using the same modified Dillman technique using a four step series of anonymous mailings and follow-up telephone calls, using separate labeled postcards for informing the investigators of completers and nonrespondents.

## Results

Of the original 2045 sample, 471 (23.0%) were ineligible as they were not primary care physicians, they were not in active practice, had moved out of the province, or had died. Of the remaining 1574 eligibles, 963 responded, giving a response rate of 61%. Nonrespondents were similar to respondents in age and gender, and respondents were representative of the national sample of FPs and general practitioners in terms of age, gender, and postgraduate education status. A detailed description of the results is published elsewhere (Tudiver & Woods, 1996). A summary of the findings is: FPs with two years of postgraduate training in Family Medicine ("certificants") were more aware of the issue of spousal abuse than those without this training; certificants were more likely to be aware of their limitations for diagnosing or treating this problem; and they were more likely to have attended continuing medical education courses than noncertificants.

### Discussion

This study took a great deal of effort, including almost two years' work to develop and test the original measure. However, a major benefit was our confidence that we had a measure with known psychometric properties, and that it was developed and tested on representative samples of the study population.

## Adapting existing self-report measures

Adapting existing measures is like working a compromise between using an existing measure and creating an original one. However, cutting, pasting, and adapting old measures to create a new one for a particular study should not be considered a light task. Investigators, in particular inexperienced ones, often take this all too lightly, borrowing items from measures, and cutting ones, that appear inappropriate for their project. The common error is to assume that the new patched together measure has the same psychometric properties as the original, with content areas and items that will be as sound as if it was a custom made measure. This is usually not true—the cut-and-pasted measure needs to be tested as thoroughly as a new one. The major advantage of adapted measures is that investigators can save a lot of time, effort, and cost on steps 1 and 2 of creating a new self-report measure. The disadvantages of cutting and pasting from existing measures are: the reconstituted measure may still not be suitable for the particular study and its intended population; or the predicted savings in time, effort, and money may not be realized.

Adapting old measures to create a new one may sometimes be a simple matter of modifying an existing measure to suit a different population. For example, a study may call for measuring the quality of life in an elderly population of people suffering from chronic severe asthma. Although there may be several high quality measures for evaluating quality of life in asthmatics, there may be none that have examined this domain in the elderly. The investigator may then have to adapt these for their specific study population. There are four essential steps in cutting and pasting existing measures from old ones. Other steps that have been described for creating original measures such as formatting are also important, but I believe the following four are necessary.

## THE FOUR STEPS IN ADAPTING EXISTING MEASURES
### (1) Selecting existing measures for your question
My suggested guidelines for selecting existing measures for adapting are similar to those described earlier in this chapter for selecting existing self-report measures. These include: knowing your question and the purpose for using the measure(s); examining the measures for how they were developed and tested; assessing the responsiveness of the measures; determining the logistical issues like how the measures have been administered in prior studies; and knowing the sorts of populations and settings where they have been tested and used in previous studies.

### (2) Ways to modify existing measures: cutting items, replacing items, combining items, modifying items, and adapting an old measure to a new population
There are several ways in which investigators modify existing measures to suit the needs of their studies. First of all, investigators often delete items from existing measures because the original measure is too long. For example, there may not be adequate time for completing an existing self-report measure in a planned study, because the study already includes a "battery" of several other instruments. Another reason could be that the resources of the study are limited, including the staff time required for data entry and analysis. Another purpose of deleting items would be because certain items were deemed unsuitable for the adapted measure. An example of this would be a measure that was originally created and used to test a physician's knowledge of clinical practice guidelines for screening breast cancer. The original measure may have been created years earlier, but the guidelines and related evidence may have changed significantly since its inception.

Secondly, items can also be replaced by new ones to make a measure more suitable for the new study population. This can be done by adapting other measures or by writing totally new ones. Further, items can be combined from different existing measures into the new measure. For example, an investigator may want to assess a population of women in their 50s in terms of menopausal symptoms and a detailed score of their level of depression. This could be accomplished more efficiently by combining items from two different measures of these domains. There is often a need for just modifying items in a measure. This is most frequently done to adapt a measure for a different population from the original sample. An example would be to alter various language terms or jargon if items were to be used for a different culture using the same language (e.g., using a UK-based measure in the US).

Finally, old measures are often adapted to suit a new population. Several examples have already been described as this is perhaps the most common reason for adapting existing measures. Common examples include conducting a study in a culture different from the original, or administering a measure to subjects with a significantly different demographic profile from the original subjects (e.g., older age, different gender, or a different setting in a similar culture like inner city versus rural).

### (3) Testing for psychometric properties

The need for rigorous testing of the psychometric properties of a cut-and-pasted measure is about the same as for a new one. Once investigators alter a measure, whether by cutting items, replacing items, or combining items, they need to assume they are dealing with a brand new and untested instrument. Unfortunately, this is frequently ignored as many assume that items cut from well tested measures are removed and pasted with their psychometric properties intact as if they were still in the original. This is rarely true. The reconstituted measure must be treated as new. The properties that can be tested are: factor structure, item characteristics, validity (construct, predictive, concurrent), reliability (internal consistency, test-retest or stability, inter-rater), norms, and replication. A detailed discussion of these properties is well beyond the scope of this chapter; I suggest the following references: Zyzanski (1992), Nunnally and Bernstein (1994), and Goddard and Villanova (1996).

Factor analysis refers to a method to determine an instrument's dimensions. Cut-and-pasted measures usually come from different old measures, each having its own dimensions. The new reconstituted measure may comprise the same or even new dimensions; it is impossible to know what these are without factor analysis testing. Once the various dimensions are known, item analysis can be done to determine the dimensions that belong to each item.

After item analysis, the relevant validity and reliability measures can be performed. These have been briefly described previously in this and Ogden's contribution (chapter 4). The development of norms is based on simple tests such as means, medians, and standard deviations that are performed on the standardized population. These norms include scoring methods of the measure, a sense of the range of scoring (large versus small values), and standard cutoff scores for distinguishing different groups or categories (Zyzanski, 1992). An example of the use of norms in a clinical medical setting would be office testing for dementia using a measure like the mini mental status examination that provides norms essential for screening patients (Folstein et al., 1975).

The last set of tests is for repeating the item analysis, validity, and reliability measures on a population separate from the one used for the original testing. This new set of tests will give a good approximation of the competence of the instrument on future studies.

### (4) Pilot testing

As with original measures, the reconstituted measure must go through preliminary testing. The reader is asked to refer to the previous description in the section on creating an original measure.

## Summary

Self-report measures are among the most useful in health research. However, the task of selecting and/or creating self-report measures for a particular study is not a simple one and should not be taken lightly. There are three choices investigators have in acquiring a measure that suits their study; they are summarized in order of effort and complexity. The first is to try and find an appropriate measure for their study. If none exist, then they can create an adapted measure by cutting and pasting items from one or more existing measures. This second option will require thorough testing of the instrument as if it was a new measure. The third option is to create an original measure from scratch. This is usually the most time consuming and costliest option, but it will ensure you have a valuable measure that can be a worthwhile contribution to health research.

# References

Albreck, P., & Settle, R. (1985). *The survey research handbook*. Homewood, IL: Irwin.

Beck A.T., & Beck R.W. (1972). Screening depressed patients in family practice: A rapid technique. *Postgraduate Medical Journal, 52*, 81–85.

Beck A.T., Ward C.H., Mendelson M.M., Mock J., & Erbaugh J. (1961). An inventory for measuring depression. *Archives of General Psychiatry, 4*, 561–571.

Culpepper, L. (1992). Symptoms: Measures of the mind. In: M. Stewart, F. Tudiver, M.J. Bass, E.V. Dunn, & P.G. Norton (Eds.), *Tools for primary care research* (pp. 115–116). Newbury Park, CA: Sage.

Del Greco, L., & Walop, W. (1987a). Questionnaire development: 1. Formulation. *Canadian Medical Association Journal, 136*, 583–585.

Del Greco, L., & Walop, W. (1987b). Questionnaire development: 5. The pretest. *Canadian Medical Association Journal, 136*, 1025–1026.

Del Greco, L., Walop, W., & Eastridge, L. (1987a). Questionnaire development: 3. Translation. *Canadian Medical Association Journal, 136*, 817–818.

Del Greco, L., Walop, W., & Eastridge, L. (1987b). Questionnaire development: 4. Preparation for analysis. *Canadian Medical Association Journal, 136*, 927–928.

Del Greco, L., Walop, W., & McCarthy, R.H. (1987c). Questionnaire development: 2. Validity and reliability. *Canadian Medical Association Journal, 136*, 699–700.

Dillman, D.A. (1978). *Mail and telephone surveys: The total design method*. New York: Wiley.

Ferris, L.E., & Tudiver, F. (1992). Family physicians' approach to wife abuse: A study of Ontario, Canada practices. *Family Medicine, 24*, 276–282.

Folstein, M.F., Folstein, S.E., & McHugh, P.R. (1975). Mini-mental state: A practical method for grading the cognitive state of patients for the clinician. *Journal of Psychiatric Research, 12*, 89–198.

Goddard, R.D.III, & Villanova, P. (1996). *Designing surveys and questionnaires for research*. Thousand Oaks, CA: Sage.

Goldberg, D. (1978). *Manual of the general health questionnaire*. Windsor, UK: NFER Pub.

Grotevant, H.D., & Carlson, C.I. (1989). *Family assessment: A guide to methods and measures*. New York: Guilford.

Henry, R. (1992). Self-report measures: Principles and approaches. In: M. Stewart, F. Tudiver, M.J. Bass, E.V. Dunn, & P.G. Norton (Eds.), *Tools for primary care research* (p. 111). Newbury Park, CA: Sage.

Marmar, C.R., Howowitz, M.J., Weiss, D.S., Wilner, N.R., & Kaltreider, N.B. (1988). A controlled trial of brief psychotherapy and mutual-help group treatment of conjugal bereavement. *American Journal of Psychiatry, 145*, 203–209.

McDowell, I., & Newell, C. (1996). *Measuring health: A guide to rating scales and questionnaires* (2nd ed.). New York: Oxford University Press.

Nunnally, J.C., & Bernstein, J.H. (1994). *Psychometric theory. Third edition.* New York: McGraw Hill.

O'Brien, K. (1993). Improving survey questionnaires through focus groups. In: D.L. Morgan (Ed.), *Successful focus groups: Advancing the state of the art* (pp. 105–117). Newbury Park, CA: Sage.

Pathman, D.E., Konrad, T.R., Freed, G.L., Freeman, V.A., & Koch, G.G. (1996). The awareness-to-adherence model of the steps to clinical guideline compliance. *Medical Care, 34,* 873–889.

Prochaska, J.O., & DiClimente, C.C. (1986). Toward a comprehensive model of change. In: W.R. Miller & N. Heather (Eds.), *Treating addictive behaviors: Processes of change* (pp. 3–27). New York: Plenum.

Sarason I.G., Levine H.M., Basham R.B., & Sarason B.R. (1983). Assessing social support: The Social Support Questionnaire. *Journal of Personality and Social Psychology, 44,* 127–139.

Spielberger, C.D. (1983). *Manual for The State-Trait Anxiety Inventory.* Palo Alto, CA: Consulting Psychologists Press, Inc.

Sudman, S., & Bradburn, N.M. (1983). *Asking questions: A practical guide to questionnaire design.* San Francisco: Jossey-Bass.

Trute, B., Sarsfield, P., & Mackenzie, D.A. (1988). Medical response to wife abuse: A survey of physicians' attitudes and practices. *Canadian Journal of Community Mental Health, 7,* 61–71.

Tudiver, F., & McQuaig, B. (1990). Handling mailed surveys the automated way. *Canadian Medical Association Journal, 146,* 1629–1631.

Tudiver, F., & Ferris, L.E. (1992). Creating an original measure. In: M. Stewart, F. Tudiver, M.J. Bass, E.V. Dunn, & P.G. Norton (Eds.), *Tools for primary care research* (pp. 86–96). Newbury Park, CA: Sage.

Tudiver, F., & Woods, J. (1996). Canadian family physicians' perceptions of and approaches to wife abuse: Does certification in family medicine make a difference? *Canadian Family Physician, 42,* 1475–1480.

Tudiver F., Hilditch J., & Permaul J. (1991). A comparison of psychosocial characteristics of new widowers and married men. *Family Medicine, 23,* 501–505.

Tudiver, F., Hilditch, J., Permaul, J., & McKendree, D. (1992). Does mutual help facilitate new widowers? Report of a randomized controlled trial. *Evaluation and the Health Professions, 15,* 147–162.

Tudiver, F., Herbert, C., Goel, V., Guibert, R., Brown, J.B.B., Katz, A., Smith, P., Campbell, S., Ritvo, P.G., & Williams, J.I. (1998). Why don't family physicians follow clinical practice guidelines for cancer screening? *Canadian Medical Association Journal, 159,* 797–798.

Vachon, M.L.S., Lyall W.A., Rogers J., Greedman-Letofsky K., & Freeman S.J. (1980). A controlled study of self-help intervention for widows. *American Journal of Psychiatry, 137,* 1380–1384.

Weissman M.M., & Bothwess S. (1976). Assessment of social adjustment by patient self-report. *Archives of General Psychiatry, 33*, 1111–1115.

Weissman M.M., Prusoff B.A., Thompson W.D., Harding P.S., & Myers J.K. (1978). Social adjustment by self-report in a community sample and in psychiatric outpatients. *Journal of Nervous and Mental Diseases, 166*, 317–326.

Wilkin, D. (1992). Selecting an instrument to measure the outcomes of health care. In: M. Stewart, F. Tudiver, M.J. Bass, E.V. Dunn, & P.G. Norton (Eds.), *Tools for primary care research* (pp. 50–63). Newbury Park, CA: Sage.

Wolff, B., Knodel, J., & Sittitrai, W. (1993). Focus groups and surveys as complementary research methods: A case example. In: D.L. Morgan (Ed.), *Successful focus groups: Advancing the state of the art* (pp. 118–136). Newbury Park, CA: Sage.

Woodward, C.A., & Chambers, L.W. (1986). *Guide to questionnaire construction and question writing*. Ottawa: Canadian Public Health Association.

Zyzanski, S.J. (1992). Cutting and pasting new measures from old. In: M. Stewart, F. Tudiver, M.J. Bass, E.V. Dunn, & P. Norton (Eds.), *Tools for primary care research* (pp. 97–111). Newbury Park, CA: Sage.

# 6 THE ASSESSMENT OF STRESSOR EXPOSURE

Elaine Wethington, David Almeida, George W. Brown,
Ellen Frank, and Ronald C. Kessler

The aim of this chapter is to review methodological research on naturalistic stressor assessment, in order to provide a framework for researchers and practitioners to choose among different categories of stressor measurement. Naturalistic stressor assessment falls into four general categories: life events; stress appraisal; chronic stress; and daily hassles. We discuss the history and current state of each of these measurement strategies, commenting on situations where their use is more appropriate. The review is necessarily brief: for more detailed information regarding methodological and technical matters, readers should consult two recent reviews of stressor measurement and theory (Herbert & Cohen, 1996; Kessler, 1997). We conclude with a look toward future development of these strategies.

Most research on stress effects is concerned with buffers in the stress process, rather than exposures to stressors. It is now generally recognized that exposure to stressors in daily life, or over the course of life, is one of the most critical factors influencing health and well-being (Kessler, 1997). Though it is long established that stress predicts ill health (Selye, 1976), there remains ambiguity about the dimensions of stress involved in this process, specifically the types of stressors that have more deleterious effects on health. Most interest in the literature concerns individual differences, specifically why some people rather than others develop ill health or disorder after exposure to stressors. To study the naturalistic stress process, the field needs equally valid and reliable measures of stressor exposure, in addition to measures of individual differences in host resistance or vulnerability. Specific research examples illustrate the utility of stressor exposure measures. The first relates to the emotional effects of job loss. One person may be depressed about a job loss while another is not. This difference in reaction could be due to objective differences in the severity of the job losses, e.g., loss of the primary household income, rather than the secondary one. To take another example, on average men are more affected by widowhood than are women, at least in the short-term.

Perhaps men are less effective at coping with widowhood. However, it is more likely that something objectively worse, on average, happens to men when they are widowed. Women lose a confidant and financial supporter. But men lose their only confidant, their primary connection to their wider social network (Umberson et al., 1992). Thus it is critical in stressor exposure research that the measures capture objective differences in stressors. Differential reactivity cannot be studied unless differential exposure is also measured.

Stressor measurement has evolved to disentangle the effects of stressor exposure from individual differences in reactivity. Four types of stressor assessment predominate: exposure to out-of-the-ordinary events that have the capacity to change the patterns of life or arouse very unpleasant feelings (life events); self-reports of perceived stressfulness and appraisals of threat posed by events (stressor appraisals); enduring or recurrent difficulties in an area of life (chronic stressors); and exposure to relatively minor, less emotionally-arousing events whose effects disperse in a day or two (hassles). No one type of measurement predominates over the other, because each of the four has evolved in response to specific types of research situations. In addition, each of the traditions has borrowed heavily from the others over time: measures of life events are often combined with measures of chronic stressors; and measures of chronic stressors overlap, in practice, with the operationalization of appraisal and hassles.

Four factors tend to guide researchers in their choices for stressor assessment: (1) variations in research question; (2) the population studied; (3) the outcome of interest to the researcher (which may have prompted the original research question); and (4) the period of time over which a particular stressor is thought to have impact, whether a few hours or many years. These four factors interact with each other to some degree, but all are important individually in establishing the choice of measure.

## Overview of the assessment of stressor exposure

In this section, we briefly discuss the history and current state of the assessment of stressor exposure.

### Assessment of life events
There are two contrasting methods of life events measurement: checklist measures (Turner & Wheaton, 1995) and personal interview

measures, that use qualitative probes in order to specify more precisely the characteristics of life events believed to produce stress, and the timing of life events in relationship to the outcome (Wethington et al., 1995). These two sorts of measures evolved from different theories of what constitutes stress and the overall stress process. Because of their ease of administration, checklist measures predominate in exploratory studies of stressor exposure.

*Checklist methods*
Checklist methods were developed from an environmental perspective on stress that asserts that events bringing about a need for readjustment are the basis of experienced stress (Holmes & Rahe, 1967). (See section below on personal interview methods for a description of alternative perspectives.) A typical checklist measure consists of a series of yes/no questions, asking participants to report if any situation like the one described has occurred over a past period of time (e.g., one month, a year). Some checklist measures have been elaborated to get more detailed information about events, such as date of occurrence, description, and self-reported stressfulness. These self-report descriptive questions are used to estimate the severity of the event, or its likely relationship to an outcome. Still the typical checklist measure does not use self-report to "rate" event severity, but assigns average ("normative") severity ratings assigned by investigators. Checklist methods yield a summary score of the estimated stressfulness of changes experienced over a period of time.

Checklist measures are popular, inexpensive and easy to administer. They also yield consistent relationships with physical health outcomes, a property making them useful for exploratory studies (Turner & Wheaton, 1995). The ancestor of most current measures is the Social Readjustment Rating Scale (SRSS: Holmes & Rahe, 1967). It included both positive and negative events because its developers believed that change *per se* was associated with changes in health status. Over time, checklists have moved toward including only negative or undesirable events, based on findings that undesirable events are more predictive of health problems than positive events (Vinokur & Selzer, 1975). Event lists intended for use in the general population have become more comprehensive and inclusive of events occurring to women, minorities, and other populations, including children and adolescents (Turner & Wheaton, 1995).

Despite their popularity, checklist measures have encountered a great deal of criticism, most of it casting doubt on their reliability and validity as measures of stressor exposure. These criticisms include the vagueness of the stimulus (broad or nonspecific questions), lack of comprehensiveness (too few or population-biased questions), inclusion of inappropriate events (too minor or not negative), and lack of attention to memory bias and failure in their administration and interpretation (Herbert & Cohen, 1996).

*Personal interview methods*
The early development of personal interview methods that use qualitative probes was driven by a perspective that assumes social and environmental changes (and anticipations of those changes) threatening the most strongly held emotional commitments are the basis of severe stress. This perspective also asserts that severe stress threatens health, rather than minor stress (Brown, 1989), distinguishing it from other stress paradigms (e.g., Lazarus & Folkman, 1984).

Interview measures are most useful if research requires one or more of the following: (1) more precise severity ratings; (2) the relative timing of exposure and disease onset; and (3) establishing that stressors are "independent" of respondent illness or behavior. Promoters of interview methods also claim that they are more reliable and valid than checklist measures. Their expense rules them out for exploratory, low budget studies.

We briefly compare and contrast extant interview measures of life events on several relevant dimensions that may be important to different investigations. (For a more detailed summary, see Wethington et al., 1995.) Table 6.1 summarizes key features of each of the measures. To make an appropriate choice researchers should take into consideration these needs: (1) severity rating; (2) precision of dating; (3) "independence" of events from disorder being studied; (4) reliability and validity; (5) comprehensiveness for the study population.

*(1) Severity.*    There are two related ways in which interviews improve severity assessment. Interviews allow investigators, when summarizing the experience of stress, to substitute real stories for brief responses to abstract phrases. The narrative material also allows investigators to rate which experiences meet set thresholds of severity rather than relying on respondent interpretation. Experiences that do not qualify as severe enough can be eliminated by investigators. Studies of responses to checklist measures have found that many respondents report relatively minor events in response to questions that are designed to elicit only severely stressful events (e.g., Dohrenwend et al., 1990). An interviewer trained in study procedures can probe to

Table 6.1. Interview measures of life events

| Instrument | Administration | Rating system | Coverage | Features |
|---|---|---|---|---|
| Life Events and Difficulties Schedule (LEDS) (Brown & Harris, 1978) | Personal interview | Contextual threat | Events, chronic stressors | Well-documented ratings |
| Psychosocial Assessment of Childhood Experience (PACE) (Sandberg et al., 1993) | Personal interview | Contextual threat | Events, chronic stressors, positive experiences | Designed for children Well-documented ratings Two-informant design |
| Structured Event Probe and Narrative Rating with Method (SEPRATE) (Dohrenwend et al., 1993) | Personal interview | Revision of contextual threat | Events | Rating not confounded vulnerability |
| Detroit Couples Study (DAS-C) (Kessler & Wethington, 1991) | Personal interview | Investigator ratings | Events, chronic stressors | Structured Life event calendar |
| Munich Events List (Wittchen et al., 1989) | Personal interview | Investigator ratings | Events, chronic stressors | |
| Brief Life Events Personal list (BLE) (Paykel, 1997) | Personal interview | Investigator ratings | Events, chronic stressors | |
| List of Recent Experiences (LRE) (Henderson et al., 1981) | Personal interview | Investigator ratings | Events | |
| Hammen Life Event Diary Interview (Hammen et al., 1986) | Personal interview | Investigator ratings | Events, chronic stressors | |
| Structured Life Events Interview partially (SLI) (Wethington et al., 1995) | Personal interview | Modified contextual threat | Events, chronic stressors | Semi- and partially structured |

determine if the event reported indeed matches the intent of the question (McQuaid et al., 1992). Reporting minor events as severe, moreover, may be related to the respondent's health status at the time of interview (Bebbington, 1986).

The purpose of the interview probing is to gather enough information to rate the objective long-term contextual threat or severity of situations. The ratings of event severity is the key component of personal interview methods, as the experience of a severely threatening situation is hypothesized to pose a risk for illness. Rating the degree of severity (threat) for objective situations has been documented over several decades. The Life Events and Difficulty Schedule (LEDS: Brown & Harris, 1978) is the best-known and best-documented interview method. Table 1 records that many interview measures use LEDS; or LEDS-like rating schemes.

The LEDS has experienced criticism for its rating and interview methods. Wethington et al. (1995) discuss these criticisms extensively. The most persistent criticism is that ratings of contextual threat include contexts many researchers would like to measure separately as modifiers of the impact of stressors on health; specifically, there is a long-standing controversy over whether LEDS ratings of contextual threat cloud the distinction between event severity and the individual's vulnerability to a stressor (Tennant et al., 1981). It is fair to say that LEDS severity ratings may be confounded with socioeconomic status and other social vulnerability factors. The Structured Event Probe and Narrative Rating Method (SEPRATE; Dohrenwend et al., 1993) uses a system of rating adjusted to remove social vulnerability factors.

Another criticism of interview measures relates to their expense. The Structured Life Events Interview (SLI; Wethington et al., 1995) is a shorter, more structured version of the LEDS, more consistent with standard survey techniques. The SLI reduced event rating and interviewer rating time.

*(2) Dating methods.*    The use of the personal interview technique is also important when the relative timing of exposure to a stressor and the onset of illness is in question. Precise dating is necessary not only to establish the relationship of stress or exposure to onset, but also to identify the aspects of the stressful experience that affect onset. This precise dating feature makes it possible to distinguish and date a series of related events and difficulties, which is useful if the disease outcome is more likely when stressors are chronic (McQuaid et al., 1992).

*(3) Independence from disorder.*    Events may also occur because of the pre-existence of a physical or mental disorder. If that pre-existing

disorder is also the outcome of a particular investigation, interpretive difficulties arise. Rating routines for most personal interview measures of stressor exposure include an assessment of whether a situation is (1) known to be related to an actual disorder the respondent reports (e.g., getting fired because of drinking), or (2) hypothetically related to symptomatology (e.g., events involving interpersonal conflict). Most interview measures rate independence.

*(4) Reliability and validity.*    Promoters of interview measures for assessing stressors claim superior validity and reliability (Brown & Harris, 1982). Checklist methods appear more prone than interview measures to the misdating of distant events into a more recent time period (McQuaid et al., 1992). Checklist methods are probably not as effective as more intensive interviewing in communicating the importance of accurate answers to the respondents (Cannell et al., 1981). An interview facilitates the use of calendars and other memory aids to improve event recall and dating (Sobell et al., 1990).

*(5) Comprehensiveness.*    All interview measures are comprehensive across types of stressors. They vary, however, in whether they include comprehensive assessment of chronic stressors as well as discrete events. This distinction is important for investigators, because chronic stress assessment is apt to be more important for some health outcomes (e.g., heart disease risk factors) in comparison to others (e.g., onset of depression).

Some concern has been raised in the past about the applicability of semi-structured interview methods to members of non-majority ethnic groups, and to children and adolescents. The fear is that events and their documented ratings are not applicable to non-majority populations, adolescents, and children, due to age, social status or racial differences in exposure or the meaning of the event. A number of LEDS studies have been conducted in racial minority groups in England and Africa (for a review of the cross-cultural studies, see Brown & Harris, 1989), as well as in Pittsburgh. Variability of meaning for different groups is approached by consensus panel and the construction of specific dictionaries of events for those groups.

Modified versions of the LEDS have been used with adolescents and children as young as eight (Goodyer et al., 1997). The LEDS adjusts for some age-related variation in meaning by applying higher severity ratings to certain events if they are a "first experience", for example, first sexual experience is distinguished as an event. (With younger children, the LEDS has also been administered to mothers, who serve as informants for their children's events as well as stressful events occurring in their lives which may have negative impact on the child.)

A semi-structured interview method that has been developed specifically for younger children is the Psychosocial Assessment of Childhood Experiences (PACE: Sandberg et al., 1993). The PACE follows the same approach as the LEDS, with several modifications. It covers events that have the most relevance for adolescents and children. The question wordings are adapted to make them effective with children. Events are rated for two types of independence: independence from the behavior or illness of the child, and independence from the behavior or illness of the parent. Finally, events and long term experiences are rated for both their positive and negative aspects. The PACE is administered to both child and parent, and the information from the two interviews is rated independently, then combined in consensus panel. Documentation for the PACE has been substantially modified by a team of American and British investigators (John D. and Catherine T. MacArthur Foundation Research Network on Psychopathology and Development, 1997).

## ASSESSMENT OF STRESSOR APPRAISAL

Appraisal plays an important part in stressor assessment, as well as in theories of the stress process, most notably the transactional model of stress (Lazarus & Folkman, 1984). Cognitive appraisal of stressors is believed to underlie the emotional experience of stress. Measures of appraisal focus on the degree to which an event threatens well-being or threatens to overwhelm resources to cope (Lazarus & Folkman, 1984). The former is referred to as primary appraisal, and the latter as secondary appraisal. Primary appraisal is further subdivided into Loss (or harm), Threat (or potential for loss), and Challenge (opportunities or potentials in the future for gain or loss). Secondary appraisal refers to evaluation of one's capability of coping with the stressor, and the availability of resources to cope. Appraisal is hypothesized to at least partially determine coping strategies that could alleviate the stressor. The distinction between primary and secondary appraisal is essentially heuristic, since they occur simultaneously and each has an effect on the other (Lazarus & Folkman, 1984). Actual measures of appraisal, however, are not as numerous or as well-established as measures of exposure to events. Many are *ad hoc*, one or two-item measures designed for particular studies (Monroe & Kelly, 1995).

Measures of stressor exposure differ in whether they include or exclude appraisal. Some measures of stressor exposure, such as the

Perceived Stress measure (Cohen et al., 1983) consist of cognitive assessments of how well one coped with stressors. Checklist and interview measures of life events for the most part aim to exclude appraisal from stressor exposure assessment, although some explicitly do not (e.g., Horowitz et al., 1977). Those that exclude appraisal do so because of concerns that stressor appraisal is confounded with the health and psychological outcomes stressor exposure is hypothesized to predict (Monroe & Kelly, 1995). Indeed, researchers have speculated that some stressor appraisals are "caused" by underlying, persistent mood disturbance, rather than vice-versa (Schwartz & Stone, 1993). The transactional model of stress (Lazarus & Folkman, 1984) posits that appraisals can be measured separately and objectively.

Measures of stressor appraisal, in our view, do not substitute for measures of stressor exposure. Their major contribution has been to test various predictions of the transactional theory of stress. Because of their importance to the psychological model of stress, we review the major multi-item measures below. Key components of the appraisal measures are summarized in Table 6.2.

Measures of stressor appraisal differ by whether they separate or combine measures of primary and secondary appraisal. They also differ

Table 6.2. Measures of stressor appraisal

| Instrument | Administration | Rating system | Theoretical basis |
| --- | --- | --- | --- |
| Stakes (Folkman et al., 1986) | Self-administration | Self-report | Transactional model |
| Stress Appraisal Measure (SAM) (Peacock & Wong, 1990) | Self-administration | Self-report | Transactional model |
| Stone's Appraisal Measure (Schwartz & Stone, 1993) | Self-administration | Self-report | Transactional model |
| Narrative Appraisal (Stein et al., 1997) | Journal method | Investigator ratings | Transactional model |
| Diary Inventory of Stressful Events (Almeida, 1997) | Telephone | Self-report | Contextual threat Transactional model |

by whether they rely on self-report from respondents, or attempt to collect more objective indicators of the components believed to underlie stressor appraisal.

Lazarus' measure of Stakes delineates dimensions of well-being, or stakes, that underlie the primary appraisal dimensions of loss, threat, and challenge (Lazarus & Folkman, 1984). Stakes include threats to health, losses of and threats to important relationships, and threats to physical safety (Folkman et al., 1986). Stakes can apply not only to a threat to the focal respondent, but also to threats to the well-being of significant others.

A strength of the Stakes measure is that it corresponds to a well-established theory of the stress process, and thus is an important research tool for establishing the dimensions of environmental exposure that are related to a negative emotional response. A weakness of the Stakes scale is the fact that it is self-report. Although worded as objectively as possible, the items may be prone to confounding with underlying mood disturbance, which could allow unmeasured individual differences to affect judgment of whether an event threatens physical safety or personal health.

The Stress Appraisal Measure (SAM; Peacock & Wong, 1990) was developed as a multi-item, multi-dimensional measure combining primary and secondary stress appraisal. Measures of secondary appraisal developed by Lazarus (Folkman et al., 1986) are primarily single-item measures (Peacock & Wong, 1990). The wordings of some of the Lazarus items also overlap with measures of coping, most notably the Ways of Coping checklist (Lazarus & Folkman, 1984). The SAM operationalizes the appraisal dimensions of threat, challenge, centrality to self, controllability (by self or others), and uncontrollability.

Stone's measure of appraisal (e.g., Schwartz & Stone, 1993) is another refinement of the transactional model. In contrast to the SAM approach, Stone's measure is designed to be used with measures of stressor exposure. The dimensions of appraisal measured are: (1) controllability; (2) meaningfulness; (3) threat to stability; and (4) perceived severity/stressfulness. The strength of the measure is its attention to the prediction of the transactional model that appraisals should vary systematically with objective characteristics of stressors (Schwartz & Stone, 1993).

A unique approach to measuring stress appraisal was recently reported by Stein et al. (1997). This team has developed a means of classifying stress appraisals from written descriptions of stressful situations. Portions of descriptions are rated for the threat and challenge that a stressful situation poses to "the state of the world and the status of valued beliefs and goals" (1997: p. 873), and the appraisal of benefit or harm to future goals. Positive and negative appraisals were found to relate to well-being in ways predicted by the transactional model of stress. A strength of this approach is its use of highly individual material to measure appraisal. A weakness is that the descriptions were collected retrospectively, after the event had occurred, rather than in the process of the stressful situation. This makes it impossible to completely rule out retrospective reassessment of situational appraisals.

Almeida (1997) has developed a structured appraisal coding scheme based on narrative descriptions of daily stressors. These ratings are based not on self-report responses to degree of Stake, but on characteristics of the events, rated by an independent coding staff. The dimensions were derived from dimensions of contextual threat developed by Brown and Harris (1978), with some additions from the transactional model (Lazarus & Folkman, 1984).

## THE ASSESSMENT OF CHRONIC STRESSORS

Traditional measures of chronic stressors rely on appraisal of stressors in the environment. A typical measure of chronic stressors is a set of questions designed to capture the more frequently occurring stressors in important life roles, such as work and marriage (e.g., Pearlin & Schooler, 1978). A great deal of research exists that has established the range of experiences in roles that may evoke stressful reactions (Moos, 1981; Moos & Moos, 1981). Researchers who pioneered this approach (e.g., Moos, 1981) were attentive to the potential difficulty of relying on self-report, and tried to make the questions as objective as possible.

A number of research approaches aim to minimize self-report bias. Semi-structured interview approaches (e.g., LEDS) claim to reduce the confounding introduced through self-report by investigator rating of chronic stressors. The traditional approach, limitations of that approach, and several alternative approaches are reviewed below.

### Traditional approaches

The traditional approach relies heavily on multi-item self-report interviews and questionnaires. The strength of the traditional instruments is their grounding in detailed, multi-dimensional assessment of environmental factors known to produce chronic stress (Lepore, 1995). Another approach is to cover a wider range, or multiple domains of life (e.g., Pearlin & Schooler, 1978), using items crafted to tap the same or similar dimensions across domains of life. Many chronic stressor measures have impressive reliability; those for work and marriage are reviewed by Lepore (1995).

The most important limitation of appraisal-based, self-report measures is that a report of severe chronic stressors might be related to the disturbed cognitions of the person reporting them (Lepore, 1995). Poor coping, or the inability of the respondent to resolve a problem, may make a stressor chronic. In addition, particular types of coping—e.g., redefinition of the situation—may cause someone to underreport the presence of a chronic stressor (Stone & Schiffman, 1992).

Another potential limitation is memory failure, specifically recency bias. Respondent reports of the current level of severity may be confounded with the recent course of this difficulty (Herbert & Cohen, 1996). This is important because the level of severity may vary across a period of time and overall assessment of the severity may be affected by the recency of the latest crisis.

*Alternative approaches to measuring chronic stressors*
One widely-used alternative to self-report structured-question assessment is the use of semi-structured interviewing techniques (Brown & Harris, 1978). Dictionaries of long-term difficulties rate exemplary cases based on objective criteria. Many interview measures that assess chronic stressors (see Table 1), such as the LEDS, also establish change-points in severity levels as part of their dating routine.

Another alternative to self-report questions is the use of objective criteria available from observation, informant report, or population-level observation of the characteristics of situations to which many individuals are exposed, such as occupational stressors (DOT; Roos & Treiman, 1980). Several examples in the literature suggest the potential of these methods, and are reviewed by Lepore (1995).

In studies using naturalistic observation, significant but modest correlations are found between observation and self-report. Observational measures, though, are less predictive of health outcomes. Although some of the lessened predictive power may be due to the elimination of self-report bias, it may also be due to observation that is less detailed or frequent than is necessary to measure true exposure to chronic stressors.

Lepore (1995) asserted that in some respects informant observation of chronic stressor exposure might prove superior to *in situ* observation. Informant data is (less) contaminated by self-report bias, less prone to influence by research subject reactivity, and better informed regarding frequency and content of exposure (Stone et al., 1991). Several groups of stress researchers (e.g., Almeida et al., 1999; Kessler & Wethington, 1991; Sandberg et al., 1993) have utilized family-level designs to collect informant data on life events, chronic stressors, and hassles.

## ASSESSMENT OF HASSLES

Early hassles assessment relied on diary methods of collection, where respondents were asked to keep records of small events occurring over a given period of time, usually a 24 hour period. Researchers took two approaches to measurement: open-ended (Eckenrode, 1984), which asked respondents to describe bothersome events of the day; and structured questions, simple yes or no response questions modeled on life events checklists (Kanner et al., 1981).

Use of these methods has evoked multiple criticisms. One of the most persistent has been that diary methods of data collection, relying on written self-report, confound objective events with psychological appraisal (Dohrenwend et al., 1984; Eckenrode & Bolger, 1995). All of these methods assume participants respond to the questions in a relatively neutral and uniform way (Schwartz & Stone, 1993). Yet it is known from research on life events and chronic stressors, that researchers have found it very difficult to communicate the meaning of an event or situation without relying on words that evoke judgment and appraisal of its stressfulness, such as "a lot of demands".

A second persistent criticism is that the self-report of hassles is confounded with coping. The argument here is that when a respondent copes successfully with small hassles, such as overloads or interruptions, (s)he is less likely to either (1) remember the occurrence, or (2) interpret the situation as a stressor (Aspinwall & Taylor, 1997).

A third criticism is that methods of data collection for hassles are too time-consuming and expensive to use in large-scale surveys of the population, particularly on a daily basis. Most research on daily events has been conducted in small, discrete, relatively homogeneous samples (Eckenrode & Bolger, 1995; Stone et al., 1991). Such samples limit generalizability of the findings. Researchers with modest budgets tend to collect large amounts of information from a relatively small number of people, rather than smaller amounts of information from a large number of people (Stone et al., 1991).

In response to these three criticisms, investigators have developed a number of new approaches. In addition to the open-ended approach, and the structured approach, researchers have also combined the two methods. The new methods have attempted to reduce confoundment of daily events with stressor appraisal and coping, and to overcome the small sample problem. Several of the most common methods are summarized in Table 6.3, along with a new telephone method applying investigator-based event rating techniques to hassles.

Many measures are particularly comprehensive. The original Daily Hassles and Uplifts Scale is a list of 117 items (Kanner & Feldman, 1991). A revised 53 item scale (DeLongis et al., 1988) is also comprehensive, but has an additional advantage. The latter version was designed not only to shorten the scale but also to respond to criticisms that many of the original items were confounded with psychological or health symptoms (Dohrenwend & Shrout, 1985; Lazarus et al., 1985). The strengths of this scale include its tight connection to the transactional model of stress, and its wide use by other researchers (Eckenrode & Bolger, 1995).

In the Daily Life Experience Checklist (DLE; Stone & Neale, 1982), participants check off whether events occurred, and are asked to rate

Table 6.3. Measures of daily hassles

| Instrument | Method | Length | Features |
| --- | --- | --- | --- |
| Hassles and uplifts (DeLongis et al., 1988) | Self-administered | 53 (orig. 117) | Positive and negative Comprehensive |
| Daily Life Experience Checklist (DLE; Stone & Neale, 1982) | Self-administered | 78 | Comprehensive open-ended component |
| Daily Stress Scale (DSS; Bolger er al., 1989) | Self-administered | 22 | Work-family focus |
| Inventory of Small Life Events (ISLE; Zautra et al., 1986) | Self-administered | 178 | Comprehensive |
| Daily Stress Inventory (DSI; Brantley et al., 1988) | Self-administered | 58 | Comprehensive |
| Unpleasant Events Schedule (UES; Lewinsohn & Talkington, 1979) | Self-administered | 320 | Includes social support assessment |
| Daily Inventory of Stressful Events (DISE; Almeida, 1977) | Telephone | 8 (plus probes) | Investigator-rated severity Open-ended |

the desirability of those they check. (They may also write in events they consider stressful, but that did not appear on the list.) One advantage of this method is that it was originally designed and validated as a comprehensive measure of daily stressors (Eckenrode & Bolger, 1995).

The Daily Stress Scale (Bolger et al., 1989) is short, enabling its use in daily diary surveys that measure multiple dimensions of the daily stress process. A strength of this scale is that it was designed to measure potentially chronic stress processes over a period of time, in the particular domains of work and family (Eckenrode & Bolger, 1995). The Daily Stress Inventory (DSI: Brantley et al., 1988) is notable because a scoring manual is available (Brantley & Jones, 1989), documenting its reliability and validity.

Other scales appear more suitable for weekly or monthly use. The Inventory of Small Life Events (ISLE) is a very comprehensive list of desirable and undesirable events (Zautra et al., 1986). The advantage of this scale is that it was composed to focus on objective, observable minor events and changes: all items are written to focus on observable change, and to exclude internal states or reactions to the environment. The Unpleasant Events Schedule (UES; Lewinsohn & Talkington, 1979), also more suitable for weekly or monthly use, contains a mixture of minor and more serious items. A potential weakness for some investigations is that several sets of items in the UES measure appraisal of social support, a concept some researchers may wish to keep separate from an event measure.

A new method is the Daily Inventory of Stressful Events (DISE; Almeida, 1997), a semi-structured survey instrument designed for telephone administration. The DISE applies investigator-based methods to rate daily events and hassles, modeled on LEDS techniques. The interview consists of a series of eight questions asking whether certain types of events (e.g., arguments, home or work events, etc.) have occurred over the past 24 hours, along with a set of guidelines for probing affirmative responses. Once an event is mentioned, the interviewer asks questions about objective circumstances surrounding the event. The purpose of the probes is to gather enough information to rate various components of the discrete events. In order to examine these events, interviews are tape-recorded, then transcribed and coded for six different aspects: (1) specific event classification; (2) focus; (3) dimension of threat; (4) event continuation; (5) connection to an ongoing situation (reported the previous day or days); and (6) severity. The ratings minimize confounding with coping to a great degree by substituting investigator judgment for respondent self-report.

# Overview and future directions

Future assessment of stressor exposure will probably rely more heavily on combinations of acute and chronic stress assessment. The majority of examples of combined measurement that we have reviewed here rely on interview assessment using qualitative probing techniques. Yet it is possible, and perhaps advisable for future innovation, to do this in several other ways, by developing more sophisticated structured interview methods, conducting focused studies of specific stressful events, utilizing quasi-experimental and intervention techniques, and paying more explicit attention to the lag between exposure and onset.

## MORE STRUCTURED AND SOPHISTICATED INTERVIEW METHODS

Some advances could be made by developing more structured interview methods for life events. Two groups of researchers have already expanded structured probing to include many of the dimensions used in semi-structured interviews, such as event duration and resolution (Turner & Avison, 1992) and objective contextual factors (SLI; Wethington et al., 1995). Almeida (1997) has applied these techniques to daily hassles.

## FOCUSED STUDIES OF SPECIFIC LIFE EVENTS

Focused studies of events combine the assessment of chronic and acute stressors, by embedding an investigation of life event effects into a larger understanding of the consequent stressors in the person's day-to-day life following the occurrence of the event (Turner et al., 1991).

Several recent studies of this sort have been conducted, each focused on a single major event such as divorce (Aseltine & Kessler, 1993), unemployment (Turner et al., 1991), and widowhood (Umberson et al., 1992). The basic approach in each study has been to start with a conceptual model of the dimensions of the event that may lead to depression in some victims and then to measure these dimensions longitudinally in a sample of people who were exposed to the event. Simultaneously, the dimensions are also measured longitudinally and in an appropriate comparison group of people who were at risk but not exposed. One then uses standard multivariate analysis procedures to examine the mediating effects of the theoretically-derived stressor dimensions on the overall relationship between the event and depression.

A consistent result of these three studies is that most of the association between the focal events and depression can be attributed to the mediating effects of role-related stressors. These three studies were unable to control for other likely confounding factors. Future work involving focused event studies should use fully prospective designs, carefully matched control groups, and intensive personal interview methods with contextual ratings to define the intervening chronic stress dimensions.

## EXPERIMENTAL AND INTERVENTION METHODS

Early work on stress was experimental (Selye, 1976), utilizing methods very unlike the naturalistic assessment methods described here. The experimental work was judged insufficient on its own because of the lack of ecological validity (mild experimental stressors used on humans) and generalizability (animal models). Naturalistic studies have to a great degree replaced experimental work, with the consequence that the rigor of experimental methods was lost. This is unfortunate, because naturalistic studies have documented that stressor exposure is not random, but often influenced by choice or behavior (Kessler, 1997). Naturalistic studies cannot, on their own, control for the nonrandom nature of stressor exposure.

Very little has been done to address this issue in naturalistic studies. A few quasi-experimental studies (e.g., Aseltine & Kessler, 1993) have attempted to take self-selection into account when estimating multi-variate models of stressor effects. Intervention studies of stress processes show the most potential for re-introducing the experimental method into more naturalistic methods of stressor assessment. The results of experimental interventions aimed at preventing depression among people exposed to particular life events demonstrate the promise of such methods (Price et al., 1992).

## LAG BETWEEN EXPOSURE AND ONSET

Techniques for assessing stressor assessment should be carefully matched to a theoretical model of what constitutes sufficient stressor exposure to lead to onset of disease. Checklist assessment methods, at both the daily and yearly level, are adequate for exploratory studies, but too often they are used in long-term prospective studies of illness course and onset where measures of chronic stressors, and long-term severity of stressor exposure may prove more beneficial. Personal interview measures, measures of daily events, and non-traditional measures of chronic stressors, combined with thoughtful prospective design, will be necessary in order to explicate more fully how long and how severe stressor exposure must be to provoke illness.

# Acknowledgement

The development of this chapter was supported by the John D. and Catherine T. MacArthur Foundation Research Network on Psychopathology and Development, the John D. and Catherine T. MacArthur Foundation Research Network on Successful Midlife Development, National Institutes of Mental Health grant R37 MH42714 (to Ronald C. Kessler), and National Institute on Aging program project 2P50 AG11711–06 (to Elaine Wethington). The first author is grateful to Nina Delligatti, Allison Kavey, and Melissa Treppicione for research assistance.

# References

Almeida, D.A. (1997). *Daily inventory of stressful events (DISE) expert coding manual*. Tucson, AZ: Division of Family Studies, University of Arizona.

Almeida, D.A., Wethington, E., & Chandler, A. (1999). Daily transmission between marital and parent-child tensions. *Journal of Marriage and the Family, 61,* 49–61.

Aseltine, R., & Kessler, R.C. (1993). Marital disruption and depression in a community sample. *Journal of Health and Social Behavior, 34,* 237–251.

Aspinwall, L.G., & Taylor, S.E. (1997). A stitch in time: Self-regulation and proactive coping. *Psychological Bulletin, 121,* 417–436.

Bebbington, P. (1986). Establishing causal links: Recent controversies. In: H. Katschnig (Ed.), *Life events and psychiatric disorder: Controversial issues* (pp. 188–200). Cambridge: Cambridge University Press.

Bolger, N., DeLongis, A., Kessler, R.C., & Schilling, E.A. (1989). Effects of daily stress on negative mood. *Journal of Personality and Social Psychology, 57,* 808–818.

Brantley, P.J., Cocke, T.B., Jones, G.N., & Goreczny, A. (1988). The daily stress inventory: Validity and effect of repeated administration. *Journal of Psychopathology and Behavioral Assessment, 10,* 75–81.

Brantley P.J., & Jones, G.N. (1989). *The daily stress inventory*. Odessa, FL: Psychological Assessment Resources.

Brown, G.W. (1989). Life events and measurement. In: G.W. Brown & T.O. Harris (Eds.), *Life events and illness* (pp. 3–45). New York: Guilford.

Brown, G.W., & Harris, T.O. (1978). *Social origins of depression: A study of depressive disorder in women*. New York: Free Press.

Brown, G.W., & Harris, T.O. (1982). Fall-off in the reporting of life events. *Social Psychiatry, 17,* 23–28.

Brown, G.W., & Harris, T.O. (1989). Summary and conclusions. In: G.W. Brown & T.O. Harris (Eds.), *Life events and illness* (pp. 439–482). New York: Guilford.

Cannell, C.F., Miller, P.V., & Oksenberg, L. (1981). Research on interviewing techniques. In: S. Leinhardt (Ed.), *Sociological methodology* (pp. 389–437). San Francisco: Jossey-Bass.

Cohen, S., Kamarck, T., & Mermelstein, R.J. (1983). A global measure of perceived stress. *Journal of Health and Social Behavior, 24*, 385–396.

DeLongis, A., Folkman, S., & Lazarus, R.S. (1988). The impact of daily stress on health and mood: Psychological and social resources as mediators. *Journal of Personality and Social Psychology, 54*, 486–495.

Dohrenwend, B.P., & Shrout, P.E. (1985). "Hassles" in the conceptualization and measurement of life stress variables. *American-Psychologist, 40*, 780–785.

Dohrenwend, B.S., Dohrenwend, B.P., Dodson, M., & Shrout, P.E. (1984). Symptoms, hassles, social supports, and life events: The problem of confounded measures. *Journal of Abnormal Psychology, 93*, 222–230.

Dohrenwend, B.P., Link, B.G., Kern, R., Shrout, P.E., & Markowitz, J. (1990). Measuring life events: The problem of variability within event categories. *Stress Medicine, 6*, 179–187.

Dohrenwend, B.P., Raphael, K.G., Schwartz, S., Stueve, A., & Skodol, A. (1993). The structured event probe and narrative rating method for measuring stressful life events. In: L. Goldberger & S. Breznitz (Eds.), *Handbook of stress: Theoretical and clinical aspects* (pp. 174–199). New York: Free Press.

Eckenrode, J. (1984). The impact of chronic and acute stressors on daily reports of mood. *Journal of Personality and Social Psychology, 46*, 907–919.

Eckenrode, J., & Bolger, N. (1995). Daily and within-day event measurement. In S. Cohen, R.C. Kessler, & L.U. Gordon (Eds.), *Measuring stress: A guide for health and social scientists* (pp. 80–101). New York: Oxford University Press.

Folkman, S., Lazarus, R.S., Dunkel-Schetter, C., DeLongis, A., & Gruen, R.J. (1986). Dynamics of a stressful encounter: Cognitive appraisal, coping, and encounter outcomes. *Journal of Personality and Social Psychology, 59*, 992–1003.

Goodyer, I.M., Herbert, J., Tamplin, A., Secher, S.M., & Pearson, J. (1997). Short-term outcome of major depression: II. Life events, family dysfunction, and friendship difficulties as predictors of persistent disorder. *Journal of the American Academy of Child and Adolescent Psychiatry, 36*, 474–480.

Hammen, C., Mayol, A., DeMayo, R., & Marks, T. (1986). Initial symptom levels and the life-event-depression relationship. *Journal of Abnormal Psychology, 95*, 114–122.

Henderson, S., Byrne, D.G., & Duncan-Jones, P. (1981). *Neurosis and the social environment.* New York: Academic Press.

Herbert, T.B., & Cohen, S. (1996). Measurement issues in research on psychosocial stress. In: H.B. Kaplan (Ed.), *Psychosocial stress: Perspectives on structure, theory, life-course, and methods* (pp. 295–332). New York: Academic.

Holmes, T.H., & Rahe, R.H. (1967). The social readjustment rating scale. *Journal of Psychosomatic Research, 11*, 213–218.

Horowitz, M., Schaefer, C., Hiroto, D., Wilner, N., & Levin, B. (1977). Life event questionnaires for measuring presumptive stress. *Psychological Medicine, 39*, 413–431.

John D. and Catherine T. MacArthur Foundation Research Network on Psychopathology and Development (1997). *The PACE/LEDS. An assessment of life events and long term experiences.* Pittsburgh: Western Psychiatric Institute and Clinic, University of Pittsburgh.

Kanner, A.D., & Feldman, S.S. (1991). Control over uplifts and hassles and its relationship to adaptational outcomes. *Journal of Behavioral Medicine, 14*, 187–201.

Kanner, A.D., Coyne, J.C., Schaefer, C., & Lazarus, R.S. (1981). Comparison of two modes of stress measurement: Daily hassles and uplifts versus major life events. *Journal of Behavioral Medicine, 4*, 1–39.

Kessler, R.C. (1997). The effects of stressful life events on depression. *Annual Review of Psychology, 48*, 191–214.

Kessler, R.C., & Wethington, E. (1991). The reliability of life event reports in a community survey. *Psychological Medicine, 21*, 723–738.

Lazarus, R.S., DeLongis, A., Folkman, S., & Gruen, R.J. (1985). Stress and adaptational outcomes: The problem of confounded measures. *American Psychologist, 40*, 770–779.

Lazarus, R.S., & Folkman, S. (1984). *Stress, appraisal, and coping.* New York: Springer.

Lepore, S. (1995). Measurement of chronic stressors. In: S. Cohen, R.C. Kessler, & L.U. Gordon (Eds.), *Measuring stress: A guide for health and social scientists* (pp. 102–120). New York: Oxford University Press.

Lewinsohn, P.M., & Talkington, J. (1979). Studies on the measurement of unpleasant events and relations with depression. *Applied Psychological Measurement, 3*, 83–101.

McQuaid, J., Monroe, S.M., Roberts, J.R., Johnson, S.L., Garamoni, G.L., Kupfer, D.J., & Frank, E. (1992). Toward the standardization of life stress assessment: Definitional discrepancies and inconsistencies in methods. *Stress Medicine, 8*, 47–56.

Monroe, S.M., & Kelley, J.M. (1995). Measurement of stress appraisal. In: S. Cohen, R.C. Kessler, & L.U. Gordon (Eds.), *Measuring stress: A guide for health and social scientists* (pp. 122–147). New York: Oxford University Press.

Moos, R.H. (1981). *Work Environment Scale manual.* Palo Alto, CA: Consulting Psychologists Press.

Moos, R.H., & Moos, B.S. (1981). *Family Environment Scale manual.* Palo Alto, CA: Consulting Psychologists Press.

Paykel, E.S. (1997). The interview for recent life events. *Psychological Medicine, 27*, 301–310.

Peacock, E.H., & Wong, P.T.P. (1990). The Stress Appraisal Measure (SAM): A multidimensional approach to cognitive appraisal. *Stress Medicine, 6,* 227–236.

Pearlin, L.I., & Schooler, C. (1978). The structure of coping. *Journal of Health and Social Behavior, 19,* 2–21.

Price, R.H, Van Ryn, N., & Vinokur, A. 1992. Impact of a preventive job search intervention on the likelihood of depression among the unemployed. *Journal of Health and Social Behavior, 33,* 158–167.

Roos, P.A., & Treiman, D.J. (1980). DOT scales for the 1970 census classification. In: A.R. Miller, D.J. Treiman, P.S. Cain, & P.A. Roos (Eds.), *Work, jobs, and occupations: A critical review of the dictionary of occupational titles* (pp. 336–389). Washington, DC: National Academy Press.

Sandberg, S, Rutter, M., Giles, S., Owen, A., Champion, L., Nicholls, J., Prior, V., McGuinness, D., & Drinnan, D. (1993). Assessment of psychosocial experiences in childhood: Methodological issues and some illustrative findings. *Journal of Child Psychology and Psychiatry and Allied Disciplines, 34,* 879–897.

Schwartz, J.E., & Stone, A.A. (1993). Coping with daily work problems: Contributions of problem content, appraisals, and person factors. *Work and Stress, 1,* 47–62.

Selye, H. (1976). *The stress of life.* New York: McGraw-Hill.

Sobell, L.G., Toneatto, T., Sobell, M.B., Schuller, R., & Maxwell, M. (1990). A procedure for reducing error in reports of life events. *Journal of Psychosomatic Research, 2,* 163–170.

Stein, N., Folkman, S., Trabasso, T., & Richards, T.A. (1997). Appraisal and goal processes as predictors of psychological well-being in bereaved caregivers. *Journal of Personality and Social Psychology, 72,* 872–884.

Stone, A.A., & Neale, J.M. (1982). Development of a methodology for assessing daily experiences. In: A. Baum & J.E. Singer (Eds.), *Advances in environmental psychology: Environment and health* (Vol. 4, pp. 49–83). Hillsdale, NJ: Erlbaum.

Stone, A.A., & Shiffman, S. (1992). Reflections on the intensive measurement of stress, coping, and mood, with an emphasis on daily measures. *Psychology and Health, 7,* 115–129.

Stone, A.A., Kessler, R.C., & Haythornthwaite, J.A. (1991). Measuring daily events and experiences: Methodological considerations. *Journal of Personality, 59,* 575–607.

Tennant, C., Bebbington, P., & Hurry, J. (1981). The role of life events in depressive illness: Is there a substantial causal relation? *Psychological Medicine, 11,* 379–389.

Turner, J.B., Kessler, R.C., & House, J.S. (1991). Factors facilitating adjustment to unemployment: Implications for intervention. *American Journal of Community Psychology, 19,* 521–542.

Turner, R.J., & Avison, W.R. (1992). Innovations in the measurement of life stress: Crisis theory and the significance of event resolution. *Journal of Health and Social Behavior, 33*, 36–50.

Turner, R.J., & Wheaton, B. (1995). Checklist measurement of stressful life events. In: S. Cohen, R.C. Kessler, & L.U. Gordon (Eds.), *Measuring stress: A guide for health and social scientists* (pp. 29–58). New York: Oxford University Press.

Umberson, D., Wortman, C.B., & Kessler, R.C. (1992). Widowhood and depression: Explaining long-term gender differences in vulnerability. *Journal of Health and Social Behavior, 33*, 10–24.

Vinokur, A, & Selzer, M.L. (1975). Desirable versus undesirable life events: Their relationship to stress and mental distress. *Journal of Personality and Social Psychology, 32*, 329–337.

Wethington, E., Brown, G.W., & Kessler, R.C. (1995). Interview measurement of stressful life events. In: S. Cohen, R.C. Kessler, & L.U. Gordon (Eds.), *Measuring stress: A guide for health and social scientists* (pp. 59–79). New York: Oxford University Press.

Wittchen, H., Essau, C.A., Hecht, H., Teder, W., & Pfister, H. (1989). Reliability of life event assessments: Test-retest reliability and fall-off effects of the Munich Interview for the Assessment of Life Events and Conditions. *Journal of Affective Disorders, 16*, 77–91.

Zautra, A.J., Guarnaccia, C.A., & Dohrenwend, B.P. (1986). Measuring small events. *American Journal of Community Psychology, 14*, 629–655.

# 7 ASSESSMENT OF COPING WITH HEALTH PROBLEMS

Norman S. Endler and Judith M. Johnson

In the context of rising expectations in relation to health, coping has come to be viewed as a critical construct in diathesis-stress models of health. Coping has been conceptualized as a conscious behavioral, affective, and cognitive attempt to mediate a perceived discrepancy between situational demands and personal capacity or competence (Endler, 1988). In the area of coping with health, there are constructs about which there is general agreement, such as on task-oriented and emotion-oriented coping. However, much remains unsettled. Perhaps the most basic disagreement is whether research should deal with interindividual coping (styles) or intraindividual coping (processes). Although many coping scales have been developed, few meet rigorous test construction standards, due to poor psychometric qualities. Many scales have a very narrow focus, being limited to particular behaviors applicable only to a single illness. Further, the coping dimensions assessed may vary from scale to scale, making comparison of results between studies and across illnesses very difficult.

There are social factors pertinent to the discussion of assessment in coping with health which must also be considered such as age, gender, social group, religious affiliation, and socioeconomic status. These will be briefly discussed. There are also moderator variables such as coping efficacy and controllability of the situation which have an influence upon coping.

Research in the area, in general, points to the adaptiveness of task-oriented (or problem-focused) coping and the frequent maladaptiveness of emotion-oriented coping in controllable situations. There is a third dimension, avoidance-oriented coping, about which a good deal has been written. However, it is well to be advised that there are two quite different conceptualizations of avoidance. It is viewed by some as efforts to suppress or deny unpleasant information and affect (denial), and by a second group as efforts to distract attention from the stressor by engaging in more pleasant activities (distraction). Some investigators take both sub-factors into consideration.

Various measures will be discussed, including general coping measures which have been applied to health questions, general coping with health measures intended for use across illnesses, and illness-specific measures. A few examples of each will be provided.

Finally, there is a brief discussion of unconscious coping processes, and of the factors which must be considered to optimize the choice of coping measure.

## Assessment of coping with health problems

In the context of rising expectations in relation to health (McDowell & Newell, 1996) coping has, since the mid 1970s (Haan, 1977), come to be seen as an important construct in behavioral medicine and health psychology (see Auerbach, 1989; Endler, 1988; Krohne, 1988, Lazarus & Folkman, 1984a, 1987; Taylor, 1990, 1999; Thomae, 1987). The belief that coping is critical to understanding the relationship of stress to health is nearly universal, although there is a good deal of disagreement about how to assess coping (Aldwin, 1994). In addition to the impact of distress on health, health problems, in and of themselves, have come to be viewed as significant stressors that place excessive demands on the person (Endler, Parker, & Summerfeldt, 1993, 1998).

Coping is a valuable construct in health psychology for a number of reasons. Firstly, it has been found to be a determinant of future health status, with relationships to both symptoms and survival times (Remien et al., 1992). According to Tross (1989), there is good evidence that the immune system is not a "headless horseman", but that it communicates with the nervous system. This may explain why maladaptive coping has been found to have a positive relationship with not only increased anxiety and depression, but also with decreased immune function. For example, in an HIV+ sample, Thomason et al. (1996) found that both interpersonal support and coping were strongly associated with symptomatology, and that anxiety and depression were associated with more rapid declines in CD4 levels. In addition, the course of the disease may be influenced by coping strategies through mechanisms such as self care and compliance with treatment regimens.

Secondly, the manner in which one copes with illness and the attendant life changes influences whether patients are able to adapt to their changed circumstances or fall victim to adjustment disorders. For example, Tross (1989) states that the HIV + patient is "vulnerable to reactive psychiatric symptoms, consisting of the triad of depression, anxiety, and preoccupation with illness" (p. 257). Research is quite clear that particular coping strategies such as task-oriented coping are negatively related, whereas emotion-oriented coping is positively related, to anxiety and depression (Carver et al., 1993; Johnson & Endler, in press).

Finally, adequate coping has been found to prevent unnecessary pain and suffering and may actually speed recovery (Levy, 1991). For example, Carver et al. (1993), in their study of optimism and coping in breast cancer patients found that acceptance was associated with reduced postsurgical distress, whereas denial and behavioral disengagement were positively related to increased postsurgical distress. This same relationship has been found with coronary artery by-pass patients (Scheier et al., 1989) and in a heterogeneous sample of cancer patients (Friedman et al., 1992). Given that coping has implications for the quality of life, mental health, pain and suffering, and disease progression of patients, coping has utility not only as a *predictor*, or *intervening variable*, but also as an *outcome measure*.

Before proceeding, it is necessary to define our terms. In Haan's model (1977), coping was seen as distinct from defense mechanisms in that coping was conscious, flexible, and purposeful. The contemporary view of coping in diathesis-stress models of stress is of a conscious response to external stressful or negative events. It comprises an individual's behavioral, affective, and cognitive attempts to mediate a perceived discrepancy between situational demands and personal capacity or competence (Cox & Ferguson, 1991; Endler, 1988; Endler & Parker, 1995; Endler et al., 1993, 1998; Folkman & Lazarus, 1988; Lazarus & Folkman, 1984a, 1987). The predisposing characteristics of a person, which facilitate a particular response to stressful situations, are the diathesis component of the model. The situational demands upon personal capacity or competence are the stress component, and when demands exceed capacity or competence, distress occurs.

Cognitive appraisal the perceived meaning of the illness to the individual and is a prerequisite of initiating coping attempts, (Schwarzer & Schwarzer, 1996). In practice, it can be very difficult to disentangle appraisal from coping, as the appraisal of the situation and the coping thought or behavior are mutually influential. In their view, although the distinction between appraisal and coping often cannot practically be made, it remains of heuristic value. Different relationships of coping with distress have been found. Coping has long been recognized as an important mediator between stressors and the ensuing psychological state (Endler, 1988; Endler et al., 1993, 1998; Lazarus & Folkman,

1984a). In the area of health psychology, coping is also seen to be an important moderator or buffer variable in the diathesis-stress models which consider environmental forces and physiological predispositions toward illness together with the influences of psychosocial factors upon resilience (Aldwin, 1994; Endler & Parker, 1995).

In order to make our understanding of coping more situationally relevant, health problems must be categorized. Most often, discussions are restricted to a particular illness and no effort is made to generalize results beyond a particular patient group (e.g., HIV; Chesney & Folkman, 1994). Occasionally, comparisons are made between illnesses such as HIV and cancer, where both would be categorized as "life-threatening". In relation to life-threatening diseases, the treatments themselves (e.g., radiation and chemotherapy) constitute an additional challenge to patients' coping resources and many induce so-called iatrogenic illness.

Where one is interested in factors common to a number of illnesses, one approach has been to classify illness as either acute or chronic (Endler et al., 1998). According to this approach, Endler et al. (1998) used two criteria to classify chronic illness. The first criterion is that it is unlikely that there will be a tangible "cure" for the health problem in the near future (at most an amelioration of symptoms). The second criterion is the duration of the illness. It must last a minimum of two months. Examples of chronic illness according to these criteria are arthritis, diabetes, and cancer. Illnesses not meeting the above criteria due to both a shorter duration and a more favorable prognosis would be classified as acute (e.g., brief respiratory infection, broken leg; Endler et al., 1998). This is pertinent not only to the stress imposed by the illness, but also to the sort of care which individuals receive. Whereas acute illnesses may bring patients into contact with health care professionals, chronic illness tends to bring the patient into regular, long-term contact with health care professionals and involve structured treatment schedules (Spirito et al., 1994).

A categorization of coping behavior is also important to this discussion. A taxonomy of specific coping behaviors could well go to several pages. Consequently, the organization of these behaviors is of importance. A good deal of debate has occurred over whether coping styles or coping processes should be the subject of study, with most of the research being conducted on coping styles (Parker & Endler, 1992). Coping styles are relatively stable sets of coping responses analogous to traits in the personality area, and coping processes are responses specific to particular situations (Aldwin, 1994) analogous to states in the personality area. These are also referred to as interindividual and intraindividual coping responses (Endler et al., 1993), or dispositional and situational coping, respectively (Schwarzer & Schwarzer, 1996).

More particularly, the interindividual approach focuses on identifying and comparing basic coping styles used by different individuals across different types of stressful situations. The intraindividual approach examines changes in coping behavior (strategies) in individuals in relation to different situations (Endler et al., 1993). It is important to note that researchers from both schools utilize paper-and-pencil self-report measures. The major difference between these approaches lies almost entirely in the instructions given to research participants (Aldwin, 1994). Interindividual measures most often ask what the participant *generally* does in the face of a stressful situation (Carver et al., 1989; Endler & Parker, 1990), an approach which assumes consistency within individuals across stressful situations. On the other hand, intraindividual measures most often ask participants to indicate their responses in particular specific stressful situations. This approach rests on the assumption that responses are consistent within, but not across, role domains (Aldwin, 1994; Pearlin & Schooler, 1978).

## Dimensions of coping

If there is consensus in the literature on coping, it is with regard to task-oriented and emotion-oriented coping (Endler & Parker, 1990; Parker & Endler, 1992). Task-oriented or problem-focused coping refers to an individual's active efforts to have an impact on, or to deal with, the stressful situation (Endler et al., 1993, 1998; Lazarus & Folkman, 1984a). Emotion-oriented or emotion-focused coping involves strategies such as rumination, daydreaming, and efforts to feel differently about the stressful situation (Higgins & Endler, 1995; Lazarus & Folkman, 1984a).

*Problem- and emotion-focused coping.* Generally speaking, the research literature supports the view that problem-focused coping is adaptive and emotion-focused coping is maladaptive, particularly when the coping effort expended can have an impact upon the stressful situation (Lazarus & Folkman, 1984b; Zeidner & Saklofske, 1996). The literature is also generally supportive of the view that emotion-focused coping can help in maintaining emotional balance in the short run (Zeidner & Saklofske, 1996), but that its utility is questionable if active efforts to manage the situation are not used either conjointly or shortly after the stressful situation arises. Task-oriented strategies have been found to be very effective in stress reduction due to their ability to confer a sense of skill in the face of the stressor, to divert attention from the stressor, and discharge energy arising from the situation (Gal & Lazarus, 1975). Emotion-oriented strategies are used when the source of stress is unclear, when the person does not know effective strategies, or when the stressful situation must simply be tolerated (Pearlin & Schooler, 1978).

*Avoidance.* In addition to task- and emotion-oriented coping, some studies also discuss a third broad coping style: avoidance-oriented coping. Avoidance-oriented coping has been conceptualized in two different ways. The most common conceptualization of avoidance coping describes it as efforts to avoid, deny, suppress or anesthetize negative feelings (Fleishman & Fogel, 1994). Generally speaking, this form of avoidance coping has been found to be maladaptive, resulting in greater distress (Aldwin, 1994; Billings & Moos, 1981; Fleishman & Fogel, 1994; Kurdek & Siesky, 1990). However, there is also evidence that avoidance coping may provide a benefit in the short term by giving the person temporary relief from the stressful situation (Carver et al., 1992).

An alternate conceptualization of avoidance is offered by Endler and Parker (1990), similar to attention diversion (Krohne, 1988). They conceive of avoidance as a dimension with two facets: distraction which includes diverting one's attention from the stressful situation by means of engaging in other activities (a task-oriented diversion) and social diversion which involves diverting attention by engaging in social activities (a person-oriented diversion). These facets have been found to be differentially related to distress with social diversion being negatively related to distress and distraction, positively related to distress for university students and unrelated to distress for HIV+ men (Higgins & Endler, 1995; Johnson & Endler, in press). In any event, caution must be exercised in the area of avoidance as it can be viewed as either a diversion of attention from the stressful situation or as a direct effort to suppress negative emotions. Therefore, caution is warranted in comparing results based on the two different conceptualizations (Johnson & Endler, 1998).

*Monitoring and blunting.* According to the monitoring-blunting hypothesis of attentional styles proposed by Miller (1987), monitoring refers to the tendency to attend to and amplify threat, whereas blunting refers to the tendency to avoid and blunt awareness of threat (Krohne, 1996). Inasmuch as these attentional styles are seen to predict particular coping strategies (e.g., avoidance, information gathering) they fall in the domain of appraisal. However, in that they are themselves a cognitive activity ensuing from the appraisal of threat, they fall into the domain of coping.

Rutherford and Endler (1999) have examined the research evidence in relation to monitoring-blunting, which tends to support the utility of the model both for the purpose of understanding the patients' situational appraisals and experiences, and for the purpose of creating treatment protocols tailored to patients' cognitive styles. Patients with a monitoring cognitive style can benefit from a treatment approach which provides detailed information about the procedures to be used, whereas patients with a blunting style may become more anxious when provided this same information. Blunting would appear to bear a strong relationship with avoidance coping. Rutherford and Endler (1999) discussed three studies (Miller et al., 1989; Miller & Mangan, 1983; Steptoe & O'Sullivan, 1986). Miller and Mangan (1983) found that when blunters were prepared for an unpleasant diagnostic procedure for cervical cancer with a distracting intervention, they demonstrated less subjective and physiological arousal than when they were given information. Monitors displayed the opposite pattern. These findings were found to extend to the individuals' desired information by Steptoe and O'Sullivan (1986) who investigated coping styles and information-seeking in a sample of women about to undergo gynecological surgery. Monitors exhibited a tendency to want more information than blunters about the upcoming surgical procedure and monitors engaged in more frequent health-related information seeking such as cervical smears and breast self-exams. In other research, it has been found that hypertensives are more apt to adopt a high-monitoring style of coping than normotensive patients (Miller et al., 1989).

## Coping efficacy and controllability

There are related constructs which may also have an important moderating effect upon the dependent variable (e.g., anxiety, depression). Coping efficacy and controllability of the situation fall into this category. Coping efficacy may refer to a retrospective perception of success or failure of the coping effort expended in the eyes of the respondent (Aldwin & Revenson, 1987). Thus, asking respondents to rate the effectiveness of the strategies employed would be presumed to account for a portion of the variance based on the assumption that the effects of stress will be removed in relation to the degree of coping efficacy experienced. For example, Aldwin and Revenson (1987) found that the impact of a little instrumental action varied depending on the success experienced. Instrumental action resulted in the fewest psychological symptoms when the individual perceived that it was an effective strategy, whereas when the effort was perceived to be ineffective, instrumental action was less effective in reducing psychological symptoms.

Alternatively, coping efficacy may refer to the patient's prospective sense that he or she has the necessary resources to be effective in dealing with the health problem (Regan et al., 1988). In the latter case, this is also termed secondary appraisal, with primary appraisal being the patient's perception of whether it is stressful, threatening, or harmful or the reverse (Lazarus & Folkman, 1984a).

Controllability of the situation is another factor which has a bearing on the success of various coping strategies to reduce stress. According to the "goodness of fit" hypothesis (Conway & Terry, 1992), problem-focused coping will be more adaptive in situations appraised as controllable, and maladaptive in uncontrollable situations. The opposite is true of emotion-focused coping. Therefore, this hypothesis asserts that the controllability of the situation will moderate the effectiveness of the coping effort employed in reducing the impact of stress. Overall, there has been support for the finding that problem-focused strategies are more adaptive when the situation is controllable, while emotion-focused coping in controllable situations is maladaptive (Carver et al., 1993; Endler et al., 1998). The results with respect to emotion-focused coping are less clear-cut (Forsythe & Compas, 1987; Vitaliano et al., 1990).

In a recent laboratory study, Endler et al. (1998) found that participants who perceived that they had more control used more task-oriented coping and reported less anxiety (for a discussion, see Endler et al., 1998). In the context of chronic illness, however, the controllability of the situation seems to have no impact (Felton & Revenson, 1984), perhaps because there is inherently an element of uncontrollability in chronic illness. This seems to be confirmed by the study of Johnson and Endler (in press), who found that the men in their sample, who had been diagnosed with HIV for a protracted interval, made significantly less use of problem-focused coping than the men in the study of Fleishman and Fogel (1994) who were diagnosed for only a short interval.

# Measurement of coping

Parker and Endler (1992) have been critical of the measures used to assess coping. They have suggested that a systematic understanding of the empirical and theoretical relationships among coping behaviors and both mental and physical health has been hampered by the type and quality of coping measures, which suffer from methodological limitations. They discuss the major weaknesses which are found in most coping scales, namely: (1) a lack of empirical validation of subscales (creation of scales based only on face validity); (2) an unstable or unsubstantiated factor structure; (3) low internal consistency; (4) scales constructed with only male or female subjects when important gender differences are reported in the coping literature; and (5) a lack of construct validity. According to Parker and Endler, methodologically inadequate coping measures make a systematic understanding of the relationship among coping strategies, personality, and health elusive (for a fuller discussion, see Parker & Endler, 1992).

Aldwin (1994) and others (Folkman, 1992; Stone et al., 1991; Stone & Kennedy-Moore, 1992) have countered that scales which assess processes should not be measured by the usual yardstick of psychometric reliability and validity, applied by interindividual researchers such as Parker and Endler (1992), because process research is inherently psychometrically messy. This results in measures that have both unstable factor structure and poor reliability. Intraindividual measures are viewed as being designed to tap variability and change in coping and this is seen to reflect reality. Researchers involved in this form of research have frequently made use of general coping measures, the most widely used of which is the Ways of Coping Questionnaire (WOCS; Folkman & Lazarus, 1988) and have altered the questionnaire instructions to fit the particular situation being measured (Aldwin, 1994). While there is evidence that coping does vary by situation (Mattlin et al., 1990) and that personality influences the use of coping strategies (Bolger, 1990), this is not seen by Parker and Endler (1992) to excuse the lowering of psychometric standards. The difficulties have been dealt with elsewhere. State anxiety is also highly reactive and yet psychometrically sound scales have been developed (Endler et al., 1991). Rather, Parker and Endler (1992) assert that researchers developing new coping scales may simply have to work harder and more efficiently than researchers assessing personality traits or attitudes, but that they should not modify or relax traditional test construction strategies (Parker & Endler, 1992). Regardless of what approach is used, coping is a construct which can account for a large portion of the variance in predicting dependent measures such as depression, anxiety, and quality of life (Aldwin, 1994).

In recent years, a wide array of coping measures has been developed (Amirkhan, 1990; Carver et al., 1989; Tobin et al., 1989). However, most have been developed in order to assess reactions to general stressors, and they are not therefore specific to illness and injury. Thus, scales may contain items irrelevant to coping with health problems. Irrelevant items can frustrate patients who can only wonder how such items can be applied to their situation (Endler et al., 1998). In addition, the inclusion of inappropriate items can undermine their psychometric merit (Waller & Reise, 1989). Conversely, scales have been developed which may be psychometrically reliable and valid, but only for a particular patient population (e.g., pain patients, cystic fibrosis patients, HIV patients). Examples of such scales which will be provided later. This latter situation makes it impossible to compare research results from one study to another or from one illness to another (Endler et al., 1998).

In all of the above scenarios, coping has been used as a predictor variable. However, coping has also been used in intervention studies as an outcome measure. In this research design, a change in coping from a less to more adaptive coping strategy or style is seen as a positive outcome of the intervention in question. The requirement here is that the instrument of choice be sensitive to change. For example Regan et al. (1988) have used this approach. They appraised the effectiveness of a cognitive behavioral intervention on the basis of an increase in a more positive strategy post- than pre-intervention. For example, in a study of rheumatoid arthritis patients, an increase in the cognitive strategy of viewing rheumatoid arthritis as a challenge was used as evidence of the success of the intervention (O'Leary et al., 1988), whereas in a second study with the same patient group, an increase in the coping factor pain control and rational thinking (Parker et al., 1988) was seen as evidence of the success.

The number of coping measures which have been used to assess coping with health problems are numerous. As previously discussed, they are of three types: (1) general coping measures; (2) general coping with health measures; and (3) measures specific to coping with a particular health problem. They will be discussed in turn, with examples provided of each type. If comparisons are made between measures of the same type, it is well to examine the strengths and weaknesses of each, and to note the fact that each scale may have different subscales. The number of coping dimensions used is wide ranging.

GENERAL COPING MEASURES

General coping measures have been developed to assess different aspects of coping and problem solving. Most of these have been developed empirically rather than theoretically, producing not only scale scores, but also operationalizing coping as a conceptual scheme and therefore influencing coping theory (Cook & Heppner, 1997).

*Ways of Coping Questionnaire (WCQ; Folkman & Lazarus, 1988)*. This is the most widely used of the general coping measures and is designed to assess intraindividual coping. In this view, coping processes have two major functions: emotional regulation, and doing something to alleviate the problem (Folkman & Lazarus, 1985). These processes may operate either cognitively or behaviorally. The scale was developed with adults, medical students, undergraduates, married couples and consists of eight subscales: problem-focused coping; wishful thinking; detachment; seeking social support; focusing on the positive; self-blame; tension reduction; and keeping to oneself (Folkman & Lazarus, 1988). Folkman and Lazarus encourage potential users to add or drop items to suit the population under study. Due to this, and other factors, Parker and Endler (1992) have noted some serious limitations. Investigators using the WCQ have often found a different number of factors depending on the sample studied and the items selected for the particular study (Parker et al., 1993). This problem is compounded in the situation of health-specific coping as the questionnaire was designed to assess coping with a stressful situation, not a stressful medical condition. In addition, the reliabilities reported (Folkman & Lazarus, 1985) were moderate and test-retest reliabilities were not reported in the manual. Nonetheless, as Parker and Endler (1992) note, the instrument is of "considerable theoretical interest, and the authors have made important theoretical and empirical contributions to the coping area. However, their coping measures have probably been used more than is justified by the psychometric properties of these scales" (pp. 333–334).

*The Coping Strategies Inventory (CSI; Tobin et al., 1984; Tobin et al., 1989)*. The difficulties associated with the WCQ are not evident in the CSI, which is based upon the WCQ, retaining 23 items from the original Ways of Coping questionnaire (Folkman & Lazarus, 1980). It does have a stable factor structure and strong evidence of reliability, reasonable stability, and evidence of construct validity (Cook & Heppner, 1997). It has eight scales: problem solving; cognitive restructuring; express emotions; social support; problem avoidance; wishful thinking; self-criticism; and social withdrawal.

*Coping Inventory for Stressful Situations (CISS; Endler & Parker, 1990).* Designed to address the psychometric weaknesses of the WCQ, and to assess interindividual coping, this scale was developed using a number of adolescent, undergraduate, adult, and clinical populations. It has three subscales: task-, emotion-, and avoidance-oriented coping. Avoidance-oriented coping is further subdivided into distraction (a task-related diversion), and social diversion (a person-related diversion). Generally speaking, results have shown emotion-oriented coping and distraction to be positively related to psychopathology, whereas task-oriented coping and social diversion have been found to be negatively related to psychopathology. Factor structure is stable; alpha reliabilities range from .83 to .90 for females and from .85 to .90 for males; and test-retest reliabilities over a 6-week interval range from .51 to .73 for males and from .59 to .72 for females.

*COPE (Carver et al., 1989).* This coping inventory is frequently used to assess coping with health. This scale was developed to assess intraindividual coping and is theoretically rather than empirically based. Its authors felt that the problem-focused, emotion-focused paradigm was too simple. Active coping was conceived to be similar to problem-focused coping.

In their study Carver et al. (1989) found that strongly associated with these tendencies were strategies which they termed adaptive. These included positive reinterpretation, planning, suppression of competing activities, restraint coping (or waiting for an appropriate opportunity to utilize a strategy), and seeking social support for instrumental reasons. They also found a cluster of strategies which they termed passive strategies, which were theoretically less adaptive. These included denial, behavioral disengagement, mental disengagement, focus on and venting of emotions, social support for emotional reasons, and alcohol use. However, the COPE was found to have four reliability values in the minimum range of adequacy (from .58 to .69). Nonetheless, this scale does have relatively good stability (Cook & Heppner, 1997).

*Factor analysis.* In an important study, Cook and Heppner (1997) factor analyzed the Coping Strategies Inventory (CSI), the Coping Inventory for Stressful Situations (CISS), and the COPE. When they explored the factor structure of the three scales together using the scaled scores as the observed variables, three factors emerged:

(1) problem engagement; (2) social/emotional; and (3) avoidance. With regard to the theoretical implications, they note that three emotion-management strategies were entwined with the first factor (problem engagement), suggesting that problem- versus emotion-focused coping is an oversimplification. The social/emotional factor included not only social support but also emotion management and express emotion (CSI). Finally, the third factor, avoidance, also included emotional activities. They conclude that a wide range of coping strategies can be conceptualized as constructs that intertwine cognitive, affective, and behavioral coping activities.

## GENERAL COPING WITH HEALTH MEASURES

Parker and Endler (1992) have discussed a number of general coping strategies with health questionnaires. The following discussion outlines portions of their discussion.

*Health Coping Modes Questionnaire (HCMQ; Feifel et al., 1987).* This scale was developed for the purpose of assessing interindividual differences in coping style between patients with life-threatening illnesses (i.e., cancer, myocardial infarction) and those with less severe illness (i.e., arthritis, dermatitis). The scale consists of three subscales: confrontation, avoidance, and acceptance-resignation. Based on factor analysis and item-total correlations the scale was developed empirically. This scale has reasonable psychometric qualities, namely, internal alpha coefficients ranging from .66 to .70, and construct validity has been established. However, before it can be recommended as a useful measure in assessing coping with health, its factor structure must be replicated. As well, it is essential that the HCMQ be validated and factor analyzed for females (as the scale was developed on men only).

*Coping with Health, Injuries, & Problems Scale (CHIP; Endler & Parker, 2000).* This scale was developed to address the psychometric weaknesses found in many scales, and the lack of congruity in the coping constructs assessed to facilitate the comparability of research results. While this scale can be used to assess interindividual coping, a particular illness is specified by the participant. The scale taps four basic coping dimensions: distraction, palliative, instrumental, and emotional preoccupation. The CHIP's factor structure, which was established with a large sample of adults reacting to a heterogeneous set of health problems has been cross validated using confirmatory factors analysis with a college sample and an adult medical patient sample. Internal alpha reliability ranged from .78 to .84 in the adult sample. Construct validity data for the CHIP was found to converge and diverge in a theoretically meaningful manner with a variety of coping styles and psychological distress measures (Endler et al., 1992, 1998; Endler & Parker, 1999). These authors note, in response to assertions that traditional methods for evaluating the psychometric properties of a scale may have to be modified or relaxed when applied to coping measures (Folkman, 1992; Stone et al., 1991; Stone & Kennedy-Moore, 1992), that the CHIP provides evidence that reliable and valid coping scales can be developed using rigorous test construction procedures. This scale can and has been used to investigate coping with specific illness and injuries such as pain, cancer (Endler et al., 1998), and HIV disease (Johnson & Endler, 1998).

## ILLNESS-SPECIFIC COPING MEASURES

There are numerous coping measures which have been designed to assess coping in patients with a particular disease or condition. For example, pain patients may be assessed with questionnaires designed specifically for pain patients, such as the Cognitive Coping Strategy Inventory (Butler et al., 1989), the Vanderbilt Pain Management Inventory (Brown & Nicassio, 1987), and the Coping Strategies Questionnaire (Rosenstiel & Keefe, 1983). The AIDS Coping Scale (Fleishman & Fogel, 1994) has been designed specifically for AIDS patients, the Tinnitus Reaction Questionnaire (Wilson et al., 1991) for tinnitus patients, and the COPD Coping Questionnaire (Ketelaars et al, 1996) for chronic obstructive pulmonary disease patients. There are also scales specific to cystic fibrosis (McCubbin et al, 1983), diabetes (Talbot et al., 1997), and arthritis (Regan et al., 1988).

Each of the scales assesses different coping dimensions. In a sample of 25 health-specific coping scales, 12 had an instrumental coping dimension, 11 an avoidance dimension, 6 an affective dimension, 5 a rumination dimension, and 4 a distraction dimension. In addition, test-retest and internal reliability values, if they are provided at all, vary widely.

To elucidate the difficulties, let us look at the case of cancer. Cancer can be assessed with the Bernese Coping Modes Questionnaire (BCMQ; Heim et al., 1993), the Mental Adjustment to Cancer Scale (MAC; Watson et al., 1988), and other measures. The BCMQ assesses action-related coping, cognition-related coping and emotion-related coping. No test-retest values or internal reliability values are provided. In contrast to the BCMQ, the MAC assesses fighting spirit, helplessness, anxious preoccupation, fatalistic coping, and avoidance. Test-retest values range from a low of .38 to a high of .65. Internal reliabilities range from a low of .34 for avoidance to a high of .76 for fighting spirit. While each scale no doubt provides much of interest, given that the coping dimensions assessed by each of these measures are different, it is apparent that it would be extremely difficult to compare the results from studies using these two questionnaires. The BCMQ assesses coping along a system dimension (i.e., behavioral, cognitive, or emotional), whereas the MAC assesses coping along a content dimension (i.e., fighting spirit, helplessness, anxious preoccupation, fatalistic coping, and avoidance). To look for a common unit of comparison, item analysis would be the only viable strategy, and this approach would in all likelihood be both cumbersome and unproductive. Further, the fact that psychometric data is not available on the former scale means that the reliability, stability, and validity of the scales are unknown and must be gathered on a study by study basis. These problems aside, it is beneficial to examine a few of the health-specific measures of coping.

*Cognitive Coping Strategies Questionnaire (CCSQ; Butler et al., 1989).* This scale was developed to assess the coping of acute pain patients by assessing the face validity of items. It contains seven coping subscales: imaginative inattention, imaginative transformation/context, imagination transformation/sensation, attention diversion/external, attention diversion/internal, somatization, and catastrophizing. Internal reliabilities for the various subscales ranged from .75 to .90. Concurrent and criterion validity data were presented. However, a second order factor analysis found six of the seven scales loaded on a single cognitive factor with all loadings above .72. Additional reliability and validity research is, therefore, required.

*Arthritis Appraisal and Ways of Coping Scale (AAWOC; Regan et al., 1988).* This scale is based upon the model of stress and coping proposed by Lazarus and Folkman (1984a) and as such is an intraindividual measure. It assesses primary and secondary appraisal, and coping. Items from the Ways of Coping Scale were assessed and modified to improve their applicability to osteoarthritis patients, with some additional items coming from a cognitive behavioral intervention, and further items from Rosenstiel and Keefe's (1983) Coping Strategies Questionnaire related to catastrophizing. Factor analysis was used to arrive at the final scales. The measure assesses five coping strategies: dependency; adapting; anger-withdrawal; distancing; and expanding thought and action, by which the authors mean "stretching as a person or thinking of others" (Regan et al., 1988, p. 143). Test-retest correlations were run and ranged from a low of .45 and a high of .72. Internal reliabilities ranged between a low of .64 and a high of .81.

The examples provided of general, health-specific, and illness-specific coping questionnaires permit a brief look at the difficulties encountered in any assessment of coping with health. Even questionnaires which have been widely used demonstrate either psychometric weakness or make generalization of results across people and illnesses problematic. Two steps are critical to clarifying our understanding of coping: agreement upon a taxonomy of coping cognition, emotion, and behavior, and agreement upon the relative contributions of the intraindividual and interindividual coping (or strategies and styles) to outcomes.

*Interviews.* Up to this point, the discussion of coping assessment has been restricted to conscious, self-reported coping strategies or styles. Aldwin (1994) discusses the "one issue that everyone acknowledges but then avoids (like the plague)" (p. 109), namely: if individuals use defense mechanisms, then coping strategies or styles are at least partially unconscious. The conscious, cognitive perspective that we have examined thus far has been criticized by some clinicians who believe that coping responses are not under conscious control. Aldwin (1994) discusses a number of problems with this unknown variable. One problem is that coping is not static. When a problem first occurs (e.g., one has a heart attack), denial may well be a relatively common response, but denial would be time limited. It would not be expected to persist indefinitely. A second problem is that if a defense mechanism is working effectively, then no problem may be reported. Aldwin (1994) states that self-report stress surveys do tend to underestimate the presence of problems which subsequent interviews reveal. Finally, participants may report the use of strategies they believe they use rather than the strategies that they actually use. Therefore, in clinical settings, paper and pencil self-report measures should be supplemented with interviews.

## Optimizing choices

Optimizing the choice of measure requires that one consider many factors. First and foremost, the population under study must be considered. Factors such as age, gender, socioeconomic status, ethnicity, religious affiliation, and social group are pertinent and may well reflect the participants' resources and capacities. Developmental studies point to the need for awareness of cohort effects (differences attributable to year of birth) (Strack & Feifel, 1996). Individuals born in a particular birth cohort have experiences similar to each other and dissimilar to other birth cohorts. This may shape some of the coping resources and strategies of individuals in the cohort. For example, elderly persons in the Western world lived through World War II and the Great Depression. As a consequence, individuals were told "don't wear your heart on your sleeve". This lesson would tend to rule out emotion-oriented coping as an admissible coping strategy. Results have tended to support the presence of these age-related differences (e.g., Feifel et al., 1987; Felton & Revenson, 1987). Therefore, it is well to be advised of these differences to be certain that the scale of choice contains items applicable to the cohort under study.

Another developmental effect concerns the cognitive ability of study participants. HIV participants may suffer from dementia, as may the elderly. Further, the tendency of cognitive performance to decline markedly in the final few years of life (known as "terminal drop") means that the proportion of participants in the "drop" phase increases gently with advancing age. These effects may well have a serious impact on research results in the area of coping with health, as the elderly are likely to experience both more illness and cognitive decline. The importance of cognitive skills for effective coping may well make this an important factor in the assessment of coping, confounding the measurement of coping (i.e., coping style may remain constant while ability declines, underestimating the presence of a particular coping style).

Not only do differences between cohorts require attention, but within cohorts, gender differences are often reported. Thoits (1991) states that gender differences are relatively infrequent, but that when they do occur, they occur within specific situational contexts. It has been found that men were more likely to use problem solving strategies than women in relation to work (Folkman & Lazarus, 1980; Pearlin & Schooler, 1978), whereas women were more likely to use problem solving strategies within marriage and as parents (Menaghan, 1982; Pearlin & Schooler, 1978). Women in general were more likely to reinterpret the situation than men and more likely than men to seek advice or support in dealing with marital or parental problems (Fleishman, 1984). Thoits (1991) concludes that "problem-solving efforts are more likely to be used when individuals perceived that they have more power, control, or responsibility in a particular role domain" (for a fuller discussion, see Thoits, 1991). Typical of within-cohort gender differences across situational contexts is the finding of Higgins and Endler (1995) that task-oriented coping was negatively related to distress, but only for males, whereas emotion-oriented coping was positively related to distress in both males and females. Therefore, care must be taken to insure that scale items allow for an assessment of the full range of coping behaviors for both men and women in the role domains affected by the illness.

Sociological factors are also of importance in the assessment of coping. Diseases may be specific to particular populations. Tuberculosis is on the increase and seems, in the Western nations, to be localized to a considerable degree among the poor and those with HIV. Further, HIV has been disproportionately a disease of gay men, although this demographic is shifting to the poor, the young, and women (Shariff, 1990). In addition, as with leprosy, a disease may stigmatize its sufferers. For example, men who are seropositive for HIV must deal with discrimination from persons, institutions, and governments, a good example of which is efforts by insurance companies to refuse them coverage (Chesney & Folkman, 1994). All of these factors have an impact upon the assessment of coping with health, magnifying the stressfulness of the situation and expanding the number of functional areas impacted by the illness.

The example of those who are HIV seropositive provides a case in point, and because the impact of this illness is so pervasive, highlights many of the issues. These patients face a devastating illness, the course of which creates a host of difficulties (Tross, 1989). In addition to the threat of loss of life, these individuals are likely to experience a wide range of losses which accrue through the course of the illness (Kiemle, 1994) including loss of a future, preferred daily activities, work, income, security, and health (Chesney & Folkman, 1994; Kiemle, 1994).

HIV is a disease with well-defined stages (Tross, 1989) which may have a bearing on the coping strategies employed. In the early stages, Fleishman and Fogel (1994) found that task-oriented coping prevented distress. However, Johnson and Endler (1998) found that among those who had been infected for a protracted interval, distraction prevented distress and that task-oriented coping did not predict distress. In this regard, Moos (1982; Moos & Schaefer, 1986) proposed the *crisis theory* to elucidate factors which may have a bearing upon how people adjust in a health crisis. Additional factors to consider which may confound results include the presence of dementia and the widespread use of many, overlapping medications (Johnson & Endler, 1998).

In addition, these patients face additional stressors not faced by most other terminally-ill patients. HIV-infected adults who are not hemophiliacs are often implicitly considered to be "guilty" for contracting the disease (Kiemle, 1994) due to the stigma resulting from the close association of HIV with both sexuality and homosexuality in the public mind. Given that HIV is a communicable disease, important changes in sexual or other practices must be made to protect others from the disease. Further, HIV-infected individuals may have to deal with the death of many associates who are also infected, and with the consequent grief (Kalichman & Sikkema, 1994). All of these factors are pertinent to the assessment of coping, seriously complicating the interpretation of results.

The second factor, which is important in selecting the instruments to be used is the purpose of the assessment. As previously discussed, if the main purpose of the study is to measure coping processes within individuals, then care must be taken to select an appropriate intraindividual measure, and if the comparison of coping across groups is the aim, then interindividual measures are appropriate. Ideally, compatible measures of intraindividual and interindividual measures would be used to facilitate the simultaneous understanding of both dimensions and the ways in which they interact.

Finally, the importance of measures of good stability, reliability, and validity cannot be overemphasized. If there is to be any consensus on the number and type of coping styles or strategies, and any understanding of coping across illness domains, then rigorous standards must be applied regardless of whether processes or styles are of interest.

## Summary and conclusions

There is a nearly universal acceptance of the critical role played by coping in diathesis-stress models of stress. The discussion has largely focused upon the conscious behavioral, affective, and cognitive aspects of coping, although lip service has been paid to possible unconscious processes. We have examined the disagreements which exist between those who would study interindividual coping (styles) or intraindividual coping (process or strategy). Some attention has been devoted to providing examples of general coping scales, general coping with health scales, and illness-specific coping scales and we have reviewed some of the difficulties which remain. Many scales have a very narrow focus, making results incomparable across different studies, and many more scales have poor psychometric properties.

There has been a brief examination of the social or contextual factors pertinent to the discussion of coping with health such as age, gender, and social group. There was also a brief discussion of coping efficacy, and controllability of the situation which may moderate the effect of coping on distress.

Research in the area, in general, points to the adaptiveness of task-oriented (or problem-focused) coping and the maladaptiveness of emotion-oriented coping. There is a third dimension, avoidance-oriented coping, about which a good deal has been written. However, it is well to be advised that there are two quite different conceptualizations of avoidance. It is viewed by some as efforts to suppress or deny unpleasant information and affect (denial), and by a second group as efforts to distract attention from the stressor by engaging in more pleasant activities (distraction). Some investigators take both sub-factors into consideration.

Various measures were discussed, including general coping measures which have been applied or adapted to health questions, general coping with health measures intended for use across illnesses, and illness-specific coping measures. A few examples of each were provided.

There was a brief discussion of unconscious coping processes, the factors which must be considered to optimize the choice of coping measure, and which measures to use for particular problems or illnesses. In brief, to optimize the choice of measure, the impact of the illness and the social characteristics of the group to be studied should be well known. Second, the purpose of the study must be clearly delineated. Finally, the psychometric quality of the assessment instrument chosen is an important consideration.

Finally, coping is an extremely important construct (both theoretically and practically) in the assessment of diathesis-stress models of health. Nonetheless, a caution is in order based upon the study of Cook and Heppner (1997), that none of the coping instruments examined may clearly assess all of the underlying coping domains, which may each include a complex of cognition, emotion, and behavior.

## Acknowledgment

Preparation of this chapter was facilitated by SSHRC grant 410–94–1473 to Norman S. Endler. Requests for reprints should be sent to Norman S. Endler, Department of Psychology, York University, Toronto, Canada, M3J 1P3.

# References

Aldwin, C.M. (1994). *Stress, coping and development: An integrative perspective*. New York: Guilford.

Aldwin, C., & Revenson, T.A. (1987). Does coping help? A reexamination of the relationship between coping and mental health. *Journal of Personality and Social Psychology, 53*, 337–348.

Amirkhan, J.H. (1990). A factor analytically derived measure of coping: The coping strategy indicator. *Journal of Personality and Social Psychology, 59*, 1066–1074.

Auerbach, S.M. (1989). Stress management and coping research in the health care setting: An overview and methodological commentary. *Journal of Consulting and Clinical Psychology, 57*, 388–395.

Billings, A.G., & Moos, R.H. (1981). The role of coping responses and social resources in attenuating the stress of life events. *Journal of Behavioral Medicine, 4*, 139–157.

Bolger, N. (1990). Coping as a personality process: A prospective study. *Journal of Personality and Social Psychology, 59*, 525–537.

Brown, G.K., & Nicassio, P.M. (1987). Development of a questionnaire for the assessment of active and passive coping strategies in chronic pain patients. *Pain, 31*, 53–64.

Butler, R.W., Damarin, F.L., Beaulieu, C., Schwebel, A.I., & Thorn, B.E. (1989). Assessing cognitive coping strategies for acute postsurgical pain. *Psychological Assessment, 1*, 41–45.

Carver, C.S., Scheier, M.F., & Weintraub, J.K. (1989). Assessing coping strategies: A theoretically-based approach. *Journal of Personality and Social Psychology, 56*, 267–283.

Carver, C.S., Scheier, M.F., & Pozo, C. (1992). Conceptualizing the process of coping with health problems. In: H.S. Friedman (Ed.), *Hostility, coping, and health* (pp. 167–199). Washington, DC: American Psychological Association.

Carver, C.S., Pozo, C., Harris, S.D., Noriega, V., Scheier, M.F., Robinson, D.S., Ketcham, A.S., Moffat, F.L. Jr., & Clark, K.C. (1993). How coping mediates the effect of optimism on distress: A study of women with early stage breast cancer. *Journal of Personality and Social Psychology, 65*, 375–390.

Chesney, M.A., & Folkman, S. (1994). Psychological impact of HIV disease and implications for intervention. *Psychiatric Clinics of North America, 17*, 163–182.

Conway, V.J., & Terry, D.J. (1992). Appraised controllability as a moderator of the effectiveness of different coping strategies: A test of the goodness of fit hypothesis. *Australian Journal of Psychology, 44*, 1–7.

Cook, S.W., & Heppner, P.P. (1997). A psychometric study of three coping measures. *Educational and Psychological Measurement, 57*, 907–923.

Cox, T., & Ferguson, E. (1991). Individual differences, stress and coping. In: C.L. Cooper & R. Payne (Eds.), *Personality and stress: Individual differences in the stress process* (pp. 7–30). Chichester: Wiley.

Endler, N.S. (1988). Hassles, health and happiness. In: M.P. Janice (Ed.), *Individual differences, stress and health psychology* (pp. 24–56). New York: Springer.

Endler, N.S., & Parker, J.D.A. (1990). Multidimensional assessment of coping: A critical evaluation. *Journal of Personality and Social Psychology, 58*, 844–854.

Endler, N.S., & Parker, J.D.A. (1995). Assessing a patient's ability to cope. In: J.N. Butcher (Ed.), *Practical considerations in clinical personality assessment* (pp. 329–352). New York: Oxford University Press.

Endler, N.S., & Parker, J.D.A. (1999). *Coping with Health, Injuries and Problems Scale (CHIP): Manual.* Toronto: Multi-Health Systems.

Endler, N.S., Edwards, J.M., & Vitelli, R. (1991). *Endler Multidimensional Anxiety Scales (EMAS) Manual.* Los Angeles: Western Psychological Services.

Endler, N.S., Courbasson, C.M.A., & Fillion, L. (1998). Coping with cancer: The evidence for the temporal stability of the French Canadian version of the Coping with Health, Injuries and Problems (CHIP). *Personality and Individual Differences, 25*, 711–717.

Endler, N.S., Parker, J.D.A., & Summerfeldt, L.J. (1993). Coping with health problems: Conceptual and methodological issues. *Canadian Journal of Behavioural Science, 25*, 384–399.

Endler, N.S., Parker, J.D.A., & Summerfeldt, L.J. (1998). Coping with health problems: Developing a reliable and valid multidimensional measure. *Psychological Assessment, 10*, 195–205.

Endler, N.S., Speer, R.L., Johnson, J.M., & Flett, G.L. (2000). Controllability, coping, efficacy, and distress. *European Journal of Personality, 14*, 245–264.

Feifel, H., Strack, S., & Nagy, V.T. (1987). Coping strategies and associated features of medically ill patients. *Psychosomatic Medicine, 49*, 616–625.

Felton, B.J., & Revenson, T.A. (1984). Coping with chronic illness: A study of illness controllability and the influence of coping strategies on psychological adjustment. *Journal of Consulting and Clinical Psychology, 12*, 343–353.

Felton, B.J., & Revenson, T.A. (1987). Age differences in coping with chronic illness. *Psychology and Aging, 2*, 164–170.

Fleishman, J.A. (1984). Personality characteristics and coping patterns. *Journal of Health and Social Behavior, 25*, 229–244.

Fleishman, J.A., & Fogel, B. (1994). Coping and depressive symptoms among people with AIDS. *Health Psychology, 13*, 156–169.

Folkman, S. (1992). Improving coping assessment: Reply to Stone and Kennedy-Moore. In: H.S. Friedman (Ed.), *Hostility, coping and health* (pp. 215–223). Washington, DC: American Psychological Association.

Folkman, S., & Lazarus, R.S. (1980). An analysis of coping in a middle-aged community sample. *Journal of Health and Social Behavior, 21*, 219–239.

Folkman, S., & Lazarus, R.S. (1985). If it changes it must be a process: Study of emotion and coping during three stages of a college examination. *Journal of Personality and Social Psychology, 48,* 150–170.

Folkman, S., & Lazarus, R.S. (1988). *Manual for the Ways of Coping Questionnaire.* Palo Alto, CA: Consulting Psychologists Press.

Forsythe, C.J., & Compas, B.E. (1987). Interaction of cognitive appraisals of stressful events and coping: Testing the goodness of fit hypothesis. *Cognitive Therapy and Research, 11,* 473–485.

Friedman, L.C., Nelson, D.V., Baer, P.E., Lane, M., Smith, F.E., & Dworkin, R.J. (1992). The relationship of dispositional optimism, daily life stress, and domestic environment to coping methods used by cancer patients. *Journal of Behavioral Medicine, 15,* 127–141.

Gal, R., & Lazarus, R. (1975). The role of activity in anticipation and confronting stressful situations. *Journal of Human Stress, 1,* 4–20.

Haan, N. (Ed.) (1977). *Coping and defending.* New York: Academic Press.

Heim, E., Augustiny, K.F., Schaffner, L., & Valach, L. (1993). Coping with breast cancer over time and situation. *Journal of Psychosomatic Research, 37,* 523–542.

Higgins, J.E., & Endler, N.S. (1995). Coping, life stress, and psychological and somatic distress. *European Journal of Personality, 9,* 253–270.

Johnson, J.M., & Endler, N.S. (in press). Coping with the immune deficiency virus. Do optimists fare better? *Current Psychology. Development, Learning, Personality, Social.*

Kalichman, S.C., & Sikkema, K.J. (1994). Psychological sequelae of HIV infection and AIDS: Review of empirical findings. *Clinical Psychology Review, 14,* 611–632.

Ketelaars, C.A.J., Schlosser, M.A.G., Mostert, R., Huyer Abu-Saad, H., Halfens, R.J.G., & Wouters, E.F.M. (1996). Determinants of health-related quality of life in patients with chronic obstructive pulmonary disease. *Thorax, 51,* 39–43.

Kiemle, G. (1994). "What's so special about HIV and AIDS?": Stresses and strains for clients and counsellors. *British Journal of Guidance and Counselling, 22,* 343–351.

Krohne, H.W. (1988). Coping research: Current theoretical and methodological developments. *German Journal of Psychology, 12,* 1–30.

Krohne, H.W. (1996). Individual differences in coping. In: M. Zeidner & N.S. Endler (Eds.), *Handbook of coping: Theory, research, application* (pp. 381–409). New York: Wiley.

Kurdek, L.A., & Siesky, G. (1990). The nature and correlates of psychological adjustment in gay men with AIDS-related conditions. *Journal of Applied Social Psychology, 20,* 846–860.

Lazarus, R.S., & Folkman, S. (1984a). *Stress, appraisal, and coping.* New York: Springer.

Lazarus, R.S., & Folkman, S. (1984b). Coping and adaptation. In: W.D. Gentry (Ed.), *The handbook of behavioral medicine* (pp. 282–325). New York: Guilford.

Lazarus, R.S., & Folkman, S. (1987). Transactional theory and research on emotions and coping. *European Journal of Personality, 1*, 141–169.

Levy, S.M. (1991) Behavioral and immunological host factors in cancer risk. In: P.M. McCabe, N. Schneiderman, T.M. Field, & J.S. Skyler (Eds.), *Stress, coping and disease* (pp. 237–252). Hillsdale, NJ: Erlbaum.

Mattlin, J., Wethington, E., & Kessler, R.C. (1990). Situational determinants of coping and coping effectiveness. *Journal of Health and Social Behavior, 31*, 103–122.

McCubbin, H.I., McCubbin, M.A., Patterson, J.M., Lauble, A.E., Wilson, L.R., & Warwick, W. (1983). CHIP—Coping Health Inventory for Parents: An assessment of parental coping patterns in the case of the chronically ill child. *Journal of Marriage and the Family, 45*, 359–370.

McDowell, I., & Newell, C. (1996). *Measuring health: A guide to rating scales and questionnaires* (2nd ed.). New York: Oxford University Press.

Menaghan, E. (1982). Measuring coping effectiveness: A panel analysis of marital problems and coping efforts. *Journal of Health and Social Behavior, 23*, 220–234.

Miller, S.M. (1987) Monitoring and blunting: Validation of a questionnaire to assess styles of information seeking under threat. *Journal of Personality and Social Psychology, 52*, 345–353.

Miller, S.M., & Mangan, C.E. (1983). The interacting effects of information and coping style in adapting to gynecologic stress: Should the doctor tell all? *Journal of Personality and Social Psychology, 45*, 223–236.

Miller, S.M., Leinbach, A., & Brody, D.S. (1989). Coping style in hypertensive patients: Nature and consequences. *Journal of Consulting and Clinical Psychology, 57*, 333–337.

Moos, R.H. (1982). Coping with acute health crises. In: T. Millon, C. Green, & R. Meagher (Eds.), *Handbook of clinical health psychology* (pp. 129–152). New York: Plenum.

Moos, R.H., & Schaefer, J.A. (1986). Life transitions and crises: A conceptual overview. In: R.H. Moos (Ed.), *Coping with life crises: An integrated approach* (pp. 3–28). New York: Plenum.

O'Leary, A., Shoor, S., Lorig, K., & Holman, H.R. (1988). A cognitive–behavioral treatment for rheumatoid arthritis. *Health Psychology, 7*, 527–544.

Parker, J., Frank, R., Beck, N., Smarr, K., Buescher, K., Smith, P.L., Anderson, S., & Walker, S. (1988). Pain management in rheumatoid arthritis patients. *Arthritis and Rheumatism, 31*, 593–601.

Parker, J.D.A., & Endler, N.S. (1992). Coping with coping assessment: A critical review. *European Journal of Personality, 6*, 321–344.

Parker, J.D.A., Endler, N.S., & Bagby, R.M. (1993). If it changes, it might be unstable: Examining the factor structure of the Ways of Coping Questionnaire. *Psychological Assessment, 5*, 361–368.

Pearlin, L., & Schooler, C. (1978). The structure of coping. *Journal of Health and Social Behavior, 19*, 2–21.

Regan, C.A., Lorig, K., & Thoresen, C.E. (1988). Arthritis appraisal and ways of coping: Scale development. *Arthritis Care and Research, 1,* 139–150.

Remien, R.H., Rabkin, J.G., Williams, J.B., & Katoff, L. (1992). Coping strategies and health beliefs of AIDS longterm survivors. *Psychology and Health, 6,* 335–345.

Rosenstiel, A.K., & Keefe, F.J. (1983). The use of coping strategies in chronic low back pain patients: Relationship to patient characteristics and current adjustment. *Pain, 17,* 33–44.

Rutherford, A., & Endler, N.S. (1999). Predicting approach-avoidance: The roles of coping styles, state anxiety and situational appraisal. *Anxiety, Stress and Coping, 12,* 63–85.

Scheier, M.F., Magovern, G.J. Sr., Abbott, R.A., Matthews, K.A., Owens, J.F., Lefebvre, R.C., & Carver, C.S. (1989). Dispositional optimism and recovery from coronary artery bypass surgery: The beneficial effects on physical and psychological well-being. *Journal of Personality and Social Psychology, 57,* 1024–1040.

Schwarzer, R., & Schwarzer, C. (1996). A critical survey of coping instruments. In: M. Zeidner & N.S. Endler (Eds.), *Handbook of coping: Theory, research, application* (pp. 107–132). New York: Wiley.

Shariff, S. (1990). Health: The hidden toll. *Macleans, 104,* 56–57.

Spirito, A., Stark, L.J., & Tye, V.L. (1994). Stressors and coping strategies described during hospitalization by chronically ill children. *Journal of Clinical Child Psychology, 23,* 314–322.

Steptoe, A., & O'Sullivan, J. (1986). Monitoring and blunting coping styles in women prior to surgery. *British Journal of Clinical Psychology, 25,* 143–144.

Stone, A.A., & Kennedy-Moore, E. (1992). Assessing situational coping: Conceptual and methodological considerations. In: H.S. Friedman (Ed.), *Hostility, coping and health* (pp. 203–214). Washington, DC: American Psychological Association.

Stone, A.A., Greenberg, M.A., Kennedy-Moore, E., & Newman, M.G. (1991). Self-report, situation-specific coping questionnaires: What are they measuring? *Journal of Personality and Social Psychology, 61,* 648–658.

Strack, S., & Feifel, H. (1996). Age differences, coping and the adult life span. In: M. Zeidner & N.S. Endler (Eds.), *Handbook of coping: Theory, research, application* (pp. 485–501). New York: John Wiley & Sons.

Talbot, F., Nouwen, A., Gingras, J., Gosselin, M., & Audet, J. (1997). The assessment of diabetes-related cognitive and social factors: The multidimensional diabetes questionnaire. *Journal of Behavioral Medicine, 20,* 291–312.

Taylor, S.E. (1990). Health psychology: The science and the field. *American Psychologist, 45,* 40–50.

Taylor, S.E. (1999). *Health psychology* (4th ed). Boston: McGraw-Hill.

Thoits, P.A. (1991). Gender differences in coping with emotional distress. In: J. Eckenrode (Ed.), *The social context of coping* (pp. 107–138). New York: Plenum Press.

Thomae, H. (1987). Conceptualizations of responses to stress. *European Journal of Personality, 1*, 171–192.

Thomason, B., Jones, G., McClure, J., & Brantley, P. (1996). Psychosocial co-factors in HIV illness: An empirically-based model. *Psychology and Health, 11*, 385–393.

Tobin, D.L., Holroyd, K.A., Reynolds, R.V., & Wigal, J.K. (1989). The hierarchical factor structure of the Coping Strategies Inventory. *Cognitive Therapy and Research, 13*, 343–361.

Tobin, D.L., Reynolds, R., Holroyd, K.A. & Wigal, J. (1984). Collecting test-retest reliability data on a measure of coping process: The problem of situational effects. Paper presented at the meeting of the Southeastern Psychological Association, New Orleans.

Tross, S. (1989). Acquired immunodeficiency syndrome (AIDS). In: J.C. Holland & J.H. Rowland (Eds.), *Handbook of psychooncology: Psychological care of the patient with cancer* (pp. 254–270). New York: Oxford University Press.

Vitaliano, P.P., DeWolfe, D.J., Maiuro, R.D., & Russo, J. (1990). Appraised changeability of a stressor as a modifier of the relationship between coping and depression: A test of the hypothesis of fit. *Journal of Personality and Social Psychology, 59*, 382–592.

Waller, N.G., & Reise, S.P. (1989). Computerized adaptive personality assessment: An illustration with the Absorption Scale. *Journal of Personality and Social Psychology, 57*, 1051–1058.

Watson, M., Greer, S., Young, J., Anayat, Q., Burgess, C., & Robertson, B. (1988). Development of a questionnaire measure of adjustment to cancer: The MAC Scale. *Psychological Medicine, 18*, 203–209.

Wilson, P.H., Henry, J., Bowen, M., & Haralambous, G. (1991). Tinnitus Reaction Questionnaire: Psychometric properties of a measure of distress associated with tinnitus. *Journal of Speech and Hearing Research, 34*, 197–201.

Zeidner, M., & Saklofske, D.H. (1996). Adaptive and maladaptive coping. In: M. Zeidner & N.S. Endler (Eds.), *Handbook of coping: Theory, research, application* (pp. 505–531). New York: Wiley.

# 8 SOCIAL SUPPORT: CONCEPTUAL ISSUES AND ASSESSMENT STRATEGIES

Eric van Sonderen and Robbert Sanderman

Since Berkman and Syme (1979) demonstrated that people with more social contacts had lower death-rates, health scientists have become interested in the phenomenon of social support. Various studies resulted in similar findings: socially isolated people appeared in general to be less healthy (Cohen & Syme, 1985; Heller & Swindle, 1983; House, 1981). In addition, it was hypothesized that social support was able to reduce or even remove the negative effects of life events and long term difficulties on mental and physical well-being. As research in the area developed, it became clear that social support was developing into a controversial concept used in models intended to describe determinants of well-being. Social support has carried this label of indistinctness to the present day. Many researchers are currently trying to disentangle the nature and function of this seemingly clear concept. Research continues to attempt to: (1) demonstrate a relationship between social support and well-being, and (2) determine whether social support has a direct effect or one that only exists under the condition of a stressor, the so called buffering effect. Some researchers have tried to settle this discussion by providing a theoretical overview of the pros and cons of both models, or by presenting meta-analyses (Cohen & Wills 1985; Lin, 1986, Chapter 10; Schwarzer & Leppin, 1991). In general these attempts did not lead to clear unequivocal conclusions. The strength of the relationship between support and well-being is generally weak. Occasionally researchers even report negative relationships between support and well-being, indicating that people with more support tend to have lower levels of well-being. Recently, more and more authors point toward conceptual and methodological problems as the cause of these peculiar findings (Barrera, 1986; Schwarzer & Leppin, 1991).

Progress in this area is seriously hampered by the great variety of instruments for measuring social support. This variety is partly induced by the conceptual confusion. Several authors present overviews of instruments used to assess social support (e.g., Bruhn & Philips, 1984;

Heitzmann & Kaplan, 1988; Orth-Gomer & Unden, 1987; Van Sonderen, 1995; Winemiller et al., 1993). Together with literature in which the problem is approached from a more theoretical perspective (Cobb, 1976; House, 1981; Thoits, 1982; Van Sonderen, 1991; Vaux, 1988), these overviews provide a list of relevant aspects of social support. However, these theoretical developments have not until now facilitated the development of new questionnaires that are based on a conceptually clear model.

But even when conceptual problems are solved, there are other features that prevent researchers from getting a clear view of the social support concept. As a result, choosing a suitable instrument to assess support is rather difficult. While people often think of explicit, supportive transactions that constitute the focal aspect of social support, both provider and receiver of this support are judging these transactions subjectively, giving way to personality characteristics and coping styles to exercise their influence. In other words, the question is to what extent social support should be considered as an *objective* feature. The other complicating factor is the fact that a lot of stressors are induced by relationships with (close) others, who are expected to give support. Moreover, the quality of relationships that are assumed to be supportive can be affected by conflicts. When a relationship ends through a serious conflict or through the death of a significant other, the change in one's social network functions as a stressor, while at the same time this network is still considered to be a provider of support.

This chapter tries to clarify some of the problems mentioned above. The most relevant conceptual problems related to the assessment of social support will be discussed. Then, by explaining the different aspects of social support, the choice of a particular approach or the selection of particular domains of social support when setting out a study is demonstrated. Finally, some operationalizations will be discussed. The enumeration of instruments is not meant to be exhaustive. Ultimately, the goal is to widen the readers' awareness of the most relevant topics that have to be considered when choosing to measure social support. Throughout the chapter the possible relationship of social support with psychological distress or physical well-being is taken into account.

## Conceptual issues

In this section three of the most important conceptual problems with respect to the definition and assessment of social support are discussed.

These are: (1) "network versus support"; (2) "actual versus perceived support"; and (3) "amount of received support versus satisfaction with received support". A distinction is often made between the social network, i.e., the people seen as providers of social support and the "transfer" of social support within these relationships. This distinction is often described as the structural versus the functional component of the concept "social support". By focussing on the functional component, we distinguish between actual received support and perceived supportiveness. Whereas actual support is provided in a real situation in the present or (recent) past, people also have a feeling of supportiveness, based on previous experiences or appraisal of the potentials of their network. The evaluation of both actual received and expected support can be viewed as perceived supportiveness of the social network. The third issue that will be discussed concerns the distinction between the amount of actual received support and the evaluation of this amount compared to the actual need for support. More specifically, the latter one is focusing more on the satisfaction with the support received, rather than with the amount of support.

## THE STRUCTURAL AND FUNCTIONAL COMPONENT OF SOCIAL SUPPORT

Social support is dependent on relationships with other people. Some researchers emphasize the social network in their approach to social support. Those who adhere to this social integration approach point to the necessity of being part of a group of related people. The mere knowledge of belonging to a group of people who are concerned about each other is considered to be beneficial for one's well-being.

Instruments assessing network or social integration typically measure number of relatives, amount of contacts among members of the social network, frequency of contacts, geographical distance of network members, and the presence or absence of specific persons in someone's network, like a spouse or friends.

One important dilemma with respect to the conceptual definition of social support concerns the delineation of the social network. This fundamental aspect is underexposed and often even overlooked in the literature. Is provision of social support by definition limited to members of the personal social network? Are fellow-sufferers part of this network? What about the support received from special trained volunteers, or from professionals, like nurses and doctors.

The question at stake is whether the type of interaction defines the belonging to the network or the type of relationship (between provider and receiver of the support). In our opinion, the adjective "social" should exclude relations with (and interactions from) professional care-givers, which is in line with the ideas of Veiel (1985). On the other hand Tardy (1985), Turner (1983) and House (1981) explicitly mention professionals as a source of social support.

We prefer to restrict the use of the label "social support" only to interactions provided by informal non-professional others. In such a relationship there is no *quid pro quo* at stake. Hence, if relationships are not incorporating these characteristics substantially, it should not be seen as *social* support. Support provided by nurses or doctors—who get paid to get in contact with a patient—or by trained volunteers or even paid employees should not be characterized as social support. An interesting example is the support patients receive in a psychosocial intervention. They do indeed receive support, but in the present con-ceptualization it is not *social* support. Yet this distinction between social and formal support will still lead to discussion with respect to the position of, for example, fellow-patients. Probably the reciprocity in these contacts is an argument to consider supportive interactions between fellow-patients as social support.

As far as network characteristics are related to indicators of well-being, this relation exists because it is mediated by the content of the contacts with network members. Therefore, it seems obvious to concentrate on these functional aspect of relationships, the provision of social support, rather than on the network characteristics.

A relevant aspect in characterizing supportive interactions is the type of support that is provided. Although few authors use the same con-cepts, some types of support often emerge. The most important and frequently made distinction is between emotional and instrumental support. Other relevant types of support are esteem support, social companionship, and informational support. Examples of these types of support are: "reassuring someone" (emotional support); "providing with help in practical everyday things" (instrumental support); "paying a compliment" (esteem support); "dropping in for a visit" (social com-panionship); and "giving someone constructive criticism" (informa-tional support). In a study by Van Sonderen (1991, 1993), it appeared that these types of support are to some extent empirically distinguish-able. However, although they factor out in the analyses, there are strong indications for one underlying concept.

## THE DIFFERENCE BETWEEN ACTUAL PROVIDED/RECEIVED SUPPORT AND EXPECTED SUPPORT

It is, from a theoretical point of view, relevant to distinguish between actual received support and support that someone is expecting to receive in case problems occur. While received support has actually been provided in the (recent) past, most probably offered to meet an actual demand, expected support is the support someone has not actually received, but expects to receive. In the latter case, two situations can be distinguished. Sometimes, someone deals with an actual stressor and is asked what amount of support (s)he expects to receive. But often there is just talk of an imaginary stressful situation, about which a person is asked to estimate the support that will be provided. Questions that measure expected support typically are formulated like "How much support do you (expect to) receive in case ... (e.g., you're ill)".

Instruments that do not distinguish between the following three aspects of support are regularly used:

(1) actual support,
(2) expected support with an actual stressor, and
(3) expected support in a hypothetical situation.

The confusion resulting from this phenomenon is strengthened by the fact that these three aspects are often given the same label: "perceived support(iveness)".

## SUPPORT AND SATISFACTION WITH RECEIVED SUPPORT

Perhaps the most important distinction concerns the amount of received support and the satisfaction with it. Often researchers only assess the amount of received support. Subsequently they fail to demonstrate a substantial positive relation between this indicator of support and well-being. The relation between the amount of received support and well-being is often not significant and sometimes even negative, indicating that higher amounts of support covary with lower levels of well-being. This phenomenon has received much attention and has given occasion to several explanations. Among them is the view that a lot of support can lead to feelings of overprotection and meddlesomeness. The most apparent cause for this phenomenon, however, is the fact that both levels of social support and well-being have a common cause, i.e., the stressor involved. In other words, the occurrence of a stressor may lead both to receiving support and to distress at the same time. So in fact we have to deal with a spurious relationship. A way to get round this pitfall is to measure the degree of satisfaction with received support instead of (or next to) the amount of received support. By asking for satisfaction, the respondent is implicitly forced to compare received support with need for support, which ensures that any differences in stressors, and thus in need for support, are taken into account.

Differentiating between the amount of supportive interactions and satisfaction with received support has another important advantage. It enables the researcher to consider satisfaction with received support no longer as an aspect of social support but as a component of quality of life, i.e., social well-being. This point will be discussed more extensively in the next section, when social support is related to outcome variables.

To summarize, the problems discussed in this section illustrate that the social support concept covers several different relevant aspects. The most important are the social network, the amount of supportive interactions, the extent to which the received support is in accordance with the need for support, and "expected" or perceived support. We limited social support to supportive interactions provided only by members of the social network, thus excluding professionals like nurses, social workers and medical doctors. The relevance of distinguishing several types of social support, for example emotional and instrumental support, was also stressed.

The next step is to decide on which of these aspects should be focal in a particular study. Simply stated the choice has to do with the research questions under study. This problem is discussed below by relating social support to outcome measures, such as physical and psychological well-being.

## Social support and outcome

The concept of social support will be now related to the presence, severity, and nature of stressors, as an important determining variable. In addition, the relationship between social support and well-being will be discussed. Figure 8.1 illustrates the relationships between these concepts. This is a very simplified model, since other relevant factors like personality characteristics or coping style are left out. The addition of

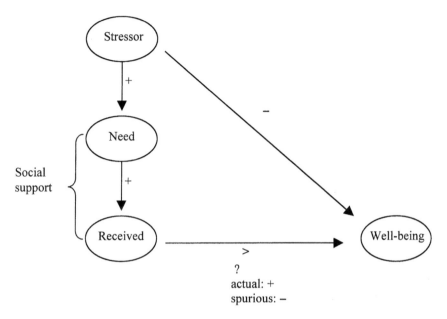

Figure 8.1. Relationship (partly spurious) between social support and well-being

these factors leads to models that are both more complete and more complicated (e.g., Sanderman et al., 1991).

It will be demonstrated that the nature and size of the relationship of social support with both determining and outcome variables depends to a great extent on which aspect of the social support concept the focus is on.

## STRESSORS AND WELL-BEING

Many stressors, like acute or chronic diseases, are well known for their negative effects on physical and psychological well-being. The stressor will keep an independent effect on well-being, regardless of the amount of social support that is provided, i.e., even if the support is aimed to neutralize (most of) the stressor, there will usually be left a negative effect of the stressor on well-being. From these considerations it can be concluded that, in general, the seriousness of the stressor is positively related to the need for social support, which in turn is often positively related to the amount of received support. At the same time however, there will be a negative relationship between the seriousness of the stressor and well-being.

Without taking methodologically precautionary measures, these two relationships will lead to a negative (spurious) relationship between amount of received support and level of well-being.

By now this phenomenon is put forth by several authors as a possible explanation of the contradictory findings in the relationship between support and well-being (Barrera, 1986; Eriksen, 1994; House et al., 1988; Schwarzer & Leppin, 1991; Tijhuis, 1994; Van Sonderen & Ormel, 1991; Vaux, 1988).

A possible solution to cope with this spurious relationship is to carry out research among subjects who all experience the same or comparable stressors. However, this approach has serious practical drawbacks, mainly due to the difficult if not impossible operationalization of "equality of stressor(s)". Another solution is to assess satisfaction with support, instead of amount of received support. Satisfaction with received support is not hampered by the problems just mentioned, when it is related to well-being. By asking for satisfaction with support received, the respondent is able to "correct" for variability in level of stressor and in need for support since the subject is explicitly asked to compare received support with the support needed. Satisfaction with support thus can be related to well-being without bothering about a possible spuriousness of the relationship. However, some questions with respect to the effect of support on well-being still remain relevant.

An important question is whether social support is directly (and always) beneficial for someone's well-being, or whether social support has an influence by reducing the effect of stressors on well-being. In our opinion this problem can only partly be solved. Therefore it is necessary to distinguish between supportive interactions aimed at a common "everyday" need and interactions that are given in the case of a stressful situation. Evidence for a direct relationship between support and well-being is then based on the relation between satisfaction with the amount of "everyday-support" received and well-being. In this way the relative, not the absolute, amount of received social support can be seen as increasing well-being.

## SOCIAL SUPPORT AS A PART OF WELL-BEING
So far we have discussed the problems that occur when relating social support to well-being or quality of life. Because of these difficulties, it is still not possible to discern from literature a clear answer with respect to the impact of social support on well-being. But social support is not the only concept that has to be made more explicit. It

seems obvious that, whatever aspect of social support is taken into account, the strength of its relationship will depend on the aspect of well-being that is measured. A very rough distinction is between physical and psychological well-being, two aspects that in turn measure something else than general well-being. It goes beyond the scope of this chapter to pay attention to the construct "well-being". One point, however, should be discussed here.

An important question that received insufficient attention is whether social support should be considered as a predictor of well-being, as is generally done. By explicitly differentiating between the amount of social support that is provided and received on the one hand and the satisfaction with received support on the other, we are able to transfer the latter aspect from the domain of support to the domain of well-being and quality of life. In this way social support is both a determinant and a part of well-being, dependent on the particular aspect of social support that is taken into account.

By distinguishing explicitly between the amount of received supportive interactions as a key concept in the social support domain, and satisfaction with the received support as one of the aspects of well-being, the function of the social network and the support it is supposed to provide becomes much clearer. Regardless of the possible benefits for physical and psychological well-being, the main task for the social network now becomes to provide exactly that amount of support necessary to comply with need for support. Whereas professional support can be considered to be primarily directed towards improvement or maintenance of physical and psychological well-being, social support should be aimed at approaching a person's needs for social well-being by providing the support that is expected. Although this might seem obvious, this point of view has some remarkable implications. All we have to concern ourselves with is the extent to which the social network succeeds in providing the support that is needed or expected. A possible beneficial effect of social support(ive interactions) on physical and psychological well-being should be considered a by-product.

In sum, in this section some guidelines are provided to help in making a selection of relevant aspects of the social support concept. The ambivalent position of one aspect of social support, satisfaction with received support, as a determinant or outcome variable, is also discussed. In the next section we will discuss several operationalizations of the most relevant aspects of social support.

## The assessment of social support

Previously, we showed that different aspects of social support were related to (pre)determining and outcome variables. Now we will discuss the assessment of several aspects of social support, in particular (1) the social network, (2) the amount of support, and (3) the satisfaction with received social support. For each of these aspects specific instruments will be evaluated. Special attention will be paid to the difference in assessing support from the social network as a whole and assessment of the supportiveness of individual network members. The last part of this section will focus on the special characteristics that are relevant when assessing social support in a clinical setting.

We will start with some general remarks with respect to selecting the most appropriate method to assess social support. As discussed earlier, the conceptual confusion with respect to social support has resulted in an enormous number of instruments, many of which are lacking a sound conceptual background. As a result, instruments are used that measure a mixture of characteristics of the social network, received support, satisfaction with support and expected support. Next, the answers to these questions are added together and summed up in order to get a single score.

Social support measures are generally designed as a questionnaire to be completed during an interview or in a mailed survey. Rarely, instruments have been developed that are based on an extensive interview. The advantage of standardized questionnaires is the reduction in the time and costs needed to gather the information. Information collected with standardized questionnaires is also easily comparable across respondents. In theory-explorating, usually large-scale surveys designed to determine the role of social support in a conceptual model, it is recommended that such instruments are used. A disadvantage of standardized questionnaires, however, is that they are not usually equipped to assess the relevant aspects of support among people in specific circumstances. For assessment of support among patients with a specific disease, standardized instruments are usually too broad. In such cases an interview, assessing very specific types of support, might be preferable. A first step to detect possible problems is to use an adapted questionnaire, skipping questions about irrelevant types of support.

Sometimes the most crucial aspect of support is not the amount that is provided by the social network as a whole, but the support that is received from one particular member of that network, typically the spouse or another confidant. With respect to confidants other than the spouse, it often suffices to determine the existence of such a person, since by definition this relationship will provide support. The presence of a partner, however, does not automatically imply that a supportive person is available, since the indication that someone has a partner merely points to the presence of a formal relationship. The supportive character of the relationship must still be established. This can be done by using standard questionnaires or by more or less tailor-made interviews.

## ASSESSMENT OF SEVERAL ASPECTS OF SOCIAL SUPPORT

In the next section instruments are presented and discussed that measure a particular aspect of social support. We have limited this overview to three aspects of social support: the social network, amount of supportive interactions, and adequacy of supportive interactions. The instruments discussed all measure only one of these aspects. This restriction has led to the omission of several instruments, even though some of them are used rather frequently. The conceptual indistinctness, however, means that the interpretation of results produced with such "hybrid" instruments is often not unequivocal.

### (1) Assessment of social network characteristics

Here we will discuss briefly the three most important ways to assess the social network. Relationships with network members can be character-ized by three properties. The first approach is the role-relationship method. Network members can be described as, for example, partner, child, parent, friend, neighbor, colleague. A study that delineated the social network by asking for so called role relationships is described by Van Sonderen et al. (1990). The advantage of this method is that network members are elicited regardless of the actual supportiveness of their relationship, although it is expected that they give some kind of support.

As discussed above, in many circumstances, in both research and in clinical settings, knowledge about the presence or absence of specific network members is relevant. This is usually restricted to the presence of a partner or children. In the latter case the geographical distance and the frequency of contact is also relevant.

Another way of evaluating the social network is by asking the focal person for people that (s)he feels affectively (strongly) related to. This network delineation method, described by Van Sonderen et al. (1990), is usually only conducted in research aimed at the further development of the relationship between the concepts of social network and social support.

The last network delineation method is to identify those network members with whom the focal person is exchanging activities. Examples of this method are the ASSIS of Barrera (1981) and the exchange instrument used by Van Sonderen et al. (1990). The number of network members delineated with these instruments is hugely dependent on the number and content of the exchange-questions that are admitted in the questionnaire. A special version of this method is often used, by determining whether the focal person has one or more network members that are able to provide them with the necessary (instrumental) support.

A consequence of social network delineation is that afterwards social support can be assessed not only from the network as a whole, but also from specific network members. Later in this section, we discuss some advantages of the assessment of "network support" and "relation specific support".

*(2) Assessment of amount of supportive interactions*
The aspect of the social support concept that is assessed most is the amount of received support. As discussed above, measuring this aspect provides little information when relating it to aspects of well-being. It is, however, indispensable for research that is aimed mainly or exclusively at the relationships between several aspects of social support. As was discussed above, when measuring supportive interactions, the main topic for the researcher is to determine which types of support are relevant. The distinction between emotional and instrumental support and social companionship seems to be particularly relevant.

Two instruments that focus solely on assessment of the amount of supportive interactions, and distinguish between the before mentioned types, are the ISSB (Barrera, 1981) and the SSL-I (Van Sonderen, 1993; Van Sonderen & Ormel, 1991). The strength and sign of the relationship between amount of supportive interactions and indicators of well-being fluctuates, as discussed earlier, due to the spuriousness of this relationship.

*(3) Assessment of adequacy of supportive interactions*
Previously in this chapter a distinction was made between actual and perceived (adequacy of) supportiveness of the social network. Perceived supportiveness was considered too complicated for many practical pur-

poses because of the intertwining of actual and hypothetical situations. We now consider the adequacy of actual received support as determined by the correspondence of the amount of received support and the need for support. Three instruments that measure adequacy of (or satisfaction with) social support are mentioned: the Social Support Questionnaire, (SSQ; Sarason et al., 1983), the ASSIS (Barrera, 1981), and the SSL-D (Van Sonderen, 1993; Van Sonderen & Ormel, 1991).

## Some considerations concerning assessment

### SOURCE OF SUPPORT: WHOLE NETWORK OR INDIVIDUAL RELATIONSHIPS

We will now discuss some advantages of assessing "network support" and "relation specific support". In general, two approaches can be followed by assessing social support. The most straightforward option is to assess the support that is received from the social network as a whole. Other methods are to assess support received from specific (categories of) network members. To measure support from individual persons it is necessary to map out these network members first. Categories of network members can be handled by asking for support received by particular role-types of network members like family, friends, and neighbors. All three sources of social support (complete network, individuals, categories of network members) have some advantages and disadvantages when assessing social support. The advantage of the latter two methods is the possibility of assessing quite accurately the source of support. However, it does not seem to balance its main drawback, which is that support from different sources has to be weighted in order to gain an understanding of the total amount of received support. Such a weighting process is hard to clarify, since it is a completely implicit and largely unaware process. The first method, assessment of the support provided by the complete network, does not have this drawback. On the other hand, this method is unable to locate the most supportive members of the social network. Another drawback of this method is the indistinct delineation of who belongs to the social network and who does not. Especially in situations where support is not only received from informal relationships but also from professionals, like doctors and nurses, it is difficult to distinguish between social and professional support.

A special provider of social support that should be mentioned explicitly is the confidant. It is generally believed that the support a confidant provides is by far the most significant. Usually this confidant is the spouse. The spouse is not only considered the most important provider of support, but is also the person whose lack of support or negative interactions, are mostly exerting influence on someone's well-being.

In sum, in our opinion the most fruitful way to determine social support is to assess both the amount of and satisfaction with the support that is received from the social network as a whole. In addition it is important to determine the support provided by the most pronounced confidant, preferably the spouse. Attention should be paid to several types of support, particularly emotional and instrumental support, esteem support and social companionship.

## ASSESSMENT IN CLINICAL SETTING

Researchers are interested in social support received by patients for two reasons. Firstly, to ground or undermine the theoretical assumption that social support is buffering against the negative effects of stressors on well-being. Acute or chronic illness is, next to divorce or loss of a relative, the most prominent example of a serious stressor. Besides, clinicians sometimes need a picture of the social support system of a patient in order to see if s/he is able to cope with the various consequences of a certain disease. For a patient to be discharged from hospital, it may be relevant to know if the social network is able to provide enough practical support at home. For patients who are just informed of a life-threatening or serious chronic disease, the presence of a confidant who can provide emotional support might be essential.

In our opinion the following reasons for assessing social support in clinical setting can be distinguished:

- to determine if the support network is able to provide enough support;
- to assess the presence of a confidant (this can be the partner);
- if there is a partner, to assess quality of the relationship;
- to assess the need for other types of support, like peer support and professional support.

Usually this information can be gathered in an informal way, during a clinical interview with the patient. Although circumstances are too heterogeneous to prescribe standardized instruments, it is often important that the topics are raised.

## SOCIAL SUPPORT AND INTERVENTIONS

When discussing the delineation of the social network an explicit distinction has been made between the social network and professional caregivers. This distinction is especially relevant in interventions focused on intensification of social support. Often, these interventions are aimed at providing additional support by peers or professionals, and should not come within the definition of social support. Some review articles that deal with different types of (chronic) diseases, like Helgeson and Cohen (1996) who describe support interventions for cancer patients, and Lanza and Revenson (1993) who aim at programs for rheumatoid arthritis patients, distinguish the support that is provided in the intervention from the support that is received from the informal, social network. Typically two types of intervention are mentioned. One of them is the educational type, mainly aimed at provision of informational support. The other type is the support offered by peers, either in group discussion sessions or by connecting new patients to another patient who has survived the disease or already has some experience in coping with it. Helgeson and Cohen (1996) provide a nice example of how formal this type of support can be: support providers were well trained and were assumed to transfer their support by making three phone calls with the patient.

Intervention programs often do not assess the need for social support, but instead assume a general need for support, not necessarily provided by the social network. The most common measure of these intervention programs is the effect this intervention has on physical and psychological well-being.

Helgeson and Cohen (1996) among others show that results of intervention programs are often indistinct because of the many methodological problems intervention programs suffer from. Beside these problems interventions often do not result in an increase in well-being. Rook and Dooley (1985) ascribe this result to the fact that peer relationships are often artificial and not intimate.

# Conclusion

The broad range of the concept of social support makes it necessary for each investigator to make choices. These choices have to be made both conceptually and with respect to the use of instruments.

It is impossible to cover all aspects of social support in one single study. In this chapter some guidelines are provided to make a well-considered choice of relevant aspects. In summary, researchers should decide if they want to assess:

- network characteristics or the supportive content of interpersonal relationships;
- the amount of support that is received or the extent to which this received support corresponds with the need for support;
- a judgment about support that is actually received or about support that someone expects to receive when confronted with (particular) problems;
- all types of support, or only some, like emotional support, instrumental support or esteem support;
- the support that is received from the social network as a whole or from specific (types of) network members;
- the support that is provided by the social network, or support that is provided by formal or even professional relationships;
- the support as it is perceived by the recipient, or (also) the evaluation of the provider(s) of the support, and particularly any discrepancy between the two "parties"; and
- the prevalence of negative interactions in relationships that are considered to be supportive; a point that has received little attention in this chapter because its relation to social support receives much attention in the literature.

Typically, these choices should lead to the development of an optimal questionnaire. There's every chance that none of the existing questionnaires are perfect for a particular piece of research. As described in this chapter, many questionnaires suffer from conceptual vagueness. Nevertheless, the conceptual problems discussed here should help those who wish to make use of an existing instrument to make a well-considered choice. And those who wish to construct a tailor-made questionnaire themselves will probably find the topics raised an aid in selecting the most suitable questions.

## References

Barrera, M. Jr. (1981). Social support in the adjustment of pregnant adolescents; assessment issues. In: B.E. Gottlieb (Ed.), *Social networks and social support* (pp. 69–96). Beverly Hills: Sage.

Barrera, M. Jr. (1986). Distinctions between social support concepts, measures, and models. *American Journal of Community Psychology, 14*, 413–445.

Berkman, L.F., & Syme, S.L. (1979). Social networks, host resistance, and mortality: A nine-year follow-up study of Alameda County residents. *American Journal of Epidemiology, 109*, 186–204.

Bruhn, J.G., & Philips, B.U. (1984). Measuring social support: A synthesis of current approaches. *Journal of Behavioral Medicine, 7*, 151–169.

Cobb, S. (1976). Social support as a moderator of life stress. *Psychosomatic Medicine, 38*, 300–314.

Cohen, S., & Syme, S.L. (Eds.) (1985). *Social support and health.* New York: Academic Press.

Cohen, S., & Wills, T.A. (1985). Stress, social support, and the buffering hypothesis. *Psychological Bulletin, 98*, 310–357.

Eriksen, W. (1994). The role of social support in the pathogenesis of coronary hearth disease: A literature review. *Family Practice, 11*, 201–209.

Heitzman, C.A., & Kaplan, R.M. (1988). Assessment of methods for measuring social support. *Health Psychology, 7*, 75–109.

Helgeson, V.S., & Cohen, S. (1996). Social support and adjustment to cancer: Reconciling descriptive, correlational, and intervention research. *Health Psychology, 15*, 135–148.

Heller, K., & Swindle, R.W. (1983). Social networks, perceived support, and coping with stress. In: R.D. Felner, L.A. Jason, J. Moritsugu, & S.S. Farber (Eds.), *Preventive psychology: Theory, research, and practice in community intervention* (pp. 87–103). New York: Pergamon Press.

House, J.S. (1981). *Work stress and social support.* Reading, MA: Addison-Wesley.

House, J.S., Umberson, D., & Landis, K.R., (1988). Structures and processes of social support. *Annual Review of Sociology, 14*, 293–318.

Lanza, A.F., & Revenson, T.A. (1993). Social support interventions for rheumatoid arthritis patients: The cart before the horse? *Health Education Quarterly, 20*, 97–117.

Lin, N. (1986). Modelling the effects of social support. In: N. Lin, A. Dean, & W.M. Ensel (Eds.), *Social support, life events, and depression* (pp. 173–209). Orlando: Academic Press.

Orth-Gomer, K., & Unden, A-L. (1987). The measurement of social support in population surveys. *Social Science and Medicine, 24*, 83–94.

Rook, K.S., & Dooley, D. (1985). Applying social support research: Theoretical problems and future directions. *Journal of Social Issues, 41*, 5–28.

Sanderman, R., van den Heuvel, W.J.A., & Langeveld, H.M. (1991). Determinants of health: A Dutch research programme. *International Journal of Health Sciences, 2*, 195–206.

Sarason, I.G., Levine, H.M., Basham, R.B., & Sarason, B.R. (1983). Assessing social support: The social support questionnaire. *Journal of Personality and Social Psychology, 44*, 127–139.

Schwarzer, R., & Leppin, A. (1991). Social support and health: A theoretical and empirical overview. *Journal of Social and personal Relationships, 8,* 99–127.

Tardy, C.H., (1985). Social support measurement. *American Journal of Community Psychology, 13,* 187–202.

Thoits, P.A. (1982). Conceptual, methodological and theoretical problems in studying social support as a buffer against life stress. *Journal of Health and Social Behavior, 23,* 145–159.

Tijhuis, M. (1994). *Social networks and health.* Thesis, University of Utrecht.

Turner, R.J. (1983). Direct, indirect, and moderating effects of social support on psychological distress and associated conditions. In: H.B. Kaplan (Ed.), *Psychosocial stress: Trends in theory and research* (pp. 105–155). New York: Academic Press.

Van Sonderen, E. (1991). *Het meten van sociale steun* [Measuring social support]. Thesis, University of Groningen.

Van Sonderen, E. (1993). *Het meten van sociale steun met de Sociale Steun Lijst-Interacties (SSL-I) en Sociale Steun Lijst-Discrepanties (SSL-D): Een handleiding* [Measuring social support with the Social Support List-Interactions (SSL-I) and Social Support List-Discrepancies (SSL-D): A manual]. NCG reeks meetinstrumenten: 2. Groningen: Noordelijk Centrum voor Gezondheidsvraagstukken.

Van Sonderen, E. (1995). Sociale steun en sociale netwerken [Social support and social networks]. In: R. Sanderman, C.M.H. Hosman, & M.Mulder (Eds.), *Het meten van determinanten van gezondheid: een overzicht van beschikbare meetinstrumenten* (pp. 162–186). Assen: Van Gorcum.

Van Sonderen, E., & Ormel, J. (1991). *Sociale steun en onwelbevinden. Een onderzoek naar de samenhang tussen aspecten van sociale steun en onwel-bevinden* [Social support and unwellbeing. A study for the relationship between aspects of social support and unwellbeing]. Groningen: Noordelijk Centrum voor Gezondheidsvraagstukken.

Van Sonderen, E., Ormel, J., Brilman, E., & Van Linden van den Heuvel, C. (1990). Personal network delineation: A comparison of the exchange, affective and role-relation approach. In: T.C. Antonucci & C.P.M. Knipscheer (Eds.), *Social network research: Methodological questions and substantive issues* (pp. 101–120). Lisse, The Netherlands: Swets & Zeitlinger.

Vaux, A. (1988). *Social support. Theory, research, and intervention.* New York: Praeger.

Veiel, H.O.F. (1985). Dimensions of social support: A conceptual framework for research. *Social Psychiatry 20,* 156–162.

Winemiller, D.R., Mitchell, M.E., Sutliff, J., & Cline, D.J. (1993). Measurement strategies in social support: A descriptive review of the literature. *Journal of Clinical Psychology, 49,* 638–648.

# 9 ASSESSMENT OF ILLNESS PERCEPTIONS

Adrian A. Kaptein, Margreet Scharloo and John A. Weinman

In the area of behavioral medicine and health psychology, research on illness perceptions represents one of the most recent developments, theoretically and empirically. Although early traces of the concept of illness perceptions of patients with somatic disorders date back to the work of Bard and Dyk (1956), the most elaborate theoretical and empirical contributions regarding illness perceptions have been published only quite recently (Petrie & Weinman, 1997; Skelton & Croyle, 1991). This chapter starts by outlining a definition of illness perceptions, and the theoretical model which incorporates illness perceptions in explaining variance in patients' adjustment to illness. This is followed by a concise chronological overview of empirical approaches to the assessment of illness perceptions. Finally, we discuss and summarize how illness perceptions have been assessed. Some suggestions for future research are presented.

## Illness perceptions: A definition and a theoretical model

Illness perceptions represent a concept in health psychology research of illness behavior. In this line of research it has been demonstrated that differences in medical and behavioral outcome of (chronic) illness cannot be explained fully by "objective" medical data (Zeidner & Endler, 1996). The response of the patient to symptoms and illness is an important determinant of outcome. Cognitive factors are viewed as an important part of the coping skills of patients (Weinman & Petrie, 1997).

Given the relatively new status of illness perceptions in health psychology research, it is hardly surprising that a clear cut definition of illness perceptions has not yet been established. Scharloo and Kaptein (1997) list a number of concepts which have been used as synonyms: for example illness perceptions, illness representations, illness beliefs, illness cognitions, and illness schemata.

Given this situation, presenting a definition of illness perceptions which encompasses the current research in this area is not easy. Lacroix's (1991) description seems the most adequate: "a distinct, meaningfully integrated cognitive structure that encompasses

(a) a belief in the relatedness of a variety of physiological and psychological functions, which may or may not be objectively accurate;
(b) a cluster of sensations, symptoms, emotions, and physical limitations in keeping with that belief;
(c) a naive theory about the mechanisms that underlie the relatedness of the elements identified in (b), and
(d) implicit or explicit prescriptions for corrective action" (Lacroix, 1991, p. 197).

Leventhal et al.'s (1980) self-regulating theory is the most elaborate work in which illness perceptions are conceptualized. Figure 9.1. depicts this theory in its most basic form. The cognitive representation of a health threat is made up by four dimensions of illness perceptions:

- *Identity*: the bodily symptoms and the label associated with the illness
- *Causality*: beliefs about factors contributing to the development of the illness
- *Time-line*: expectations about the length of time for the illness to develop, as well as its duration
- *Consequences*: immediate or long-term consequences of the illness (Baumann et al., 1989).

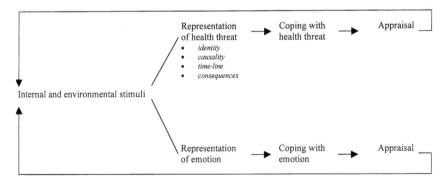

**Figure 9.1.** Leventhal et al.'s (1980) self-regulating theory

# Assessing illness perceptions

In this section nine approaches to the assessment of illness perceptions will be outlined. These approaches are ordered chronologically in order to illustrate how the concept of illness perceptions has developed over the past 40 years. For each approach we will summarize the type of research in which the concept of illness perceptions was assessed, the operationalization of illness perceptions, and the purpose for which the illness perceptions are considered to be relevant or useful.

## (1) PSYCHOANALYTIC BEGINNINGS

One of the first studies on illness perceptions focused on the beliefs of patients with cancer about causes of their illness (Bard & Dyk, 1956). These beliefs were elicited with an extensive open interview. It was demonstrated that assigning culpability or responsibility for the illness, in particular self-blame or projection of blame, were the dominant themes in the patients' beliefs. Assessment and data-analysis of the illness beliefs or perceptions in this study were guided by psycho-analytic theoretical notions. The authors speculate about the potential implications that illness beliefs have with regard to complaints, seeking medical care, doctor-patient interaction, illness behavior and resumption of life's activities. In addition, they point at the importance of congruence between illness beliefs in physicians with those of patients. In this study, there is no attention on relationships between patients' beliefs and health outcomes. We are unaware of additional research by these authors or psychoanalytically oriented colleagues concerning patients with physical disorders.

## (2) SEMANTIC DIFFERENTIAL FOR HEALTH

The second approach to studying perceptions of illnesses was developed from a public health perspective by Jenkins and colleagues (Jenkins 1966a, 1966b; Jenkins & Zyzanski, 1968). Jenkins' work on studying beliefs (or perceptions, ideas, qualities, attributes, thoughts, feelings, attitudes, to sum up the terms used in the paper) about various illnesses, employed the semantic differential for health (SDH) as the questionnaire with which beliefs about various illnesses were assessed in various groups of respondents. The SDH was based on the work by Osgood and colleagues on the semantic differential (Osgood et al., 1957). Specifically, Jenkins set out to capture 11 dimensions of beliefs about various illnesses. These 11 dimensions comprised general public susceptibility, personal susceptibility, salience, three aspects of severity (i.e., pain, risk of death, amount of residual disability), difficulty of prevention, feelings of mystery about the disease, clean–dirty, proud–disgraced, a moral judgment about the kind of people attacked by the disease, speed and power (Jenkins, 1966a, p. 418). Factor analysis with varimax rotation yielded one factor labeled "ideas of personal involvement and power of impact of the disease" (p. 423).

Jenkins suggests using the SDH when evaluating the effects of health education with regard to changing beliefs and feelings about a disease, when planning preventive or case-finding programs, or when studying differential responses of communities or certain groups to programs of health agencies.

Antonovsky (1972) and Ben-Sira (1977) continued Jenkins' line of research in studying the image of diseases. Antonovsky asked respondents to indicate their position with respect to four diseases (cancer, heart disease, mental illness, and cholera) on the following four dimensions: seriousness, control, susceptibility, and salience. The items were scored on a Likert-type scale with 9 response categories (e.g., usually causes death (9) to rarely causes death (1)). Ben-Sira's (1977) study essentially applied Jenkins' and Antonovsky's methodology.

None of these studies in which the SDH was applied focused on relationships between beliefs and health outcome.

## (3) EXPLANATORY MODELS

The medical anthropologist and psychiatrist Kleinman studied people's perceptions concerning aspects of physical and psychiatric disorders. Central to Kleinman's work are the explanatory models, described as "the notions about an episode of sickness and its treatment that are employed by all those engaged in the clinical process" (Kleinman, 1988, p. 121). Questions used to assess these perceptions about illness include the following:

> What is the nature of this problem?
> Why has it affected me?
> Why now?
> What course will it follow?
> How does it affect my body?
> What treatment do I desire?

Notice that these questions show a remarkable correspondence to the dimensions of illness representations as described in the work of Leventhal et al. (1980), e.g., identity, causality, course, consequences.

Kleinman's line of writing has a rather qualitative emphasis. His operationalization of the concept "explanatory model" is based on interviews with a limited number of respondents from various cultural backgrounds, especially from Asian countries. As far as is known, this investigator has not reported on relations between explanatory models and health outcomes found in empirical studies with a substantial sample size. The relevance of Kleinman's work, in our view, lies in drawing attention to the ubiquity of illness perceptions over cross-cultural boundaries, and in his pointing out the importance of concordance between the views of patients and health care providers in achieving effective delivery of medical care.

## (4) HEALTH LOCUS OF CONTROL

The concept of "control" in relation to health and illness has been the subject of a wealth of studies, inspired by earlier work on assessing people's beliefs about whether or not their health is determined by their behavior (Wallston, 1989; Wallston et al., 1978). In health promoting behaviors in healthy persons, and in illness behavior which helps coping with chronic illness in patients, beliefs of control are assumed to play a positive role (Norman & Bennett, 1996). In addition, control is one of the five dimensions in Leventhal's self-regulating theory, which adds to the relevance of this concept for this chapter.

The Multidimensional Health Locus of Control (MHLC) scale is an 18-item questionnaire with three 6-item subscales. The "Internal Health Locus of Control (IHLC)" subscale represents beliefs that health is the result of one's own behavior (e.g., When I get sick I am to blame); The "Powerful Others Health Locus of Control (PHLC)" (e.g., Health professionals control my health) subscale assesses beliefs that health is determined by powerful others, while the "Chance Health Locus of Control (CHLC)" subscale (e.g., No matter what I do, if I am going to get sick, I will get sick) represents beliefs about health being a consequence of chance or fate.

Norman and Bennett (1996) provide an excellent review of the applications of the Health Locus of Control construct with respect to preventive health behavior.

## (5) IMPLICIT MODELS OF ILLNESS

By referring to the authors whose work was discussed previously in this chapter (i.e., Antonovsky, Ben-Sira, Jenkins, Kleinman, Leventhal), Turk et al. (1986) make explicit the link between their Implicit Models of Illness and Leventhal's theory on self-regulation.

Their study is relevant and highly interesting as it attempts "to determine whether there is a generic illness representation that is consistent across the diversity of populations, different diseases, and actual experience with a specific illness and to describe the characteristics of this generic model" (p. 456). The concepts of identity, time-line, consequences, cause and cure (dimensions in Leventhal et al.'s 1980 model), personal responsibility (Jenkins, 1966a) and disruptiveness (Jones et al., 1981) were assessed with 38 illness statements on a 9-point scale. Turk et al. thus used a priori dimensions, operationalized them, and tested whether the dimensions identified by previous researchers could be replicated.

Their respondents were students, diabetic nurse educators and diabetic patients. Factor analysis produced four dimensions: (1) seriousness (9 items; e.g., "goes away on its own", "requires medical attention"); (2) personal responsibility (8 items; e.g., "caused by one's behavior", "cured by reduced stress"); (3) controllability (5 items; e.g., "controllable by the individual"); (4) changeability (2 items; e.g., "changes over time").

This study failed to identify the dimensions "time line" and "symptom identity" of Leventhal et al.'s (1980) model. Rather, dimensions that have direct personal and affective consequences were uncovered. The authors stress also that attention should be paid to affective aspects of illness schema or illness models in addition to cognitive aspects. We are unaware of empirical papers in which these four dimensions have been used to evaluate their potential value as predictors of health/medical outcomes.

## (6) SCHEMA ASSESSMENT INSTRUMENT

The approach of Lacroix (1991) to assessing illness schemata represents a unique one. In his work, the extent to which patients' illness schemata correspond to objective medical and psychological evidence is used as a predictor of outcome variables such as return to work (cf. Petrie et al., 1996) and level of adaptive functioning. Also notable is that illness schemata are thought of as interacting dynamically with the symptoms which constitute the content of these schemata.

Stimulated by clinical work with patients with low back pain, Lacroix noted the discrepancy between "objective" measures of severity of this condition, and outcome variables such as return to work. The cognitive views the patients held were implicated as contributing to the concordance or divergence with these objective measures of severity. Using Pennebaker's (1982) and Leventhal et al.'s (1980) theoretical notions about symptom perception, Lacroix developed an instrument to assess the accuracy of illness schemata in various patient groups and in analogue studies.

The Schema Assessment Instrument (SAI) is an open ended interview aimed to assess "the patient's presenting physical and psychological symptoms and how these may be related to one another, the patient's understanding of his or her medical condition(s) and prognosis, and the patient's understanding of the relationship between his or her medical condition and the presenting symptoms" (Lacroix, 1991, p. 199).

These "assessed schemata" are then contrasted to the "expected schemata". Expected schemata are constructed by the patient's treating physician on the basis of medical, psychological and other available information. Dimensions in the SAI are: severity and prognosis (based on the medical records), differentiation (the degree to which overall symptom groupings concur), content (the degree to which the content of each of the assessed clusters concurs with the medical/psychological evidence), aetiology (the degree to which the patient's understanding of the causes for each assessed cluster accurately represents the medical, and psychological evidence), and "global" (an overall rating of the patient's understanding of the condition).

The SAI and empirical studies with this measure can be found in Lacroix (1991); an illustration of the application of the SAI (procedure, scoring system) is given in Lacroix et al. (1991).

## (7) ILLNESS REPRESENTATIONS

Elaborating on the model of the self-regulating theory, as printed in Figure 9.1, Leventhal and Nerenz (1985) give a detailed history of why and how illness perceptions have been assessed within the model. It is quite difficult to trace exactly how Leventhal and colleagues assess illness perceptions. In their 1985 chapter, they describe how a combination of open-ended questions and checklists yielded four dimensions: identity, causality, time line, and consequences (Baumann et al., 1989). The paper by Cameron et al. (1993) is one of the few publications from which insight can be gained into how the illness perceptions were assessed. In this study with a community-dwelling sample of middle aged and older adults, identity was assessed by asking the respondents: "Is there a disease name you would give to this problem?". Meyer et al. (1985) examined common sense models of hypertension with a 45-minute structured interview to assess identity, time line, and causes. Details on scoring, reliability or validity, however, were not given.

In a third study (Prohaska et al., 1985), 15 items were included in a questionnaire which "tapped the respondent's representation of the illness. It included questions about the individual's perceived vulnerability to the illness, judgements of its severity, ratings of emotional responses to the disease, evaluations of self-affectance, and ability to monitor changes in conditions over brief (1 week) and longer (5 years) periods of time" (p. 571).

Hampson and Glasgow (1996) used an interview when assessing illness representations in patients with diabetes mellitus and with osteoarthritis. In addition, they used a card-sorting task in which patients were asked to sort cards with adjectives into piles "that describe different aspects of arthritis (diabetes) ... that contain words that go together, have something in common" (p. 51).

## (8) A FIFTH DIMENSION

Three publications make a case for adding a fifth component or dimension "cure" to the four illness representations identified by Leventhal's group: Lau and Hartman (1983), Lau et al. (1989) and Lau (1997). Lau and his research group did not focus on chronic conditions such as hypertension or breast cancer, as was the case in Leventhal et al.'s (1980) work, but rather on acute conditions (e.g., a cold). Included in a questionnaire on health behaviors and health beliefs, three questions were asked: "Now please think back to the last time you had a cold. When was this? Please, tell us everything you remember about this illness. Now considering this same cold, please think for a minute about why you got sick on the specific occasion. To what extent was the reason for your getting sick controllable? And considering this same cold again, think for a moment about why you recovered from this illness. Was your recovery due to your own efforts?" (Lau et al., 1989, p. 201).

The second and third questions were 5-point closed-ended scales. Responses were coded into five categories (identity, time line, consequence, cause, and cure). "Cure" turned out to be a consistent category in the answers of the respondents to the question of reasons for getting better following an acute illness (Lau & Hartman, 1983).

Lau (1997) not only reviews the subject of cognitive representation of health and illness, he also pleads for the development of an instrument which measures illness representations. The paper on the Illness Perception Questionnaire by Weinman et al. (1996) answered his plea.

---

## Box 9.1   Illness perception as predictors of cardiac rehabilitation

The study by Petrie and colleagues (1996) is a nice illustration of the relevance of assessing illness perceptions. In 143 patients with a confirmed first myocardial infarction, the associations between IPQ dimensions scores and admission to and attendance at a cardiac rehabilitation program, the time taken to return to work, functioning outside work, and sexual difficulties three and six months later were studied. Results showed that irrespective of medically-determined severity of illness, illness perceptions reflecting cure/control, time-line, and consequences predicted attendance at the cardiac rehabilitation program and time to return to work.

As pointed out by the authors of the study, it appears relevant to focus in future studies on the efficacy of brief psychological interventions designed to elicit, and, if necessary, modify specific illness perceptions as a basis for improving attendance at rehabilitation as well as facilitating adaptation and return to work.

---

### (9) ILLNESS PERCEPTION QUESTIONNAIRE

Weinman et al. (1996) described the development of the Illness Perception Questionnaire (IPQ). Items for the IPQ were derived from Leventhal et al.'s theory and address the five components of Leventhal et al.'s and Lau and Hartman's (1983) conceptualizations. Items from symptom checklists, generated by patients, or by the investigators themselves formed the sources for the 12 core symptom items which make up the "identity" subscale. The "cause" subscale has 10 items, the "time line" subscale 3, the "consequences" subscale 7, and the "control/cure" subscale has 6 items (the full IPQ with extensive details on psychometric characteristics can be found in Weinman et al., 1996).

Empirical work with the IPQ has been and is being performed by various research groups. Petrie and Moss-Morris demonstrated how IPQ scores predicted medical and behavioral outcomes in patients with myocardial infarction and with chronic fatigue syndrome (Moss-Morris et al., 1996; Petrie et al., 1996). Dutch investigators (Heijmans, 1998; Scharloo et al., 1998, 1999, 2000) have reported on this issue in

Table 9.1. The nine approaches to assessing illness perceptions.

| First author & year | Theoretical approach | Dimension(s) | N items | Mode of assessment | Nature of concept |
|---|---|---|---|---|---|
| Bard 1956 | psychoanalysis | cause | – | open interview | beliefs predict illness behavior |
| Jenkins 1966 | public health | personal involvement; impact of disease | 16 | questionnaire | beliefs contribute to theories of health behavior |
| Kleinman 1988 | medical anthropology | identity course cause; consequences | – | open interview | purpose: descriptive |
| Wallston 1978 | health behavior | internal powerful others; chance | 18 | questionnaire (MHLC) | predictor and outcome variable |
| Turk 1986 | illness behavior | seriousness; personal; responsibility; controllability; changeability | 38 | questionnaire (IMIQ) | predictor and outcome variable |
| Lacroix 1991 | social medicine | assessed vs. expected schemata | 20 | interview (SAI) | predictor and outcome variable |
| Leventhal 1985 | health psychology | identity; causality; time-line; consequences | – | open ended questions and checklists | predictor and outcome variable |
| Lau 1983 | health psychology | cure | – | questionnaire/ interview | predictor and outcome variable |
| Weinman 1996 | health psychology | identity; causality; time-line; consequences; cure | 12 + 26 | questionnaire/ interview (IPQ) | predictor and outcome variable |

patients with chronic fatigue syndrome, and in patients with COPD, RA and psoriasis, respectively.

Petrie (1999, personal communication) is currently involved with an intervention study in which the effects of changing illness cognitions on the medical and behavioral outcomes in patients with a myocardial infarction are examined. Scharloo et al. (2000) are investigating the course in time of illness cognitions in COPD patients. Horne et al. (1999) used the illness perceptions approach to develop a questionnaire which assesses perceptions about medications. Finally, the designers of the IPQ are currently working on a revision of the IPQ (IPQ-R; Weinman, 1998, personal communication) which involves adding subscales that assess emotional aspects as well (Moss-Morris et al., 2001).

In conclusion, the IPQ has been used in studies on various illnesses (e.g., diabetes, asthma, myocardial infarction, chronic fatigue, psoriasis). In some cases, authors have reported rather low reliability coefficients for some of IPQ dimensions (e.g., Scharloo et al., 1999). However, the designers are aware of these problems and are currently searching for adequate solutions.

Table 9.1. summarizes the nine approaches to the assessment of illness perceptions.

## Discussion

The current review of how illness perceptions have been assessed in theoretical and empirical work allows the following preliminary conclusions. We use the word preliminary since the field of illness perceptions is still in its infancy.

(1) In various scientific disciplines, illness perceptions have been described, discussed and assessed, for example in medical anthropology, sociology, public health, and (cognitive) health psychology (Weinman & Petrie, 1997). It seems safe to state that clinical reality inspired researchers and theoreticians in these disciplines to discuss, assess and apply the topic of illness perceptions to patients with physical disorders. Psychologists represent the largest group in this area, and cognitive health psychology appears to be the dominant theoretical approach.

(2) Assessment methods used in research with illness cognitions are mainly questionnaires and interviews. Most questionnaires are relatively concise.

(3) In the majority of the more recent instruments for assessing illness perceptions, four to five dimensions are measured: identity, cause, time line, consequence, and cure.

(4) Only recently has the relationship between illness perceptions and medical and/or behavioral outcome come into focus (e.g., Petrie et al., 1996; see also Box 9.1).

(5) The history of assessing illness perceptions seems quite comparable to the history of assessing other concepts in the (health) psychology field (cf. "quality of life", (Spilker, 1996; chapter 16), "coping" (De Ridder, 1997; chapter 7) or "social support" (chapter 8). Initially, quality of life was a concept which enjoyed enormous popularity, especially in the medical field. However, not only did theoretical underpinnings lag behind the wealth of empirical studies which included quality of life as a concept, the assessment of the elusive concept of quality of life was a free for all. Quality of life became a buzz-word, which was received with enthusiasm by journal editors. Only very recently have books been published which try to bring some degree of order and scientific basis to the theoretical founda-tions of quality of life, and to the assessment of quality of life (Bowling, 2001; McGee & Jenkinson, 1997; Spilker, 1996). A com-parable situation seems to exist with regard to illness perceptions.

The Illness Perception Questionnaire apparently fills the need for an adequate assessment tool to measure illness perceptions. Current research with this instrument increases our knowledge of illness per-ceptions and their predictive value with respect to health outcomes. Current theoretical developments with respect to this concept make us feel confident about future applications and theoretical refinements.

It is important to be aware of a number of limitations of the present review. One pertains to our selection of the investigators whose work has been discussed. As described by Scharloo and Kaptein (1997), the literature on pain and illness perceptions includes other authors whose work could or should have been discussed in this chapter as well. However, we feel that the selected approaches represent the most rele-vant ones, because they each represent a unique contribution to the assessment of illness perceptions. Another limitation pertains to the fact that it was not always possible to derive detailed information about the used assessment techniques. We expect that in the near future, additional research will result in new and more sophisticated assessment methods.

Future research should also focus on perceptions about illness of health care providers (physicians, nurses, pharmacists), spouses of patients (e.g., Helder et al., 2001; Richardson et al., 2001), and the public at large (e.g., on AIDS, Landrine & Klonoff, 1992). A most exciting topic in illness perception research concerns the effects of interventions in illness perceptions on medical and behavioral outcomes in patients with physical disorders (cf. Petrie's work). A further interesting area for study are illness perceptions of psychiatric patients. The degree of concordance between illness perceptions of these patients and their health care providers and partners could be considered to be an important predictor of success of psychiatric treatment.

One final comment: investigations in this area should not be restricted to scientific work. Poems and novels about health and illness can also be used to study illness perceptions. Trautmann and Pollard (1982) discuss hundreds of books and novels on literature and medicine. The plague, tuberculosis, prostate cancer and cancer in general are the subjects of books by Camus (1984), Mann (1952), Broyard (1992) and Solzhenitsyn (1971). These books and many others (see the journal *Literature and Medicine*) contain accounts by patients about their symptoms and their illness perceptions, each of which merits a study of its own. In short, there is a rich literature that may be helpful for stimulating and inspiring research and clinical work concerning illness perceptions.

## Acknowledgment

The authors are grateful for the excellent technical support from Aliek Uijlenbroek.

## References

Antonovsky, A. (1972). The image of four diseases held by the urban Jewish population of Israel. *Journal of Chronic Disease, 25*, 375–384.

Bard, M., & Dyk, R.B. (1956). The psychodynamic significance of beliefs regarding the cause of serious illness. *Psychoanalytic Review, 43*, 146–162.

Baumann, L.J., Cameron, L.D., Zimmerman, R.S., & Leventhal, H. (1989). Illness representations and matching labels with symptoms. *Health Psychology, 8*, 449–469.

Ben-Sira, Z. (1977). The structure and dynamics of the image of diseases. *Journal of Chronic Disease, 30*, 831–842.

Bowling, A. (2001). *Measuring disease (2nd ed.)*. Buckingham: Open University Press.

Broyard, A. (1992). *Intoxicated by my illness*. New York: Clarkson Potter Publishers.

Cameron, L., Leventhal, E.A., & Leventhal, H. (1993). Symptom representations and affect as determinants of care seeking in a community-dwelling, adult sample population. *Health Psychology, 12*, 171–179.

Camus, A. (1948). *The plague*. New York: Alfred A. Knopf.

De Ridder, D. (1997). What is wrong with coping assessment? A review of conceptual and methodological issues. *Psychology & Health, 12*, 417–431.

Hampson, S.E., & Glasgow, R.E. (1996). Dimensional complexity of older patients' illness representations of arthritis and diabetes. *Basic and Applied Social Psychology, 18*, 45–59.

Heijmans, M.J.W.M. (1998). Coping and adaptive outcome in chronic fatigue syndrome: Importance of illness cognitions. *Journal of Psychosomatic Research, 45*, 39–51.

Helder, D.I., Kaptein, A.A., Kempen, G.M.J. van, & Roos, R.A.C. (2001). Huntington's Disease: A review of psychological aspects. *Psychology & Health* (in press).

Horne, R., Weinman, J., & Hankins, M. (1999). The beliefs about medicines questionnaire: The development and evaluation of a new method for assessing the cognitive representation of medication. *Psychology & Health, 14*, 1–24.

Jenkins, C.D. (1966a). Group differences in perception: A study of community beliefs and feelings about tuberculosis. *The American Journal of Sociology, 71*, 417–429.

Jenkins, C.D. (1966b). The Semantic Differential for Health: A technique for measuring beliefs about diseases. *Public Health Reports, 81*, 549–558.

Jenkins, C.D., & Zyzanski, S.J. (1968). Dimensions of belief and feeling concerning three diseases, poliomyelitis, cancer, and mental illness: A factor analytic study. *Behavioral Science, 13*, 372–381.

Jones, R.A., Wiese, H.J., Moore, R.W., & Haley, J.V. (1981). On the perceived meaning of symptoms. *Medical Care, 19*, 710–717.

Kleinman, A. (1988). *The illness narratives*. New York: Basic Books.

Lacroix, J.M. (1991). Assessing illness schemata in patient populations. In: J.A. Skelton & R.T. Croyle (Eds.), *Mental representation in health and illness* (pp. 193–219). New York: Springer.

Lacroix, J.M., Martin, B., Avendano, M., & Goldstein, R. (1991). Symptom schemata in chronic respiratory patients. *Health Psychology, 10*, 268–273.

Landrine, H., & Klonoff, E.A. (1992). Culture and health-related schemas: A review and proposal for interdisciplinary integration. *Health Psychology, 11*, 267–276.

Lau, R.R. (1997). Cognitive representations of health and illness. In: D.S. Gochman (Ed.), *Handbook of health behavior research I: Personal and social determinants* (pp. 51–69). New York: Plenum Press.

Lau, R.R., & Hartman, K.A. (1983). Common sense representations of common illnesses. *Health Psychology, 2,* 167–185.

Lau, R.R., Bernard, T.M., & Hartman, K.A. (1989). Further explorations of common-sense representations of common illnesses. *Health Psychology, 8,* 195–219.

Leventhal, H., & Nerenz, D.R. (1985). The assessment of illness cognition. In: P. Karoly (Ed.), *Measurement strategies in health psychology* (pp. 517–554). New York: Wiley.

Leventhal, H., Meyer, D., & Nerenz, D.R. (1980). The common sense representation of illness danger. In: S. Rachman (Ed.), *Contributions to medical psychology*, vol. II (pp. 7–30). Oxford: Pergamon Press.

Mann, T. (1952). *The magic mountain.* New York: Modern Library.

McGee, H.M., & Jenkinson, C. (Eds.) (1997). Quality of life: Recent advances in theory and methods. *Psychology & Health (special issue), 12,* 733–854.

Meyer, D., Leventhal, H., & Gutmann, M. (1985). Common-sense models of illness: The example of hypertension. *Health Psychology, 4,* 115–135.

Moss-Morris, R., Weinman, D., Petrie, K.D., Horne, R., Cameron, L.D. & Buick, D. (2001). *The Revised Illness Perception Questionnaire (IPQ-R).* Psychology & Health (in press).

Moss-Morris, R., Petrie, K.J., & Weinman, J. (1996). Functioning in chronic fatigue syndrome: Do illness perceptions play a regulatory role? *British Journal of Health Psychology, 1,* 15–25.

Norman, P., & Bennett, P. (1996). Health locus of control. In: M. Conner & P. Norman (Eds.), *Predicting health behaviour* (pp. 62–94). Buckingham: Open University Press.

Osgood, C.E., Suci, G., & Tannenbaum, P. (1957). *The measurement of meaning.* Urbana, Ill.: The University of Illinois Press.

Pennebaker, J.W. (1982). *The psychology of physical symptoms.* New York: Springer.

Petrie, K.J., & Weinman, J.A. (Eds.) (1997). *Perceptions of health & illness.* Reading: Harwood Academic Publishers.

Petrie, K.J., Weinman, J.A., Sharpe, N., & Buckley, J. (1996). Role of patients' view of their illness in predicting return to work and functioning after myocardial infarction: Longitudinal study. *British Medical Journal, 312,* 1191–1194.

Petrie, K.J. (1999). Personal communication, Auckland, September.

Prohaska, T.R., Leventhal, E.A., Leventhal, H., & Keller, M.L. (1985). Health practices and illness cognition in young, middle aged, and elderly adults. *Journal of Gerontology, 40,* 569–578.

Richardson, R.D., Engel, C.C., McFall, M., McKnight, K., Boehnlein, D.K. & Hunt, S.C. (2001). Clinician attributions for symptoms and treatment of Gulf War-related health concerns. *Archives of Internal Medicine, 161,* 1289–1294.

Scharloo, M., & Kaptein, A.A. (1997). Measurement of illness perceptions in patients with chronic somatic illness: A review. In: K.J. Petrie & J.A. Weinman (Eds.), *Perceptions of health & illness* (pp. 103–154). Reading: Harwood Academic Publishers.

Scharloo, M., Kaptein, A.A., Weinman, J., Hazes, J.M., Willems, L.N.A., Bergman, W., & Rooijmans, H.G.M. (1998). Illness perceptions, coping and functioning in patients with rheumatoid arthritis, chronic obstructive pulmonary disease and psoriasis. *Journal of Psychosomatic Research, 44,* 573–585.

Scharloo, M., Kaptein, A.A., Weinman, J.A., Hazes, J.M., Breedveld, F.C., & Rooijmans, H.G.M. (1999). Predicting functional status in patients with rheumatoid arthritis. *Journal of Rheumatology, 26,* 1686–1693.

Scharloo, M., Kaptein, A.A., Weinman, J.A., Willems, L.N.A., Rooijmans, H.G.M., & Dijkman, J.H. (2000). Physical and psychological correlates of functioning in patients with chronic obstructive pulmonary disease. *Journal of Asthma, 37,* 17–29.

Skelton, J.A., & Croyle, R.T. (Eds.) (1991). *Mental representation in health and illness.* New York: Springer.

Solzhenitsyn, A. (1971). *Cancer ward.* Harmondsworth: Penguin.

Spilker, B. (Ed.) (1996). *Quality of life and pharmacoeconomics in clinical trials (2nd ed.)* Philadelphia: Lippincott-Raven.

Trautmann, J., & Pollard, C. (1982). *Literature and Medicine.* Pittsburgh: Pittsburgh University Press.

Turk, D.C., Rudy, T.E., & Salovey, P. (1986). Implicit models of illness. *Journal of Behavioral Medicine, 9,* 453–474.

Wallston, K.A. (1989). Assessment of control in health-care settings. In: A. Steptoe & A. Appels (Eds.), *Stress, personal control and health* (pp. 85–105). Chichester: Wiley.

Wallston, K.A., Wallston, B.S., & DeVellis, R. (1978). Development of the multidimensional health locus of control (MHLC) scales. *Health Education Monographs, 6,* 160–170.

Weinman, J., Petrie, K.J., Moss-Morris, R., & Horne, R. (1996). The Illness Perception Questionnaire: A new method for assessing the cognitive representation of illness. *Psychology & Health, 11,* 431–445.

Weinman, J., & Petrie, K.J. (1997). Illness perceptions: A new paradigm for psychosomatics? *Journal of Psychosomatic Research, 42,* 113–116.

Weinman, J. (1998). Personal communication, Vienna, September.

Zeidner, M., & Endler, N.S. (Eds.) (1996). *Handbook of coping.* New York: Wiley.

# 0 ASSESSING PERSONALITY TO EXPLORE RELATIONS WITH HEALTH

Leslie R. Martin and Howard S. Friedman

Much as perceptions, diagnoses, and treatments of disease are influenced by the society and culture in which they occur (Payer, 1988), the personality-to-health links we observe are strongly influenced by how both personality and health are defined and measured. In terms of health assessment, traditional medical methods identify organic diseases by locating tissue damage, viruses, fungi, and the like, but biopsychosocial methods focus on illness as opposed to disease, recognizing the importance of various social, cultural, and individual factors that influence symptom perception, seeking of treatment, and entrance into the sick role. Analogously, personality assessment techniques typically refer to self-reports of personality, or trait ratings of behavior, but broader assessments may include others' reports of personality, long-term habits and habit changes, projective tests, interviews, and dynamic judgments of various sorts that allow the researcher to draw deeper conclusions about basic patterns of the individual's personality, as motivations interact with life situations.

Such distinctions directly affect how we approach the relationship between personality and health. Consider, for example, the case of neuroticism, which has most often been linked to reports of illness symptoms and feelings rather than organic disease (Costa & McCrae, 1985b; Watson & Pennebaker, 1989). That is, the trait of neuroticism may not be simply and directly linked to disease. Although neurotic people are indeed more likely to enter the (social) sick role, at least some neurotic people are also more likely to: feel sick; change their behavior in unhealthy ways because they feel sick (such as disrupting their work schedules); receive more medical tests (including dangerous medical tests that may make them sick); avoid healthy behaviors (by overeating, finding excuses not to exercise, etc.); experience depression, which is correlated with impaired immune function; over-medicate (both prescription and nonprescription); and decrease their social support, and so in general may be more likely to become ill. What it means to be healthy is complex, and an understanding of the relationships of both narrower and broader aspects of health to personality is vital to achieving a clear conception of personality-health links.

This chapter will first present several models which can be used to organize and understand the personality-health relationship. Often two or more of these processes may be at work simultaneously. This will be followed by a review of specific personality factors which have been linked to health outcomes, and ways to measure these personality constructs. We will end with a brief discussion of disease-prone and self-healing personalities.

## Models of personality and health

First, physiological reactivity models posit a direct, causal link between personality and health (Suls & Rittenhouse, 1990; Smith & Anderson, 1986) although even in this type of model, personality is unlikely to be the sole contributor to the disease (Weiner, 1977). According to this view, individuals vary along a continuum of physiological reactivity, with some people being hyper-responsive or vulnerable to stressful environmental stimuli. These individuals are influenced in their interactions with the environment by their psychological makeup—how they view and interpret the world, their emotional responses to the world, and the coping mechanisms and social supports they have at their disposal. Someone who is easily aroused emotionally, who tends to perceive threats-to-self in the environment, and whose coping resources are taxed is likely to respond to stressful events with high levels of unhealthy physiological arousal—including increased heart rate, blood pressure, and other symptoms of chronic catecholamine release.

Diathesis-stress models derive from Selye's (1956) general adaptation syndrome in which an organism encountering a stressful stimulus becomes physiologically aroused for fight or flight but cannot maintain this state continuously and eventually becomes exhausted. According to this type of model, individuals experiencing psychological distress also become hyper-aroused and exhausted; illness is likely to follow, occurring at the individual's area of weakness. For example, someone prone to lung problems might experience breathing distress or respiratory infections more frequently during times of stress.

Second, constitutional disposition models posit that personality and health are linked by an underlying biological third variable. According to this type of model, a biological predisposition increases the likelihood of demonstrating certain personality characteristics and of developing certain health problems. Thus, an individual might have heart disease and be highly anxious, not because the anxiety contributed directly to the heart disease (nor that the disease made the person anxious), but because an overactive nervous system contributed to both the anxiety and the disease (Krantz & Durel, 1983). More complexly, early temperament or innate ability might set a person down certain paths which have somewhat predictable outcomes in both personality and health, but treating the anxiety would have no direct effect on heart health.

Third, interactional or bio-behavioral models posit that personality is related to health through various health-related behaviors (Suls & Rittenhouse, 1990; Bolger & Zuckerman, 1995). According to this view, an individual's personality plays a causal role in determining a host of health-impacting behaviors including diet, exercise, smoking, alcohol consumption, drug use, and creating stressful situations. A conscientious person might maintain good health by exercising, eating plenty of fruits and vegetables, and not smoking.

Other personality-disease models are more specific to certain disease processes. For example, health problems can influence personality characteristics. Hypoxia has been linked to depression (Katz, 1982) and it is not uncommon for cancer patients to become depressed (Dunkel-Schetter & Wortman, 1982). Another model posits that ultimate health outcomes given a particular threatening disease or medical crisis are influenced by personality factors like coping. For instance, optimism has been linked to quicker recovery from coronary bypass surgery (Scheier & Carver, 1987).

None of these models is completely explanatory, and they are not mutually exclusive. The relationships they attempt to explain are complicated and not yet fully understood. In an effort to understand the processes involved in the personality-disease relationship, small pieces of the puzzle are often first pursued individually. In the next section, some of the specific personality factors and assessments which have been found to be relevant to health are reviewed.

## Personality factors relevant to health

### BIG THREE AND BIG FIVE

Hans Eysenck (1967; 1990), working from Ivan Pavlov's framework, described links among biology, three basic aspects of personality (neuroticism, psychoticism, and extroversion), and health. Neuroticism was characterized as describing how easily and often an individual was distressed, with more moodiness indicative of a higher level of emotional instability. This conception has been expanded by others to include the facets of anxiety, angry hostility, depression, self-consciousness, impulsiveness, and vulnerability (Costa & McCrae, 1985a). Both encoding and recall of symptoms may be influenced by neuroticism (Larsen, 1992; Costa & McCrae, 1987a). Neuroticism is also linked to health through a variety of health behaviors (Booth-Kewley & Vickers, 1994; Vingerhoets et al., 1990), including adherence to medical recommendations (Christensen & Smith, 1995).

An often-used measure of neuroticism is the neuroticism subscale from Costa and McCrae's (1992) NEO PI-R which is an extensively validated and normed measure of the Big Five factors of personality (McCrae & Costa, 1987). Other popular measures of neuroticism include the neuroticism subscale from Eysenck's Revised Personality Inventory (Eysenck et al., 1985), the Taylor (1953) Manifest Anxiety Scale (TMAS), and the trait form of the State-Trait Anxiety Inventory (A-Trait; Spielberger et al., 1970).

Eysenck's Big Three construct of psychoticism (Eysenck, 1992; Eysenck & Eysenck, 1976) describes a predisposition toward sociopathic or psychotic behavior (but high scorers are not necessarily psychotic in the clinical sense). Individuals high on this dimension are hostile, solitary, impulsive, novelty-seeking, manipulative, and without fear. This dimension may be linked to health in a number of ways—through health-related behaviors and psychophysiologically (see also "Hostility" below). For instance, Fontaine (1994) has found that psychoticism is correlated with risky sexual behavior. Might Psychoticism also be related to increased levels of testosterone which is related to health behaviors? Dabbs and colleagues (Banks & Dabbs, 1996; Dabbs et al., 1987) have linked testosterone levels with violence and other behaviors, which may in turn influence health. Psychoticism is assessed with the Eysenck Personality Questionnaire (Eysenck & Eysenck, 1975), or with a combination of hostility and impulsivity measures.

The remaining Big Three factor (Extroversion) and the Big Five factors of Extraversion, Agreeableness, and Openness are also seen as important. Extraversion includes warmth, gregariousness, assertiveness, activity, excitement-seeking, and positive emotions; agreeableness incorporates the concepts of trust, straightforwardness, altruism, modesty, and tender-mindedness; openness is often described as including creativity, aesthetics, ideas, and values (Costa & McCrae, 1992). All have been proposed as positively related to good health. Friedman et al. (1993) did not find any evidence that sociability (which is corre-lated .40 with NEO PI-R Extraversion in a study by Martin and Friedman, 2000) in childhood was related to life span mortality risk, but social ties are characteristic of good health (Schwarzer & Leppin, 1991). Smith and Williams (1992) found that agreeableness predicted health behaviors and that openness to experience seemed to lead to less stressful appraisals of novel situations, which may in turn impact health. Additionally, insofar as openness is correlated with risk-taking behaviors (through enjoyment of novel activities) it might correlate with health; this has not yet been explored, however. And even if this were the case, it is unclear that measuring openness would contribute anything over simply measuring conscientiousness which is also related to health partially via risk-taking. Costa and McCrae's (1992) NEO PI-R is also widely used for measuring these three personality factors. Other measures include Eysenck et al.'s (1985) Revised Personality Inventory for assessing extraversion.

The fifth Big Five factor exhibits perhaps the simplest links with physical health. Conscientiousness includes the facets of competence, order, dutifulness, achievement-striving, self-discipline, and delibera-tion (Costa & McCrae, 1992) and Friedman et al. (1993) found that conscientious children (rated by parents and teachers as conscientious, truthful, free of vanity/egotism, and having prudence/forethought) were at a decreased risk for early mortality throughout their adult years compared to their less conscientious peers. In a follow-up, Friedman et al. (1995) demonstrated that conscientious children grew up to be adults who smoked less, drank less, and took fewer risks, but that these behavioral factors did not fully explain the personality-health link observed. Other studies have also demonstrated links between conscientiousness and health-related behaviors, such as fewer auto accidents (Arthur & Graziano, 1996). Costa and McCrae's (1992) NEO PI-R measure of conscientiousness is widely used to assess consci-entiousness and its facets, but behavioral observation and peer ratings are also valuable here.

The five factor model provides an overarching structure which can aid organization and understanding of the personality-health relation-ship (Costa & McCrae, 1987b; Smith & Williams, 1992; Van Heck, 1997), though it is used in different ways. Marshall et al. (1994) identified three major health-related personality dimensions: (1) opti-mistic control which seems linked to neuroticism, extraversion, and conscientiousness; (2) anger expression which seems related to agree-ableness and neuroticism; and (3) inhibition which seems to indicate, to some degree, neuroticism and openness. Most of the health psychology constructs currently in use do not map clearly and cleanly onto a single Big Five dimension, and the Big Five and Big Three may be too broad to be related to health in any simple ways.

## EXPLANATORY STYLE AND DEPRESSION

Learned helplessness (Seligman, 1975), which describes the outlook of an individual who has learned that s/he cannot control outcomes and thus stops trying, has been studied in both humans and animals. Depression is a common result of learned helplessness and is often characterized by withdrawal from friends and family, loss of appetite, and cessation of most normal activities. Abramson et al. (1978) describe a learned helplessness model of depression which incorporates the interrelationships of depressed mood, feelings of helplessness, and feelings of hopelessness.

A number of animal studies have demonstrated links between helplessness and health outcomes such as rate of tumor growth (Greenberg et al., 1984; Shavit et al., 1984) although not all studies agree, and some indicate a reverse effect (Keast, 1981). Similar results have been found in studies with humans (DiClemente & Temoshok, 1985; Greer et al., 1985). There are also studies which link depression to decreased immunocompetence (Weiss, 1992), cancer prognosis (Levy & Schain, 1987; Temoshok, 1985), and coronary heart disease (Barefoot & Schroll, 1996), although again, not all studies support the existence of such a link (Cassileth et al., 1985; Jamison et al., 1987). Depression is popularly assessed with the Beck Depression Inventory (BDI; Beck, 1967), the Self-Rating Depression Scale (Zung, 1965), and the Carroll Rating Scale for Depression (Carroll et al., 1981).

The corresponding cognitive personality construct to helplessness involves explanatory style—how people typically explain the causes of negative events in their lives. It includes the dimensions of internality/externality, stability/instability, and globality/specificity (Abramson et al., 1978; Peterson & Seligman, 1984). Each of the three dimensions correlates with depression (Sweeney et al., 1986) and various studies have linked individual dimensions of explanatory style to poor health. For instance, Peterson and Bossio (1991) found that stability and globality predicted poor health, but that internality did not; and Peterson et al. (1998) found that globality was a risk factor for premature mortality, but that stability and internality were not. Explanatory style factors may be linked to health via an immunological pathway (e.g., by their relationship to hopelessness; Eysenck, 1988), through a cardiovascular pathway (by their link with stress; Dykema et al., 1995), or through a behavioral pathway (by association to risky decision-making and poor problem-solving skills; Peterson et al. [1993]; or to injury; Peterson et al. [1998]).

Explanatory style may be measured with the Attributional Style Questionnaire (Peterson & Villanova, 1988); or may also profitably be assessed from already-available writing samples such as letters and essays, using the Content Analysis of Verbatim Explanations (CAVE; Peterson et al., 1992).

Conversely, optimism (having positive expectancies for future outcomes) is generally viewed as beneficial to health. Optimism has been linked to effective coping (Taylor, 1989) and to various physical health factors (Peterson et al., 1988) including rate of recovery following joint-replacement surgery (Chamberlain et al., 1992) and coronary artery bypass surgery (Scheier et al., 1989), and successful completion of an alcoholism after-care treatment program (Strack et al., 1987). Some studies suggest, however, that optimism may not always be beneficial. For instance, Tennen and Affleck (1987) present evidence that there are both health benefits and risks associated with optimism. Bauman and Siegel (1987) found that denial and *unrealistic* optimism were major factors in causing a sample of gay men to underestimate the riskiness of their behaviors, and Friedman et al. (1993) found that childhood cheerfulness (comprised of cheerfulness/optimism and a sense of humor) was inversely related to longevity. Thus, optimism cuts both ways, and simple links to health have not been established.

Optimism is commonly measured using Scheier and Carver's (1985) Life Orientation Test (LOT), although some have argued that this measure is confounded with neuroticism (Smith et al., 1989). An alternative measure is Fibel and Hale's (1978) Generalized Expectancy for Success Scale (GESS). The concept is still vague.

## LOCUS OF CONTROL, HARDINESS, AND COHERENCE
Related constructs, sometimes associated with optimism and lack of depression, include hardiness, locus of control, and sense of coherence. Hardy individuals demonstrate a sense of commitment to their work, a sense of control over their lives, and see changes as challenging rather than threatening (Kobasa, 1979). Hardiness has been linked to health outcomes in both retrospective and prospective studies (Kobasa, 1979; Kobasa et al., 1982), although some researchers have voiced criticisms of the construct itself (Funk & Houston, 1987; Hull et al., 1987). Hardiness is most commonly measured with the Hardiness Test

(Maddi, 1987), which was created, in part, by combining six other (earlier) hardiness scales from the literature on hardiness. Funk (1992) provides an evaluation of a number of hardiness scales, as well as a critique of the hardiness construct itself.

Locus of control describes a person's generalized beliefs about what determines various outcomes, with internals placing emphasis on personal efforts and externals viewing outcomes as primarily influenced by external forces (Rotter, 1966). Individuals with an internal locus of control have been found to seek more information about their health and to take more steps to protect their health than those with an external locus of control (Kelly et al., 1990; Seeman & Evans, 1962). An internal locus of control seems inversely related to depression and hopelessness (Rabkin et al., 1990), at least in Western cultures.

Locus of control may be measured using the Internal-External Locus of Control Scale (Rotter, 1966), Levenson's (1981) Internality, Powerful Others, and Chance Scales, Paulhus' (1983) Spheres of Control, and Nowicki and Duke's (1974; 1983) Adult Nowicki-Strickland Internal-External Control Scale.

Sense of coherence is a construct defined by Antonovsky (1987) as a tendency to believe that stimuli are comprehensible, manageable, and meaningful; it thus employs a series of appraisals (of situations, resources, etc.). Sense of coherence has been linked to positive health outcomes (Chamberlain et al., 1992), and it is hypothesized that a sense of coherence may be related to health through neuroimmunological pathways (that is, a high sense of coherence might lead to more general bodily homeostasis) as well as through influences on healthy behaviors, environments, and coping (Antonovsky, 1990). Sense of coherence can be measured using Antonovsky's (1987) Orientation to Life Questionnaire, but sometimes Neal and Groat's (1974) Meaninglessness Scale or Crumbaugh's (1968) Purpose in Life Test, or combinations are used.

## REPRESSION AND ALEXITHYMIA

Repression is a construct describing an individual's tendency to inhibit emotional expression or to harbor unconscious troubling feelings. It is not the same, however, as simple low expressivity, which can be benign in some individuals (Friedman & Booth-Kewley, 1987a). Early attempts to link this personality style with health have shown that repression may be linked to cancer (Derogatis et al., 1979; Kissen, 1966), elevated blood pressure (Davies, 1970), and physical disease in general (Blackburn, 1965) but the specific evidence for repression as a cause is weak. Pennebaker and colleagues have found that people who talk about (express feelings about) traumatic events have fewer subsequent health problems than those who repress their feelings (Berry & Pennebaker, 1993; Pennebaker, 1985).

Alexithymia is related to repression, but it includes difficulty identifying and describing one's own feelings along with an impaired ability to fantasize and imagine (Nemiah et al., 1976); that is, there is a deficit in abilities rather than a conscious or unconscious defense against emotional experience or expression (Myers, 1995; Taylor et al., 1997). Alexithymia has been linked with depression and anxiety (Hendryx et al., 1991), with ego overcontrol and brittleness (Haviland & Reise, 1996), and Bagby et al. (1994) determined that alexithymia was inversely correlated with openness and extraversion, and positively with neuroticism. In their review of the literature, Lumley et al. (1996) found that alexithymia was associated with physiological hyperarousal, unhealthy behaviors, and increased symptom perception. Alexithymia's link with health has previously been shown to be somewhat similar to that of neuroticism, in that it is positively associated with medically unexplained symptoms (Deary et al., 1997) and hypochondriasis (Kauhanen et al., 1991). Alexithymia may be measured with the Twenty-Item Toronto Alexithymia Scale (TAS-20; Bagby et al., 1994), the Alexithymia Prototype which utilizes Q-sort methodology (Haviland & Reise, 1996), or observation of nonverbal affect.

Two personality types which seem to show a close correspondence to repression and alexithymia are so-called Type C and Type D. Type C individuals typically suppress or repress negative emotions and are passive in the face of stress; this type is sometimes referred to as the "cancer prone personality" (Eysenck, 1995; Temoshok, 1987). Type D has been identified as describing those who are both distressed and who inhibit expression of these negative emotions (Denollet, 1997). Type D also has been linked to mortality risk in patients with CHD (Denollet et al., 1996). Type D can be measured using a combination of two measures to assess the experience of negative emotions and the tendency to inhibit the expression of these emotions (Denollet et al., 1996), such as the State-Trait Anxiety Inventory (Spielberger et al., 1970) and the social inhibition scale of the Heart Patients Psychological Questionnaire (Erdman, 1982). However, it is important to note the difference between Type C and Type D, on the one hand,

and repression on the other hand. Whereas repression refers to *low negative affect*/high defensiveness and an *unconscious* process, wherein negative emotions are excluded from awareness, Type D, and probably Type C too, refers to *high negative affect*/high social inhibition and the *conscious* suppression of emotions/behavior in order to avoid disapproval by others. These seemingly subtle differences once more illustrate the importance of clear construct validation and model-building in this field.

## TYPE A AND HOSTILITY

The Type A behavior pattern, which was first identified by Friedman and Rosenman (1974), describes an individual who is aggressively pushing to achieve too much in too little time, with excessive competition. It was proposed to explain the observable links between a tense stress and coronary heart disease. Recent studies indicate that it is the hostility component of Type A that is most closely related to coronary health (Miller et al., 1996), although it seems that Type A, as it was originally defined, reflected some degree of conscientiousness, neuroticism, extraversion, and lack of agreeableness (Barefoot et al., 1983; Booth-Kewley & Friedman, 1987; Smith & Williams, 1992). Some argue that aspects of Type A are a form of neuroticism (Costa, 1986).

There is a vast literature on these matters, and there is significant progress in measuring hostility, Type A, and related dimensions (Barefoot, 1992; Friedman et al., 1995b). Studies predicting health from chronic negative patterns may want to include at least four measures: aggressive overt hostility, alienated bitterness, introversion, and anxiety/depression. The many measures vary in their conceptualization of the construct. These include the Jenkins Activity Survey of Type A (JAS; Jenkins et al., 1974), the Framingham Type A Scale (FTAS; Haynes et al., 1980), and the Type A Structured Interview (SI; Rosenman, 1978). Structured interviews generally provide more valid information. Scales which focus on the hostility component include the Buss-Durkee Hostility Inventory (Buss & Durkee, 1957) and the Cook-Medley Hostility (Ho) Scale, which is derived from the MMPI (see Barefoot, 1992).

Type B was the term used to describe the absence of Type A behavior patterns, that is, those who are calm and relaxed and have low levels of competitive drive. However, these notions are better and more comprehensively conceived in terms of the self-healing personality.

# The self-healing personality

It is now clear that personality plays an important role in health and illness. Unfortunately, studies often examine the relationship of one narrow personality dimension to a single health outcome, thereby fragmenting the field and precluding the discovery of more basic causal processes. Friedman and Booth-Kewley (1987b), in the first broad meta-analysis in this field, found that there seems to be a general personality type which is predictive (but not necessarily causative) of a host of diseases, but that there is no strong evidence that specific diseases are related to specific personality factors. They thus asked whether there is a more general disease-prone personality.

Overall, there is substantial evidence that chronic depression, hostility, and repression (and their various cognitive and behavioral concomitants) affect physical health and recovery from illness. Some of the mechanisms are psychophysiological: chronic stress disrupts the neurohormonal system that regulates metabolic and immune functions. Many of the other mechanisms are behavioral: emotional disruption is associated with homicides, suicides, smoking, alcoholism, drunken driving, and various failures to take prophylactic measures. Other problems are somewhere in between such as sleep disturbances, eating disturbances and exercise disturbances. These patterns occur, however, in a socio-cultural and developmental context, and so cannot be simply assessed.

Considering the reverse, over the past dozen years there has been increasing evidence that there is also a generally healthy or resilient pattern, which Friedman (1991, 1998) termed "the self-healing personality." Individuals with a self-healing emotional style have a match between the individual and the environment, which maintains a physiological and psychosocial homeostasis, and through which good mental health promotes good physical health. Self-healing people are alert, responsive, and energetic, but may also be calm and conscientious. They are not ecstatic nor manic but are generally curious, secure, and constructive. They are also people one likes to be around. Multipronged assessments are therefore most useful here.

Just as we do not have a personality-meter that we can stick into a person to measure personality, neither do we have a simple set of personality concepts and scales that we can use to know the course of health. Nevertheless, with sufficient effort and continually-refined concepts, we do have a good sense of who is more disease prone and who is more self-healing.

## Acknowledgment

Supported in part by grants AG08825 and AG15188–01A1 from the National Institute on Aging. The views expressed are those of the authors.

## References

Abramson, L., Seligman, M., & Teasdale, J. (1978). Learned helplessness in humans: Critique and reformulation. *Journal of Abnormal Psychology, 87,* 49–74.

Antonovsky, A. (1987). *Unraveling the mystery of health.* San Francisco, CA: Jossey-Bass.

Antonovsky, A. (1990). Personality and health: Testing the sense of coherence model. In: H.S. Friedman (Ed.), *Personality and disease* (pp. 155–177). New York: Wiley.

Arthur, W. Jr., & Graziano, W.G. (1996). The five factor model, conscientiousness, and driving accident involvement. *Journal of Personality, 64,* 593–618.

Bagby, R.M., Taylor, G.J., & Parker, J.D.A. (1994). The Twenty-Item Toronto Alexithymia Scale—II: Convergent, discriminant, and concurrent validity. *Journal of Psychosomatic Research, 38,* 33–40.

Banks, T., & Dabbs, J.M. Jr. (1996). Salivary testosterone and cortisol in a delinquent and violent urban subculture. *Journal of Social Psychology, 136,* 49–56.

Barefoot, J.C. (1992). Developments in the measurement of hostility. In: H.S. Friedman (Ed.), *Hostility, coping, and health* (pp. 13–31). Washington, DC: APA.

Barefoot, J.C., Dahlstrom, W.G., & Williams, R.B. Jr. (1983). Hostility, CHD incidence, and total mortality: A 25-year follow-up study of 255 physicians. *Psychosomatic Medicine, 45,* 59–63.

Barefoot, J.C., & Schroll, M. (1996). Symptoms of depression, acute myocardial infarction, and total mortality in a community sample. *Circulation, 93,* 1976–1980.

Bauman, L., & Siegel, K. (1987). Misperceptions among gay men of the risk for AIDS associated with their sexual behavior. *Journal of Applied Social Psychology, 17,* 329–350.

Beck, A.T. (1967). *Depression: Causes and treatment.* Philadelphia, PA: University of Pennsylvania Press.

Berry, D.S., & Pennebaker, J.W. (1993). Nonverbal and verbal emotional expression and health. *Psychotherapy and Psychosomatics, 59*, 11–19.

Blackburn, R. (1965). Emotionality, repression-sensitization, and maladjustment. *British Journal of Psychiatry, 111*, 399–400.

Bolger, N., & Zuckerman, A. (1995). A framework for studying personality in the stress process. *Journal of Personality and Social Psychology, 69*, 890–902.

Booth-Kewley, S., & Friedman, H.S. (1987). Psychological predictors of heart disease: A quantitative review. *Psychological Bulletin, 101*, 343–362.

Booth-Kewley, S., & Vickers, R.R. Jr. (1994). Associations between major domains of personality and health behavior. *Journal of Personality, 62*, 282–298.

Buss, A.H., & Durkee, A. (1957). An inventory for assessing different kinds of hostility. *Journal of Consulting Psychology, 21*, 343–349.

Carroll, B.J., Feinberg, M., Smouse, P.E., Rawson, S.G., & Greden, J.F. (1981). The Carroll Rating Scale for Depression: Development, reliability, and validation. *British Journal of Psychiatry, 138*, 205–209.

Cassileth, B., Lusk, E., Miller, D., Brown, L., & Miller, C. (1985). Psychosocial correlates of survival in advanced malignant disease? *New England Journal of Medicine, 312*, 1551–1555.

Chamberlain, K., Petrie, K., & Azariah, R. (1992). The role of optimism and sense of coherence in predicting recovery following surgery. *Psychology and Health, 7*, 301–310.

Christensen, A.J., & Smith, T.W. (1995). Personality and patient adherence: Correlates of the five factor model in renal dialysis (pp. 127–144). *Journal of Behavioral Medicine, 18*, 305–313.

Costa, P.T. Jr. (1986). Is neuroticism a risk factor for CAD? Is Type A a measure of neuroticism? In: T. Schmidt, T. Dembroski, & G. Blumchen (Eds.), *Biological and psychological factors in cardiovascular disease* (pp. 127–144). New York: Springer.

Costa, P.T. Jr., & McCrae, R.R. (1985a). *The NEO Personality Inventory manual.* Odessa, FL: PAR.

Costa, P.T. Jr., & McCrae, R.R. (1985b). Hypochondriasis, neuroticism, and aging: When are somatic complaints unfounded? *American Psychologist, 40*, 19–28.

Costa, P.T. Jr., & McCrae, R.R. (1987a). Neuroticism, somatic complaints, and disease: Is the bark worse than the bite? *Journal of Personality, 55*, 299–316.

Costa, P.T. Jr., & McCrae, R.R. (1987b). Personality assessment in psychosomatic medicine: Value of a trait taxonomy. *Advances in Psychosomatic Medicine, 17*, 71–82.

Costa, P.T. Jr., & McCrae, R.R. (1992). *The Revised NEO Personality Inventory professional manual*. Odessa, FL: PAR.

Crumbaugh, J. (1968). Cross-validation of a purpose-in-life test based on Frankl's concepts. *Journal of Individual Psychology, 24*, 74–81.

Dabbs, J.M. Jr., Frady, R.L., Carr, T.S., & Besch, N.F. (1987). Saliva testosterone and criminal violence in young adult prison inmates. *Psychosomatic Medicine, 49*, 174–82.

Davies, M. (1970). Blood pressure and personality. *Journal of Psychosomatic Research, 14*, 89–104.

Deary, I.J., Scott, S., & Wilson, J.A. (1997). Neuroticism, alexithymia, and medically unexplained symptoms. *Personality and Individual Differences, 22*, 551–564.

Denollet, J. (1997). Non-expression of negative emotions as a personality feature in coronary patients. In: A.J.J.M. Vingerhoets, F.J. van Bussel, & A.J.W. Boelhouwer (Eds.), *The (non)expression of emotions in health and disease* (pp. 181–192). Tilburg, Netherlands: Tilburg University Press.

Denollet, J., Sys, S.U., Stroobant, N., Rombouts, H., Gillebert, T.C., & Brutsaert, D.L. (1996). Personality as independent predictor of long-term mortality in patients with coronary heart disease. *Lancet, 347*, 417–421.

Derogatis, L.R., Abeloff, M.D., & Melisaratos, N. (1979). Psychological coping mechanisms and survival time in metastatic breast cancer. *Journal of the American Medical Association, 242*, 1504–1508.

DiClemente, R.J., & Temoshok, L. (1985). Psychological adjustment to having cutaneous malignant melanoma as a predictor of follow-up clinical status. *Psychosomatic Medicine, 47*, 81.

Dunkel-Schetter, C., & Wortman, C. (1982). The interpersonal dynamics of cancer. In: H.S. Friedman & M.R. DiMatteo (Eds.), *Interpersonal issues in health care* (pp. 69–100). New York: Academic Press.

Dykema, J., Bergbower, K., & Peterson, C. (1995). Pessimistic explanatory style, stress, and illness. *Journal of Social and Clinical Psychology, 14*, 357–371.

Erdman, R.A. (1982). *HPPQ: Heart Patients Psychological Questionnaire*. Lisse, Netherlands: Swets & Zeitlinger.

Eysenck, H.J. (1967). *The biological basis of personality*. Springfield, IL: Charles C. Thomas.

Eysenck, H.J. (1988). Personality and stress as causal factors in cancer and heart disease. In: M.P. Janisse (Ed.), *Individual differences, stress, and health psychology* (pp. 129–145). New York: Springer.

Eysenck, H.J. (1990). Biological dimensions of personality. In: L.A. Pervin, (Ed.), *Handbook of personality: Theory and research* (pp. 244–276). New York: Guilford Press.

Eysenck, H.J. (1992). Four ways five factors are not basic. *Personality and Individual Differences, 13*, 667–673.

Eysenck, H.J. (1995). The causal role of stress and personality in the aetiology of cancer and coronary heart disease. In: C.D. Spielberger, I.G. Sarason, J.M.T. Brebner, E. Greenglass, P. Laungani, & A.M. O'Roark, (Eds.), *Stress and emotion: Anxiety, anger, and curiosity* (pp. 3–12). Washington, DC: Taylor & Francis.

Eysenck, H.J., & Eysenck, S.B.G. (1975). *Manual for the Eysenck Personality Questionnaire*. San Diego, CA: Educational and Industrial Testing Service.

Eysenck, H.J., & Eysenck, S.B.G. (1976). *Psychoticism as a dimension of personality*. London: Hodder & Stoughton.

Eysenck, S.B.G., Eysenck, H.J., & Barrett, P. (1985). A revised version of the Psychoticism Scale. *Personality and Individual Differences, 6*, 21–29.

Fibel, B., & Hale, W.D. (1978). The Generalized Expectancy for Success Scale: A new measure. *Journal of Consulting and Clinical Psychology, 46*, 924–931.

Fontaine, K.R. (1994). Personality correlates of sexual risk-taking among men. *Personality and Individual Differences, 17*, 693–694.

Friedman, H.S. (1991). *The self-healing personality: Why some people achieve health and others succumb to illness*. New York: Henry Holt.

Friedman, H.S. (1998). Self-healing personalities. In: H.S. Friedman (Ed.), *The encyclopedia of mental health* (Vol. 3, pp. 453–459). San Diego: Academic Press.

Friedman, H.S., & Booth-Kewley, S. (1987a). Personality, Type A behavior and coronary heart disease: The role of emotion and expression. *Journal of Personality and Social Psychology, 53*, 783–792.

Friedman, H.S., & Booth-Kewley, S. (1987b). The disease-prone personality: A meta-analytic view of the construct. *American Psychologist, 42*, 539–555.

Friedman, H.S., Tucker, J.S., & Reise, S.P. (1995b). Personality dimensions and measures potentially relevant to health: A focus on hostility. *Annals of Behavioral Medicine, 17*, 245–253.

Friedman, H.S., Tucker, J.S., Tomlinson-Keasey, C., Schwartz, J.E., Wingard, D.L., & Criqui, M.H. (1993). Does childhood personality predict longevity? *Journal of Personality and Social Psychology, 65*, 176–185.

Friedman, H.S., Tucker, J.S., Schwartz, J.E., Martin, L.R., Tomlinson-Keasey, C., Wingard, D.L., & Criqui, M.H. (1995a). Childhood conscientiousness and longevity: Health behaviors and cause of death. *Journal of Personality and Social Psychology, 68*, 696–703.

Friedman, M., & Rosenman, R.H. (1974). *Type A behavior and your heart*. New York: Knopf.

Funk, S.C. (1992). Hardiness: A review of theory and research. *Health Psychology, 11*, 335–345.

Funk, S.C., & Houston, B.K. (1987). A critical analysis of the hardiness scale's validity and utility. *Journal of Personality and Social Psychology, 53*, 572–578.

Greenberg, A., Dyck, D., & Sandler, L. (1984). Opponent processes, neurohormones, and natural resistance. In: B. Fox & B. Newberry (Eds.),

*Psychoneuroendocrine systems in cancer and immunity* (pp. 27–52). Toronto: C.J. Hogrefe.

Greer, S., Petingale, K., Morris, T., & Haybittle, J. (1985). Mental attitudes to cancer: An additional prognostic factor. *Lancet, 3,* 750.

Haviland, M.G., & Reise, S.P. (1996). A California Q-set alexithymia prototype and its relationship to ego-control and ego-resiliency. *Journal of Psychosomatic Research, 41,* 597–608.

Haynes, S.G., Feinleib, M., & Kannel, W.B. (1980). The relationships of psychosocial factors to coronary heart disease in the Framingham Study: Eight-year incidence of coronary heart disease. *American Journal of Epidemiology, 111,* 37–58.

Hendryx, M.S., Haviland, M.G., & Shaw, D.G. (1991). Dimensions of alexithymia and their relationships to anxiety and depression. *Journal of Personality Assessment, 56,* 227–237.

Hull, J.G., Van Treuren, R.R., & Virnelli, S. (1987). Hardiness and health: A critique and alternative approach. *Journal of Personality and Social Psychology, 53,* 518–530.

Jamison, R.N., Burish, T.G., & Wallston, K.A. (1987). Psychogenic factors in predicting survival of breast cancer patients. *Journal of Clinical Oncology, 5,* 768–772.

Jenkins, C.D., Zyzanski, S.J., & Rosenman, R.H. (1974). Prediction of clinical coronary heart disease by a test for the coronary-prone behavior pattern. *New England Journal of Medicine, 23,* 1271–1275.

Katz, I.R. (1982). Is there a hypoxic affective syndrome? *Psychosomatics, 23,* 846–853.

Kauhanen, J., Julkunen, J., & Salonen, J.T. (1991). Alexithymia and perceived symptoms: Criterion validity of the Toronto Alexithymia Scale. *Psychotherapy and Psychosomatics, 56,* 247–252.

Keast, D. (1981). Immune surveillance and cancer. In: K. Bammer & D.H. Newberry (Eds.), *Stress and cancer* (pp. 172–186). Toronto: C.J. Hogrefe.

Kelly, J.A., St. Lawrence, J.S., Brasfield, T.L., Lemke, A., Amidei, T., Roffman, R.E., Hood, H.F., Smith, J.E., Kilgore, H., & McNeill, C. (1990). Psychological factors that predict AIDS high-risk versus AIDS precautionary behavior. *Journal of Consulting and Clinical Psychology, 58,* 117–120.

Kissen, D.M. (1966). The significance of personality in lung cancer in men. *Annals of the New York Academy of Science, 125,* 820–826.

Kobasa, S.C. (1979). Stressful life events, personality and health: An inquiry into hardiness. *Journal of Personality and Social Psychology, 37,* 1–11.

Kobasa, S.C., Maddi, S.R., & Kahn, S. (1982). Hardiness and health: A prospective study. *Journal of Personality and Social Psychology, 42,* 168–177.

Krantz, D.S. & Durel, L.A. (1983). Psychobiological substrates of the Type A behavior patterns. *Health Psychology, 2,* 393–411.

Larsen, R.J. (1992). Neuroticism and selective encoding and recall of symptoms: Evidence from a combined and concurrent-retrospective study. *Journal of Personality and Social Psychology, 62*, 480–488.

Levenson, H. (1981). Differentiating among internality, powerful others, and chance. In: H.M. Lefcourt (Ed.), *Research with the locus of control construct* (Vol. 1, pp. 15–63). New York: Academic Press.

Levy, S. & Schain, W. (1987). Psychological response and breast cancer: Direct and indirect contributions to treatment outcome. In: M. Lippman, A. Lichter, & D. Danforth (Eds.), *Diagnosis and treatment of breast cancer* (pp. 18–27). New York: Saunders.

Lumley, M.A., Stettner, L., & Wehmer, F. (1996). How are alexithymia and physical illness linked? A review and critique of pathways. *Journal of Psychosomatic Research, 41*, 505–518.

Maddi, S.R. (1987). Hardiness training at Illinois Bell Telephone. In: J.P. Opatz (Ed.), *Health promotion evaluation.* Stevens Point, WI: National Wellness Institute.

Marshall, G.N., Wortman, C.B., Vickers, R.R. Jr., Kusulas, J.W., & Hervig, L.K. (1994). The five-factor model of personality as a framework for personality-health research. *Journal of Personality and Social Psychology, 67*, 278–286.

Martin, L.R., & Friedman, H.S. (2000). Comparing personality scales across time: An illustrative study of validity and consistency in a life span archival data. *Journal of Personality, 68*, 85–110.

McCrae, R.R., & Costa, P.T. Jr. (1987). Validation of the five factor model of personality across instruments and observers. *Journal of Personality and Social Psychology, 52*, 81–90.

Miller, T.Q., Smith, T.W., Turner, C.W., Guijarro, M.W., & Hallet, A.J. (1996). Meta-analytic review of research on hostility and physical health. *Psychological Bulletin, 119*, 322–348.

Myers, L.B. (1995). Alexithymia and repression: The role of defensiveness and trait anxiety. *Personality and Individual Differences, 19*, 489–492.

Neal, A., & Groat, H.T. (1974). Social class correlates of stability and change in levels of alienation. *Sociological Quarterly, 15*, 548–558.

Nemiah, J.C., Freyberger, H., & Sifneos, P.E., (1976). Alexithymia: A view of the psychosomatic process. In: O.W. Hill (Ed.), *Modern trends in psychosomatic medicine* (Vol. 3, p. 430–439). London: Butterworths.

Nowicki, S., & Duke, M.P. (1974). A locus of control scale for noncollege as well as college adults. *Journal of Personality Assessment, 38*, 136–137.

Nowicki, S., & Duke, M.P. (1983). The Nowicki-Strickland life span locus of control scales: Construct validation. In: H.M. Lefcourt (Ed.), *Research with the locus of control construct* (Vol. 2, pp. 9–43). New York: Academic Press.

Paulhus, D. (1983). Sphere-specific measures of perceived control. *Journal of Personality and Social Psychology, 44*, 1253–1265.

Payer, L. (1988). *Medicine and culture: Varieties of treatment in the United States, England, West Germany, and France.* New York: Henry Holt.

Pennebaker, J.W. (1985). Traumatic experience and psychosomatic disease: Exploring the roles of behavioural inhibition, obsession, and confiding. *Canadian Psychology, 26,* 82–95.

Peterson, C. & Seligman, M.E.P. (1984). Causal explanations as a risk factor for depression: Theory and evidence. *Psychological Review, 91,* 347–374.

Peterson, C., & Villanova, P. (1988). An expanded Attributional Style Questionnaire. *Journal of Abnormal Psychology, 97,* 87–89.

Peterson, C., & Bossio, L.M. (1991). *Health and optimism.* New York: Free Press.

Peterson, C., Seligman, M.E.P., & Vailliant, G.E. (1988). Pessimistic explanatory style is a risk for physical illness: A thirty-five-year longitudinal study. *Journal of Personality and Social Psychology, 55,* 23–27.

Peterson, C., Maier, S.F., & Seligman, M.E.P. (1993). *Learned helplessness: A theory for the age of personal control.* New York: Oxford University Press.

Peterson, C., Schulman, P., Castellon, C., & Seligman, M.E.P. (1992). CAVE: Content analysis of verbatim explanations. In: C.P. Smith (Ed.), *Motivation and personality: Handbook of thematic content analysis* (pp. 383–392). New York: Cambridge University Press.

Peterson, C., Seligman, M.E.P., Yurko, K.H., Martin, L.R., & Friedman, H.S. (1998). Catastrophizing and untimely death. *Psychological Science, 9,* 127–130.

Rabkin, J.G., Williams, J.B.W., Neugebauer, R., Remien, R.H., & Goetz, R. (1990). Maintenance of hope in HIV-spectrum homosexual men. *American Journal of Psychiatry, 147,* 1322–1326.

Rosenman, R.H. (1978). The interview method of assessment of the coronary-prone behavior pattern. In: T.M. Dembroski, S.M. Weiss, J.L. Shields, S.G. Haynes, & M. Feinleib (Eds.), *Coronary-prone behavior* (pp. 55–70). New York: Springer.

Rotter, J.B. (1966). Generalized expectancies for internal versus external control of reinforcement. *Psychological Monographs, 80,* (no. 609).

Scheier, M.F., & Carver, C.S. (1985). Optimism, coping, and health: Assessment and implication of generalized outcome expectancies. *Health Psychology, 4,* 219–247.

Scheier, M.F., & Carver, C.S. (1987). Dispositional optimism and physical well-being: The influence of generalized outcomes expectancies on health. *Journal of Personality, 55,* 169–210.

Scheier, M.F., Magovern, G., Abbott, R., Matthews, K., Owens, J., Lefebvre, R., & Carver, C. (1989). Dispositional optimism and recovery from coronary artery bypass surgery: The beneficial effects on physical and psychological well-being. *Journal of Personality and Social Psychology, 57,* 1024–1040.

Schwarzer, R., & Leppin, A. (1991). Social support and health: A theoretical and empirical overview. *Journal of Social and Personal Relationships, 8,* 99–127.

Seeman, M., & Evans, J.W. (1962). Alienation and learning in a hospital setting. *American Sociological Review, 27,* 772–783.

Seligman, M.E.P. (1975). *Helplessness: On depression, development, and death.* San Francisco, CA: Freeman.

Selye, H. (1956). *The stress of life.* New York: McGraw-Hill.

Shavit, J., Lewis, J., Terman, G., Gale, R., & Liebeskind, J. (1984). Opioid peptides mediate the suppressive effect of stress on natural killer cytotoxicity. *Science, 223,* 188–190.

Smith, T.W., & Anderson, N.B. (1986). Models of personality and disease: An interactional approach to Type A behavior and cardiovascular risk. *Journal of Personality and Social Psychology, 50,* 1166–1173.

Smith, T.W., & Williams, P.G. (1992). Personality and health: Advantages and limitations of the five-factor model. *Journal of Personality, 60,* 395–423.

Smith, T.W., Pope, M.K., Rhodewalt, F., & Poulton, J. (1989). Optimism, neuroticism, coping, and symptom reports: An alternative interpretation of the Life Orientation Test. *Journal of Personality and Social Psychology, 56,* 640–648.

Spielberger, C.D., Gorsuch, R.L., & Lushene, R.E. (1970). *Manual for the State-Trait Anxiety Inventory.* Palo Alto, CA: Consulting Psychologists Press.

Strack, S., Carver, C., & Blaney, P.H. (1987). Predicting successful completion of an aftercare program following treatment for alcoholism: The role of dispositional optimism. *Journal of Personality and Social Psychology, 53,* 579–584.

Suls, J., & Rittenhouse, J.D. (1990). Models of linkages between personality and disease. In: H.S. Friedman (Ed.), *Personality and disease* (pp. 38–64). New York: Wiley.

Sweeney, P.D., Anderson, K., & Bailey, S. (1986). Attributional style in depression: A meta-analytic review. *Journal of Personality & Social Psychology, 50,* 974–991.

Taylor, G.J., Parker, J.D.A., & Bagby, R.M. (1997). Relationships between alexithymia and related constructs. In: A.J.J.M. Vingerhoets, F.J. van Bussel, & A.J.W. Boelhouwer (Eds.), *The (non)expression of emotions in health and disease* (pp. 103–113). Tilburg, The Netherlands: Tilburg University Press.

Taylor, J.A. (1953). A personality scale of manifest anxiety. *Journal of Abnormal and Social Psychology, 48,* 285–290.

Taylor, S. (1989). *Positive illusions: Creative self-deception and the healthy mind.* New York: Basic Books.

Temoshok, L. (1985). Biopsychosocial studies on cutaneous malignant melanoma: Psychosocial factors associated with prognostic indicators, progression, psychophysiology and tumor-host response. *Social Science and Medicine, 20*, 833–840.

Temoshok, L. (1987). Personality, coping style, emotion, and cancer: Towards an integrative model. *Cancer Surveys, 6*, 545–567.

Tennen, H., & Affleck G. (1987). The costs and benefits of optimistic explanations and dispositional optimism. *Journal of Personality, 55*, 377–393.

Van Heck, G.L. (1997). Personality and physical health: Toward an ecological approach to health-related personality research. *European Journal of Personality, 11*, 415–443.

Vingerhoets, A.J.J.M., Croon, M., Jeninga, A.J., & Menges, L.J. (1990). Personality and health habits. *Psychology & Health, 4*, 333–342.

Watson, D., & Pennebaker, J.W. (1989). Health complaints, stress, and distress: Exploring the central role of negative affectivity. *Psychological Review, 96*, 234–254.

Weiner, H. (1977). *Psychobiology and human disease*. New York: Elsevier.

Weiss, C.S. (1992). Depression and immunocompetence: A review of the literature. *Psychological Bulletin, 111*, 475–489.

Zung, W.W.K. (1965). A self-rating depression scale. *Archives of General Psychiatry, 12*, 63–70.

# 1 MEASUREMENT OF PATIENT COMPLIANCE WITH DRUG THERAPY: AN OVERVIEW

Erik de Klerk

In modern medicine, consultation with a physician results more often than not in a drug prescription. Prescribing a drug does not ensure optimal intake, however. Most readers will have at least some experience with a drug regimen, and chances are one can recall that during the execution phase of such a prescribed regimen one or more doses were omitted, or that the timing of the ingestion of the drug was not quite as prescribed. This phenomenon is known as variable patient compliance, and this chapter will review various aspects associated with this phenomenon.

This is not a new subject: "Keep a watch also on the faults of the patients which often makes them lie about the taking of things prescribed", Hippocrates stated over 2,500 years ago. Compliance can be studied for all medical advice, as indicated by Sackett and Haynes (1976) who defined patient compliance as: "the extent to which a person's behavior (in terms of taking medications, following diets, or executing lifestyle changes) coincides with medical or health advice."

However, the optimal execution of a drug prescription is substantially different from following a diet or a program to quit smoking. Once acceptance of the therapy is established, the actual ingestion of a tablet or capsule is a very small act, requiring only memory and willingness to interrupt briefly ongoing activities to do so. Lifestyle changes ask much more of the recipient, for example, strong determination, a constant rejection of impulses to do whatever the recipient would prefer to do (such as eating or smoking) and a much more rigid execution of the correct regime. Smoking a few cigarettes will by many be regarded as a total treatment failure, while missing one or a few tablets in most instances would not have such a dramatic impact. However, the consequences of missed doses are directly related to the type of diseases. Whereas for most diseases it holds that missing a few doses will not be a problem, in the case of, for example, HIV, non-compliance to any degree can have serious consequences for the patients. In other words, the main errors made in drug regimen compliance are errors of omission, whereas the main errors made in following a special diet or a smoking cessation program are errors of commission.

Therefore we propose to make a clear distinction between compliance on drug regimen, the focus of this chapter, and compliance on other medical advice. For the purpose of *measurement of patient compliance on drug therapy* the definition: "patient compliance is the extent to which the prescribed (and presumably optimal) regimen conforms to the actual dosing history" from Urquhart and Chevalley (1988), is preferred.

## Terminology

A short note on the use of the word "compliance" is considered appropriate here. Several early authors in this field found the word authoritarian (the doctor tells the patient what to do) and to some it implies obeisance or servility. Opponents of the word have therefore proposed a variety of alternative words including adherence, fidelity, maintenance (Feinstein, 1990), obedience (Joyce, 1962), cooperation and, more recently, concordance (Dolan-Mullen, 1997).

Although optimal therapy requires cooperation of both physician and patient, preferably on a basis of equality, none of the other proposed words appear to have any evident advantage over "compliance". Therefore we opted to follow the choice of the National Library of Medicine which maintains the term patient compliance as Mesh index, and indexes papers that prefer adherence or other definitions under the Mesh term patient-compliance.

### ASPECTS OF NON-COMPLIANCE

Variable compliance in drug therapy includes taking too many or not enough pills (so called taking-compliance) and/or altering the intervals between consecutive doses (timing-compliance). It makes sense pharmacologically to take the interdose interval as a starting point to describe the effects of various forms of non-compliance.

Short interdose intervals (e.g., when extra tablets are taken) usually result in an increased efficacy but also in a higher probability for adverse drug reactions and toxicity.

Longer interdose intervals (e.g., after omission of one or more doses) can result in loss of efficacy, but also, in selected cases such as B-blockers in an increase in safety problems such as rebound effects. Usually restarting therapy occurs in full-dose, and if a particular drug requires careful up-titration first-dose effects may re-occur during "steady state therapy" for someone not informed about the actual pattern of drug intake.

Non-compliance can thus result in a variety of effects. From a clinical point of view, an important aspect is to distinguish non-responders (patients who receive adequate therapy but do not show the clinically desirable result) from non-compliers (those that do not receive adequate therapy). Non-responders should be treated with higher doses, other drugs, or a combination of drugs while non-compliers should be helped in assuring intake. Certain adverse drug reactions and drug-related toxicity, as well as symptoms resulting from rebound effects, can be labeled as drug related, while in fact they may be compliance related.

## Short review

From an historical perspective, 1962 stands out as the year when two seminal papers discussed several important concepts related to patient compliance. Even 40 years later, several of their findings and conclusions still hold. Moulding (1962) described the first special-purpose device to measure timing aspects of patient compliance. The device was "a wedding of a clock to a pill dispenser", resulting in a cabinet that stored drug dosage forms in small individual trays, with special photographic film exposed to a radioactive source until the drug was removed from the tray. The patient had to press a button to remove the drug, and such an event was thus recorded by the occurrence of evidence of radiographic rays (black notches) on the film. Omissions of dosing would be detected by the absence of black notches, in essence creating a bar-code of individual patient compliance. The idea was years ahead of its time, and consequently it has never been used.

Joyce (1962) described the results of three different compliance measurements (interview, pill-count, and the use of phenol red as a chemical marker of ingestion) in a trial comparing phenylbutazone, a compound labeled C2041 and placebo, in patients with rheumatoid arthritis. Substantial non-compliance was noted: only 35% of all urine samples that should have contained marker were labeled marker present and the frequency distribution of dosing discrepancies between returned tablets and prescribed dosing ranged from zero to almost maximal, thus showing that compliance varied markedly between individuals.

When the results of the intention-to-treat analyses were corrected for variable compliance the new compound showed a higher efficacy while at the same time showing higher toxicity. The author at that time felt the need to apologize for "presenting a result that is so agreeably acceptable to common-sense" but noted that there had been very few attempts to confirm that patients are following treatment as prescribed in diverse conditions, and that no one had tried to use this type of data to a scientific advantage (Joyce, 1962). Although written over 35 years ago, unfortunately this statement still holds true.

Since it is not possible to review all research addressing the many aspects of compliance three prototypical studies are described in detail to illustrate the important issues regarding the measurement of patient compliance.

### (1) The Coronary Drug Project

In 1980 the data of the Coronary Drug Project, a randomized, placebo-controlled, double-blinded, multicenter trial to evaluate the efficacy and safety of several lipid-influencing drugs in the secondary preven-tion of coronary heart disease (CHD), (CDP, 1973; 1974) were re-analyzed (CDP, 1980). Compliance was operationalized as the estimated number of capsules taken per day divided by the number of capsules dictated by the protocol dosage (nine per day) for each four-month period for each patient—multiplied by 100. The cumulative percentage of compliance was then computed for each patient for the first five years of follow-up or until death, if death occurred before the fifth anniversary of entry.

The good compliers in the active drug group had a substantially lower five-year mortality than the poor compliers (15.0 vs 24.6%). However, surprisingly, the placebo group yielded similar results: 15.1% mortality for good compliers vs 28.3% mortality for poor compliers. The authors concluded that "these findings show the serious difficulty, if not impossibility, of evaluating treatment efficacy in subgroups deter-mined by patient responses such as compliance" (CDP, 1980).

This publication has since then served as the standard literature ref-erence that compliance data could not be used in statistical analyses since it is a variable that is assessed post-randomization and, given the CDP re-analyses, it must be confounded by treatment-efficacy, side-effects or other factors under scrutiny.

There are three important arguments against the generalization of the conclusion of this article. The first, and perhaps strongest, is that the CDP was a secondary prevention trial, implying that all patients who were enrolled had evidence of at least one myocardial infarction prior to study entry. The drug studied in the CDP, clofibrate, is expected to have only a minor effect on mortality reduction, given the severe disease state that many of the enrolled patients had (reflected by the almost 21% mortality in the placebo group) (CDP, 1974). Most, if not almost all patients were treated with much stronger mortality decreasing drugs such as loop-diuretics, digitalis, etc., regardless of whether randomized in the treatment- or placebo-group. Since it is reasonable to assume that compliance on one drug reflects compliance on another drug (see, for example Cramer et al., 1995), it is likely that the reduction in mortality in the good compliers in the placebo group actually reflects good compliance on other, powerful drugs as well.

The second argument against the conclusion is related to the fact that it makes no sense pharmacologically to divide patients into groups of good or bad compliers based on a "more or less than 80% of all drugs taken rule". A good example is the comparison to another field of medicine where compliance is recognized as important when looking at efficacy of the drug, that is oral contraceptives. Timing errors alone (taking all prescribed doses but with variable intervals) can allow for breakthrough of ovulation, and thus allow pregnancy to occur despite 100% compliance (Guillebaud, 1993). This shows the inappropriateness of the use of artificial boundaries like "more or less then 80% of all drugs taken".

Another strong argument against the use of dichotomous cut-offs is the possible emergence of resistant strains of the Human Immunodeficiency Virus (HIV) as a result of just one 5-day drug holiday for AZT (Vanhove et al., 1996). Again, any attempt to organize data in x% more or less groups is likely to fail if the appropriate mechanism of action and the pharmaco-kinetics and pharmaco-dynamics are not taken into account. Compliance should be defined with the relevant pharmacological aspects in mind, and it should preferably be treated as a continuous variable instead of being dichotomized.

The third argument against the validity of the conclusions of the CDP re-analyses concerns the vague measurement instrument for compliance. Presumably the measure consisted of a pill-count, though this is not described in detail in the original publication, and we know by now that pill-counts are not very accurate as a compliance measurement instrument (Pullar et al., 1989).

Interestingly, Feinstein (1991) noted that "the investigators failed to suitably investigate the most powerful agent noted in the study: compliance". Compliance on placebo yielded a large reduction in mortality and thus provided a major clue to prognostic susceptibility, but this was given no further attention.

Therefore, the conclusion of this article cannot be generalized beyond secondary prevention trials, and certainly cannot be taken as proof that compliance data should never be used to explain drug effects. A comprehensive discussion of the "smart" use of compliance data in the analyses of clinical trials can be found in Hasford (1991).

*(2) The Lipid Research Clinics Primary Prevention Trial*
The Lipid Research Clinics Coronary Primary Prevention Trial (LRCCPPT), also is a very large, randomized, placebo-controlled, double-blinded multicenter trial to test the effectiveness of cholestyramine in reducing CHD in middle-aged men with primary hypercholesterolemia (LRCPPT, 1984a; 1984b). Since there is a well-established relation between total cholesterol levels and the incidence of CHD on the one hand, known efficacy of cholestyramine resin on total cholesterol lowering on the other hand, and the possibility of an individualized tolerance for cholestyramine, the primary intention-to-treat analyses (LRCPPT, 1984a) were accompanied by an analysis of the relationship between cholesterol lowering and reduction in incidence of CHD (LRCPPT, 1984b). Compliance to the prescribed doses (6 packets per day) was estimated for each participant at bimonthly visits by packet count. A Cox proportional hazards model was used to quantify the parameters relating changes in lipid levels to incidence of CHD in each treatment group.

The results (Figure 11.1) showed that a patient who could tolerate the six packets (24 gram) of cholestyramine per day could expect a 49% reduction of CHD incidence, contrasting with the average, Intention To Treat based estimate of a reduction of 19% in CHD, influenced by the average tolerability of approximately 3.5 packets per day. Many patients could not tolerate the full dose and therefore had a lower reduction in risk of CHD, whereas those who could tolerate the full dose benefitted from more than twice the reduction in risk of CHD.

When looking at placebo compliance, reduction in lipid levels, and reduction of CHD, the authors found no effect among the placebo group for either of these variables. Since this was a primary prevention trial, where one would expect little or no concomitant "strong", non-trial drug use, these findings thus support the argument against the conclusions of the CDP-re-analyses discussed in the previous paragraphs.

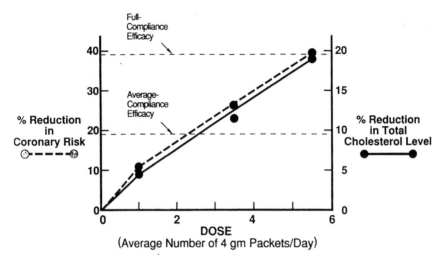

Figure 11.1. Compliance related reduction in CHD incidence.

*(3) The Leuven experience*
A successful heart transplantation, one of the miracles of modern medicine, can only be successful if there is sufficient post-operative immunosuppression. This regimen, usually consisting of a combination of drugs including corticosteroids and cyclosporine, has to be maintained lifelong. Unfortunately, to ensure sufficient action pharmacologic properties of cyclosporine require it to be taken every day, with no or almost no mistakes. The transplant team in Leuven, Belgium, therefore decided to study compliance on cyclosporine in more detail (de Geest, 1996) in 101 transplant patients who were followed for an average of 90 days with an electronic monitoring system, described in detail below. Various compliance variables were recorded, all showing excellent compliance on group level: 99.4% of all tablets were taken, of which 98.8% were on schedule. Seven of the eight rejection periods, however, were related to a few skipped doses. Compliance was therefore considered an important factor in the maintenance therapy posttransplantation, and a reason to focus the management program in Leuven on optimization of patient compliance (de Geest, 1997). It is noteworthy that the success of such a remarkable achievement of modern medicine almost completely depends on the daily act of taking medication at the right moment.

# Compliance measurement and statistical analyses

The standard "intention-to-treat analyses" (ITT), where all patients who were randomized are analyzed as having had a full treatment (thus including non-compliers, drop-outs and other protocol violations) in a trial where there is substantial variation in compliance, are likely to generate a distorted estimate of both efficacy and safety of the drug. This distortion can in selected cases be both scientifically and ethically unacceptable (Feinstein, 1991; Lasagna & Hutt, 1991). Therefore, as Cox (1998) noted: "The statistical challenge will be to develop methods of analysis that take due account of the complex character of compliance without analysis becoming too complicated conceptually."

Among the recent attempts to incorporate compliance data into statistical analyses is the award winning method on the recovery of the true dose-response curve from the compliance-response curves (Efron & Feldman, 1991). Bayesian analyses lead to new estimates of the effect of receipt of treatment, and to new randomization-based procedures that yield more powerful results than those obtained by intention-to-treat analyses (Rubin, 1998). Markow chain, probability based simulation models provide accurate methods to predict compliance (de Klerk et al., 1997b) and may lead to more effective population pharmacokinetic analyses (Girard et al., 1996), and high-dimensional models enable comparisons of the full pattern of daily dosing indicators for subjects between groups (Vrijens & Goetghebeur, 1997). A more extensive overview of progress in the statistical analyses of compliance data can be found in Goetghebeur & Shapiro (1996). It is likely that this work will eventually lead to the incorporation of compliance data in the analyses of clinical trials in the future.

# A "gold standard" for compliance measurement?

If one wants to measure patient compliance, it is wise to consider which measurement method is optimal for the given situation. The minimum requirements of a "gold standard" for compliance measurement would ask for: (1) validity—proving ingestion of the medication and giving detailed overview of the timing of the ingestion; (2) reliability and sensitivity to change—stable results under stable compliance and differential results under variable compliance and (3) feasibility—

the patient should not be aware of compliance measurement and should not be able to censor the results, the method should not be invasive nor require special equipment to collect and process that data, and the researcher/physician should always have access to the data.

Unfortunately, no single instrument currently available has all these properties, and none is foreseeable. Therefore we must consider the instruments that are now available and describe them in terms of these requirements.

## Overview of assessment methods

It has become the custom to distinguish patient compliance measurement instruments in direct methods, those that prove that the drug reached the site of action, and indirect methods, those that do not prove ingestion.

These measurement methods, including their advantages and disadvantages are summarized in Table 11.1.

INDIRECT METHODS
*(1) Patient interviews*
Patient interviews, although easy to perform, should be discarded as a scientific method for patient compliance. It is very easy for patients to censor the number of pills actually taken, and even with totally honest patient reports, the influence of poor memory is too large to be ignored.

Note that the criticism only applies to scientific research, however. In everyday clinical practice, when patients admit non-compliance, it is of course good practice to inquire about potential barriers, and to offer practical advice to enhance compliance.

*(2) Questionnaires*
Questionnaires designed to measure compliance and related issues such as barriers, beliefs, regimen-knowledge and other compliance-influencing concepts can provide useful information. The advantages over interviews are: standardized questions for every patient; the possibility to validate the results against other compliance measurement methods such as chemical markers or electronic monitoring; and the possibility to do standardized across-group comparisons of the results. In addition, questionnaires are in general easy to administer, analyze

Table 11.1. Patient compliance measurement methods.

| Method[1] | Proves ingestion of medication | Gives detailed overview on timing of ingestion | Stable result under stable compliance | Differential result under variable compliance | Patient is aware of compliance measurement | Invasive method | Measurement method requires |
|---|---|---|---|---|---|---|---|
| 1. Interviews | no | no | yes | possible | yes | no | staff |
| 2. Questionnaires | no | no | yes | possible | possible | no | questionnaire |
| 3. Diary method | no | possible | yes | possible | yes | no | diary |
| 4. Physician estimate | no | no | possible | possible | no | no | consultation |
| 5. Counting returned medication | no | no | yes | possible | possible | no | consultation |
| 6. Electronic monitoring | no | yes | yes | yes | usually | no | electronic monitors |
| 7. Concentration measurement | yes | no | possible | possible | possible | yes | drawing blood/ urine sample and laboratorium analyses |
| 8. Clinical outcome | no | no | possible | possible | no | no | measurement of clinical outcome |
| 9. Direct observation | yes | yes | yes | yes | yes | no | staff, consultation |
| 10. Duration of treatment | no | no | yes | possible | no | no | data collection of prescriptions |

[1] Description of the method can be found in the text.

and report from. The biggest disadvantage is of course the possibility that patients censor their report.

### (3) Diary method

Diary methods require consistent patient cooperation, especially when applied on a daily basis. Some technical aids, such as digital organizers that remind the patient when the diary has to be completed, make the diary method slightly more reliable and valid. When applied frequently over a longer period the results can provide interesting data, and make it possible to relate self-report to clinical events. Apart from this desirable property, the same advantages and disadvantages as questionnaires apply.

### (4) Physician estimate

Physicians' estimates of compliance of their patients, though a little better then a gamble, fail to provide accurate data. In one study testing physicians' ability to predict their patients' medication compliance after hospital discharge (Mushlin & Appel, 1977), physicians at best accurately predicted 35% of the non-compliers and one half of their predictions were incorrect. Less than half of the physicians' predictions correctly discriminated between compliant and non-compliant patients and three quarters of their predictions of non-compliance were inaccurate. In this particular study the measure that was used to compare physicians' estimates was an extensive effort of the hospital staff to collect data on patients' maintenance of the schedule of return clinical visits, hand-counted medications given out at the hospital pharmacy, and routinely done pill-counts over a four week period. The resulting data obviously lack both sensitivity and precision, and therefore cannot be used as a scientific measurement instrument.

### (5) Counting returned tablets

The so-called pill-counts have been used extensively as a routine compliance measure in clinical trials, and continue to be used, despite the widespread evidence that the data substantially over-estimate patient compliance (Pullar et al., 1989; Waterhouse et al., 1993). A consistent finding in these studies is that compliance reports as indicated by pill-counts are almost always higher than the reliable measures provided by low-dose phenobarbitone or electronic monitoring.

One study in which returned tablets were compared to phenobarbitone level-to-dose ratios concluded that "although return tablet count may seem attractive, simple, cheap and non-invasive, the findings of this analysis suggest that it is very inaccurate. Its continued use in clinical trials cannot be justified" (Pullar et al., 1989).

### (6) Electronic monitoring

Electronic monitors, i.e., normal pill-bottles fitted with a special cap that contains micro-electronics designed to register the time and date when the cap is opened, were developed for commercial use in the late 1980s, and have since been widely used in many fields of medicine. Under the assumption that every opening reflects the ingestion of one dose this method has the advantage of giving an unobtrusive, difficult to censor and very precise dosing history. In the absence of better methods, this instrument is regarded as the "gold standard" by experts. The disadvantages are: compared to most other methods they are relatively expensive; the fact that they do not prove ingestion of the medication; and the requirement that the bottle has to be returned in order to get a read-out of the data.

## DIRECT METHODS

### (7) Measured concentrations of drugs in plasma

Only a few drugs exhibit pharmaco-kinetic and pharmaco-dynamic properties that allow for a good estimation of compliance from their concentrations in plasma. This conclusion is based on the large intra- and inter-patient variability between drug absorption, metabolism and excretion characteristics, and the relatively short half-life of many drugs (up to 24 hours) that do not allow accurate estimates of patient compliance over a longer period than a few days. In fact, some anecdotal evidence exists of patients in a clinical trial who only took a few doses immediately prior to the clinical visit (de Klerk, 1997), but who always maintained plasma levels in the low-normal range.

Several drugs and metabolites have been studied that, as markers, could overcome the above-mentioned problems, e.g., phenobarbitone, digoxin, phenol red or disulfiram. Of these, only phenobarbitone has proved to be a valuable addition to the chemical markers' arsenal.

## OTHER METHODS

### (8) Clinical outcome

Some authors have suggested clinical outcome as a measure of compliance, starting at the notion that compliance determines plasma levels, and plasma levels determine clinical outcome. It has the attractive property of looking at the most significant parameter of compliance, but is not very precise, and hardly offers a useful concept to study com-

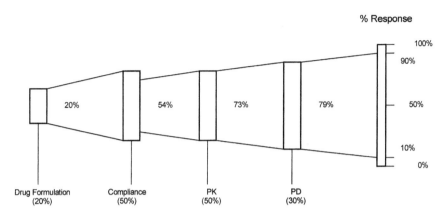

Figure 11.2. Sources of variability in drug response in the individual patient.

pliance. Although clinical outcome as a surrogate for compliance may be of some use in large epidemiological surveys, the complex interaction of the many factors relating to improved or deteriorating clinical condition generally renders this method of limited value as a stand-alone measurement of compliance (McGavock, 1996).

The interaction between various factors contributing to clinical outcome has been nicely described for theophylline (Harter & Peck, 1991), a drug that was widely used in the treatment of asthma. Figure 11.2 shows the cumulative effect of several known sources of variability in outcome of drug therapy based on data from experience with theophylline.

The percentages in the boxes are the relative contribution of various sources of variability to the cumulative total variability in clinical outcome, modeled as the % response. The drug formulation, the chemical substances that are necessary to deliver the drug in an indigestible form (chemical buffers, materials for the capsule, etc.) contributes 20% of the overall variation. Variations in compliance, with the addition of 50% to the overall variation in clinical outcome, is together with the pharmaco-kinetic (PK) properties of the drug (the combined process of absorption, distribution, metabolization and excretion of the drug in the body) the largest source of variation. Pharmaco-dynamic (PD) properties (drug-receptor interactions and intra-cellular mechanisms responsible for the clinical effect) contribute only 30% of the overall variation.

The theory was that reducing variance due to minor sources resulted in a small impact on the overall variability. For example: elimination of the variance due to drug formulation (by giving the drug intravenously) reduces overall variability by only 2.19%. Elimination of the variability of compliance (e.g., by directly observed therapy) would in this model result in a reduction of 17% of overall variability in clinical outcome (Harter & Peck, 1991).

*(9) Direct observation*

Direct observation of drug intake is a technique that has been developed in the United States to ensure long-term medication compliance with tuberculosis treatment. It is a combination of intervention and a measurement instrument at the same time. A large retrospective analysis of all available data in one US city before and after directly observed therapy (DOT) was introduced showed that despite a higher prevalence of tuberculosis (TBC) in the population and a higher percentage of intravenous drug users and homeless among TBC patients, a rigorously executed DOT system reduced both the primary resistance (from 13 to 6.7%) and the acquired resistance (from 14 to 2.1%) compared to the period before DOT. This remarkable result was accomplished with the same hospital staff as before the DOT was started (Weis et al., 1994).

*(10) Duration of treatment*

Some authors have suggested using the duration of treatment, for example as established in pharmacy databases by counting the number of consecutive prescriptions, as a measure of compliance (van Wanghe & Dequeker, 1982). Although the data that are collected in this way do not comply with either of the above mentioned definitions, it is notable that drop-out of therapy is the ultimate form of non-compliance. However, the data can only be used to compare continuation of drug use between different kinds of drugs, not related to individuals, and therefore will not be considered as a compliance measurement instrument here.

# Choosing the best compliance measurement instrument

It should be clear by now that the ideal compliance measurement instrument does not exist. Given the preceding discussion, however, it is possible to choose the method that fulfills the desired criteria.

To this end, the following questions should be answered:

- What is the objective of measuring compliance? For example, is it to: ensure that the drug is approximately ingested as prescribed; to compare compliance between two different formulations of the same drug; compare "forgiveness" for non-compliance between two drugs with the same actions but different PK and PD profiles; to assess the impact of a compliance intervention?

- What is the desired level of precision of the instrument: Is an average over a longer period of time sufficient, are exact interdose intervals needed?

- How important is it that ingestion is actually proven: If it is very important, then direct measurement instruments are the only choice, but, fortunately, many situations do not need the proof of ingestion *per se*.

- How important is it that the patient is unaware of the compliance measurement? There is often a trade-off between having an unaware

---

**Box 11.1    Some guidelines for choosing the optimal instruments based on Urquhart (1997)**

The researcher who is focused on:

- determining the impact of variable compliance on bulk pharmaceutical consumption will concentrate on the percentage of prescribed doses taken.

- determining the adequacy of therapeutic response, or on distinguishing between pharmacological nonresponse and non-compliance, or on determining the limits of compliance needed for good outcome, will concentrate on dosing chronologies, long intervals between doses and the clinical events that occur in their wake.

- predicting the likelihood of adverse reactions will concentrate on clusters of short-interval dosing and on occurrence of drug-holidays that may trigger adverse rebound or recurrent first-dose effects.

- the patient's behavior and ways to improve compliance, or on minimizing the impact of persistent partial compliance, will concentrate on the chronology of dosing to see within-day patterns, e.g., morning-evening; to see between-day patterns, e.g., weekday-weekend and proximate-remote from scheduled visits, and to see changes with the treatment duration.

- modeling drug dosing behavior will concentrate on the probabilities of transition between correct and incorrect dosing.

patient versus a lack of precision of the method such as the use of pharmacy databases and physician estimates.

# Examples of application of compliance measurement methodology

With the preceding discussion on advantages and disadvantages of the various methods in mind we will discuss three practical applications of compliance measurement chosen to cover a broad range of instruments: questionnaires, chemical markers and electronic monitoring.

*Example 1: questionnaires*
Examples of well-designed questionnaires developed specifically for measuring patient compliance are the Long Term Medication Behavior Scale (LTMBS; de Geest et al., 1994), the Wisconsin Brief Medication Questionnaire (BMQ; Svarstad et al., 1999) and the Compliance Questionnaire Rheumatology (CQR-19; de Klerk et al., 1997a, 1999). Both the LTMBS and the BMQ have been validated against electronic monitoring data, and will be discussed in detail below. The CQR still has to be validated against electronic monitoring data and is therefore not discussed in detail in the present chapter.

The development of the LTMBS questionnaire consisted of in-depth patient interviews targeted on the questions: (a) which knowledge and skills do you think are necessary in order to take your medication correctly? and (b) can you describe situations in which it is more difficult for you to take your medication correctly ? The responses on the interviews were taped and transcribed, and qualitatively analyzed. This approach yielded 13 themes, which were subsequently organized in Bandura's (1977) three dimensions: (1) personal attributes, (2) environmental factors, and (3) task-related and behavioral factors (Table 11.2).

The 26-item LTMBS applies a 5-point Likert scale, and the total score is calculated by averaging the scores on all items so that higher scores reflect higher levels of self-efficacy, defined as the perception that one can master a certain task or perform adequately in a given situation. The internal consistency in one study with 150 renal transplant recipients, measured by Cronbach's alpha, was 0.88 (de Geest, 1996).

The BMQ is a 25-item questionnaire divided into several sections assessing different types of compliance and patient perceived barriers

Table 11.2. Organization of themes into dimensions of personal attributes in the Long Term Medication Behavior Scale (LTMBS; de Geest et al., 1994).

| Personal attributes | Environmental factors | Task-related and behavioral factors |
| --- | --- | --- |
| —emotional distress | —routine | —medication aids |
| —perceived health scores | —distraction | —medication schedule |
| —normalcy | —cost of medication | —drug delivery system |
| —confidence in the physician | —social support | —knowledge |
| | | —side-effects |

From: De Geest et al., (1994).

to compliance. Item writing was based on the authors' experience. Six sections, or "screens", are distinguishable and are referred to as Dose-, Knowledge-, Outcome-, Recall-, Access- and Other Barriers screens. Svarstad et al. (1996) used the BMQ to assess compliance in 98 patients on phosphate binders used in dialyses protocols, and validated it against electronic monitoring data. The results showed that one in four patients took less then 20% of the prescribed doses, and of this subgroup 80% were identified as non-compliers by the BMQ Dose Screen. The BMQ also clarified several potential (practical) barriers to non-compliance that can be starting points for intervention. In addition the authors found a significant negative association between compliance as measured by electronic monitoring and the BMQ Knowledge, Outcome, Recall and Access screens.

The potential advantage of a measure like the BMQ is its applicability in any field of medicine, instead of being targeted to one specific field such as the LTMBS to transplant patients. The disadvantage is that specific aspects of therapy in a given field are not explored in detail, such as the discomfort of frequent toilet visits on diuretics, negative beliefs regarding the long-term effects of steroids, for example, and so on. If this is desirable, general measures like the BMQ may lack validity and sensitivity to change. In such situations, the investigators should develop medication-specific modules to assess adequately such specific problems, analogous to the disease-specific measures developed for quality of life (see also chapter 16 in this volume).

*Example 2: chemical markers*
A good example of what can be done with validated markers is the work of the group in Leeds (Feely et al., 1987; Peaker et al., 1989;

Pullar et al., 1988a; 1989). These investigators used low-dose phenobarbitone added to the active drug to test the intake of these drugs. Phenobarbitone in a dose of 2 mg has no pharmacological or clinical activity, has a long half-life (approximately four days), and there are very sensitive measurement methods available to determine very low phenobarbitone plasma levels such as enhanced immuno-assays and HPLC (Peaker et al., 1989). The intra- and inter-patient variability is relatively low when age is taken into account. Therefore, low dose phenobarbitone, when added to another drug, reflects intake for a relatively long period (2 weeks), challenging the detection capabilities for the majority of drugs currently in the market. This minimizes the sampling effect, the phenomenon that plasma levels only reflect the drug intake during a very brief period prior to the taking of the blood sample.

One accomplishment of this method was revealing the great discrepancies between phenobarbitone data and pill-counts. Results of three studies were combined in one analysis: (1) a study with 179 patients with type II diabetes mellitus given their usual drugs and, in addition, 2 mg phenobarbitone randomized to be taken once, twice, or three times daily (Pullar et al., 1988a); (2) a study with 26 rheumatoid arthritis patients; who had inadequate therapeutic response despite high-dose penicillamine (Pullar et al., 1988b); and (3) a study with 20 poorly controlled type II diabetes mellitus patients receiving glibenclamide (Feely et al., 1989). All patients were given an excess of pills to allow for detection of pill-dumping. Pill counts and level-to-dose ratios were compared; the results are described in Table 11.3.

Table 11.3. Comparison of pill-counts and phenobarbitone level to dose ratios (PB, LDE).

| | Compliance by pill-count | | | | | |
| | <30% | 30–59% | 60–89% | 90–109% | >110% | failed to return container |
|---|---|---|---|---|---|---|
| **PB LDR** | | | | | | |
| <30% | 1 | 4 | 1 | 2 | 1 | 0 |
| 30–59% | 0 | 6 | 8 | 9 | 0 | 2 |
| 60–89% | 0 | 0 | 9 | 66 | 5 | 4 |
| 90% or more | 0 | 0 | 4 | 84 | 4 | 6 |

From: Pullar et al. (1989)

From this table it becomes clear that pill-counts tend to overestimate compliance compared to the marker data. It is also clear that the phenobarbitone method is capable of detecting "pill-dumping". In fact, the authors were so convinced by these results that they concluded that "return tablet count grossly overestimates compliance".

### Example 3: electronic monitoring

One particularly well worked out example of a study with electronic monitoring data was a randomized, double blinded phase III study to compare the efficacy and effectiveness of once daily 20 mg piroxicam vs once daily 20 mg tenoxicam in ankylosing spondylitis, a painful inflammatory disorder of predominantly the spine (de Klerk & van der Linden, 1996). Sixty-five patients were followed for an average duration of 225 days with electronic monitoring. Analysis of the clinical results showed that both drugs performed equally with respect to efficacy and safety. The initial summary of compliance data is shown in Table 11.4.

A subsequent effort to capture the wide variability of compliance in that trial resulted in a table summarizing both frequency and duration of drug holidays (Table 11.5). The columns in the table reflect some basic patient identifiers, followed by the frequency of dosing omissions in drug holidays of variable length: 1–10 days, and the frequency of longer holidays. All data for individuals are shown, and the patients are rank-ordered by percentage of days in which the prescribed number of drugs were taken (labeled "compliance"). To emphasize the amount of variation in the table, a fictitious "average complier" was added to the table.

Table 11.4. example of compliance data gathered with electronic monitoring

|  | All patients  (n=65) |
| --- | --- |
| Days monitored | 14.607 |
| % days of which at least one dose taken | 81 |
| % days of which dose taken as prescribed | 78 |
| % days with extra doses | 3 |
| % days with missed doses | 19 |

From: de Klerk & van der Linden (1996).

Table 11.5. Listing of individual patient's frequency of drug holidays rank-ordered by compliance.

| Patient number | Treatment | Duration of drug holidays (in days) | | | | | | | | | | Total | Number of monitored days | Compliance |
|---|---|---|---|---|---|---|---|---|---|---|---|---|---|---|
| | | 1 | 2 | 3 | 4 | 5 | 6 | 7 | 8 | 9 | 10 or more | | | |
| *100% compliance (n=5)* | | | | | | | | | | | | | | |
| 138 | tenoxicam | . | . | . | . | . | . | . | . | . | . | 0 | 373 | 100 |
| 122 | piroxicam | . | . | . | . | . | . | . | . | . | . | 0 | 345 | 100 |
| 134 | tenoxicam | . | . | . | . | . | . | . | . | . | . | 0 | 233 | 100 |
| 130 | tenoxicam | . | . | . | . | . | . | . | . | . | . | 0 | 107 | 100 |
| 84 | piroxicam | . | . | . | . | . | . | . | . | . | . | 0 | 55 | 100 |
| *95–99% compliance (n=15):* | | | | | | | | | | | | | | |
| 133 | piroxicam | 3 | . | . | . | . | . | . | . | . | . | 3 | 298 | 99 |
| 128 | tenoxicam | 2 | . | . | . | . | . | . | . | . | . | 2 | 119 | 98 |
| 58 | tenoxicam | 4 | 1 | . | . | . | . | . | . | . | . | 6 | 352 | 98 |
| 93 | tenoxicam | 2 | . | . | . | . | . | . | . | . | . | 2 | 111 | 98 |
| 3 | tenoxicam | 5 | . | . | . | . | . | . | . | . | . | 5 | 223 | 98 |
| 124 | piroxicam | 5 | . | . | . | 1 | . | . | . | . | . | 10 | 369 | 97 |
| 66 | piroxicam | 2 | 1 | . | . | . | . | . | . | . | . | 4 | 126 | 97 |
| 140 | piroxicam | 2 | 2 | . | . | 1 | . | . | . | . | . | 11 | 332 | 97 |
| 59 | piroxicam | 8 | . | . | . | . | . | . | . | . | . | 8 | 227 | 96 |
| 78 | tenoxicam | 4 | 2 | . | . | . | . | . | . | . | . | 8 | 223 | 96 |
| 96 | piroxicam | 4 | . | . | . | . | . | . | . | . | . | 4 | 111 | 96 |
| 137 | tenoxicam | 5 | . | . | . | . | . | . | . | . | . | 5 | 127 | 96 |
| 123 | piroxicam | 6 | . | . | . | . | . | . | . | 1 | . | 15 | 375 | 96 |

(to be continued)

Table 11.5. Listing of individual patient's frequencies of drug holidays rank-ordered by compliance (*continued*).

| Patient number | Treatment | Duration of drug holidays (in days) | | | | | | | | | | Total | Number of monitored days | Compliance |
|---|---|---|---|---|---|---|---|---|---|---|---|---|---|---|
| | | 1 | 2 | 3 | 4 | 5 | 6 | 7 | 8 | 9 | 10 or more | | | |
| 108 | tenoxicam | 9 | . | . | . | . | . | . | . | . | . | 9 | 224 | 96 |
| 23 | tenoxicam | 8 | 1 | . | . | . | . | . | . | . | . | 10 | 223 | 96 |
| *91–95% compliance (n=13)* | | | | | | | | | | | | | | |
| 94 | tenoxicam | 3 | 1 | . | . | . | . | . | . | . | . | 5 | 111 | 95 |
| 51 | piroxicam | 10 | . | . | . | . | . | 1 | . | . | . | 17 | 372 | 95 |
| 139 | piroxicam | 2 | . | . | 2 | . | . | 1 | . | . | . | 17 | 345 | 95 |
| 68 | tenoxicam | 7 | 2 | . | . | . | . | . | . | . | . | 11 | 223 | 95 |
| 1 | piroxicam | 5 | . | 1 | 1 | . | . | . | . | . | . | 12 | 223 | 95 |
| 6 | tenoxicam | 1 | 1 | . | . | . | . | . | . | . | . | 3 | 55 | 95 |
| 45 | piroxicam | 10 | 2 | . | . | . | . | . | . | . | . | 14 | 223 | 94 |
| 104 | piroxicam | 7 | 1 | . | 1 | . | . | . | . | . | 11 | 24 | 357 | 93 |
| 90 | piroxicam | 9 | 1 | . | . | . | . | . | . | . | . | 11 | 158 | 93 |
| 116 | piroxicam | 13 | 2 | . | . | . | . | . | . | . | . | 17 | 216 | 92 |
| 129 | piroxicam | 9 | 1 | 2 | . | . | . | . | . | . | . | 17 | 215 | 92 |
| 97 | tenoxicam | 16 | 1 | . | . | . | . | . | . | . | . | 18 | 213 | 92 |
| 14 | tenoxicam | 17 | . | . | 1 | . | . | . | . | . | . | 21 | 223 | 91 |
| *80–90% compliance (n=9):* | | | | | | | | | | | | | | |
| 67 | tenoxicam | 17 | 2 | . | . | . | . | . | . | . | 13 | 34 | 351 | 90 |
| 12 | piroxicam | 13 | . | . | . | . | . | . | . | . | . | 13 | 124 | 90 |
| 25 | piroxicam | 14 | 3 | . | 1 | . | . | . | . | . | . | 24 | 223 | 89 |

(to be continued)

**Table 11.5.** Listing of individual patient's frequencies of drug holidays rank-ordered by compliance (*continued*).

| Patient number | Treatment | Duration of drug holidays (in days) | | | | | | | | | | Total | Number of monitored days | Compliance |
|---|---|---|---|---|---|---|---|---|---|---|---|---|---|---|
| | | 1 | 2 | 3 | 4 | 5 | 6 | 7 | 8 | 9 | 10 or more | | | |
| 87 | tenoxicam | 8 | 2 | 1 | . | . | . | . | . | . | . | 15 | 131 | 89 |
| 39 | piroxicam | 23 | 2 | . | . | . | . | . | . | . | . | 27 | 223 | 88 |
| 28 | tenoxicam | 11 | 1 | . | . | . | . | . | . | . | 16 | 29 | 223 | 87 |
| 88 | tenoxicam | 29 | 3 | 1 | . | . | . | . | . | . | 18 | 56 | 369 | 85 |
| 105 | piroxicam | 11 | 2 | . | . | . | 1 | 1 | . | . | 13 | 41 | 223 | 82 |
| 111 | tenoxicam | 17 | 4 | 2 | 1 | . | . | . | 1 | . | . | 43 | 223 | 81 |

*60–80% compliance (n=11):*
average patient

| Patient number | Treatment | 1 | 2 | 3 | 4 | 5 | 6 | 7 | 8 | 9 | 10 or more | Total | Number of monitored days | Compliance |
|---|---|---|---|---|---|---|---|---|---|---|---|---|---|---|
| 91 | piroxicam | 12 | 3 | 1 | 1 | 0 | 0 | 0 | 0 | 0 | 19 | 44 | 225 | 79 |
| 46 | piroxicam | 9 | . | . | . | . | 1 | . | . | . | 13  24 | 52 | 221 | 77 |
| 135 | piroxicam | 36 | 8 | 3 | . | . | . | . | . | 1 | 16 | 86 | 350 | 75 |
| 18 | piroxicam | 35 | 6 | . | 1 | 1 | . | . | . | . | . | 56 | 223 | 75 |
| 43 | tenoxicam | 31 | 2 | 4 | 1 | 1 | . | . | . | . | . | 56 | 223 | 75 |
| 103 | tenoxicam | 9 | 2 | 2 | 1 | . | . | 1 | . | . | . | 30 | 111 | 73 |
| 60 | tenoxicam | 42 | 7 | 3 | . | . | . | . | . | . | . | 65 | 229 | 72 |
| 24 | piroxicam | 13 | 3 | 1 | . | . | . | . | . | . | 30 | 52 | 167 | 69 |
| 126 | piroxicam | 42 | 15 | 6 | . | 1 | . | . | . | . | 13  19 | 127 | 379 | 66 |
| 114 | piroxicam | 26 | 2 | 2 | 2 | 1 | . | . | . | . | 31 | 80 | 216 | 63 |
| 19 | piroxicam | 11 | 4 | 1 | . | . | . | . | . | . | 14  27 | 63 | 169 | 63 |

(to be continued)

**Table 11.5.** Listing of individual patient's frequencies of drug holidays rank-ordered by compliance (*continued*).

| Patient number | Treatment | Duration of drug holidays (in days) | | | | | | | | | | Total | Number of monitored days | Compliance |
|---|---|---|---|---|---|---|---|---|---|---|---|---|---|---|
| | | 1 | 2 | 3 | 4 | 5 | 6 | 7 | 8 | 9 | 10 or more | | | |
| *0–60% compliance (n=11)* | | | | | | | | | | | | | | |
| 57 | tenoxicam | 8 | 2 | 1 | 2 | 2 | 1 | . | . | . | 10  13 13 37 . | 112 | 245 | 54 |
| 95 | tenoxicam | 22 | 4 | 3 | 1 | . | . | 1 | 1 | . | 13  13 33 . . | 104 | 227 | 54 |
| 7 | tenoxicam | 27 | 13 | 1 | 7 | 2 | . | 2 | . | 1 | .  . . . . | 117 | 223 | 48 |
| 121 | tenoxicam | 28 | 6 | 5 | 1 | 4 | 7 | 3 | . | . | 10  12 14 39 . | 217 | 372 | 42 |
| 42 | piroxicam | 18 | 8 | 4 | 7 | 1 | 6 | 1 | . | . | 10  . . . . | 132 | 225 | 41 |
| 102 | piroxicam | 11 | 6 | 4 | . | 1 | 2 | 1 | 1 | 1 | 10  27 . . . | 113 | 191 | 41 |
| 131 | tenoxicam | 20 | 11 | 3 | 5 | . | 1 | . | . | 1 | 15  19 25 33 52 | 230 | 350 | 34 |
| 9 | piroxicam | 6 | 5 | 2 | 4 | 2 | . | . | . | . | 12  13 . . . | 81 | 122 | 34 |
| 83 | tenoxicam | 11 | 3 | 2 | 1 | . | 2 | . | 1 | . | 12  111. . . | 162 | 222 | 27 |
| 106 | piroxicam | 5 | 8 | 3 | . | . | . | . | . | . | 24  29 . . . | 83 | 111 | 25 |
| 4 | piroxicam | 2 | 1 | . | 1 | . | . | . | . | . | 12  82 . . . | 102 | 126 | 19 |
| 32 | tenoxicam | 1 | 2 | . | . | . | 1 | . | . | . | 16  31 37 . . | 95 | 105 | 10 |

The diversity of drug exposure revealed by electronic monitoring data when arranged in this format is astonishing. It captures not only the wide variability of compliance over the whole group (from almost 0 to 100% when measured as number of drugs taken correctly), but also shows that patients in the lower regions of the table not only have longer holidays, but also more frequent shorter holidays.

Given the long measurement period (average 225 days), another obvious question arises: can these patients be identified at an early stage during trial planning, such as a run-in period, and be either excluded or stratified (depending on trial goals and strategy)? No adequate answers to this question exist yet, but projects are under way to explore this important issue.

A perhaps surprising finding with the spreading use of electronic monitoring is the similarity of compliance distribution in various fields of medicine, and between very different drugs. Figure 11.3 is one such example, being a histogram showing the distribution of patient compliance in bands of 10% for Non Steriodal Anti Inflammatory Drug (NSAIDs) in ankylosing spondylitis (de Klerk & van der Linden, 1996), β-blocker eye-drops for open angle glaucoma (Kass et al., 1987) and anti-epileptic medication for epilepsy (Cramer et al., 1989).

Though there seems to be a small difference in distributions in the high region, all three studies show a wide distribution of compliance in the middle and lower regions. Note, however, that these are three entirely different diseases in terms of symptoms and medication, expectation of the therapy, and typical age distribution of the patients.

## Conclusion

This chapter has reviewed several aspects related to the measurement of patient compliance on drug regimen. Measurement of patient compliance in clinical trials has long been ignored, following the re-analyses of the Coronary Drug Project. However, it is now clear that the findings of this trial were not conclusive, and subsequent research has shown the great importance of accurate compliance measurement for drawing adequate results.

No "gold standard" for compliance measurement exists, and none is foreseeable. Therefore we have discussed the advantages and disadvantages of ten different measurement methods, and the objective of compliance measurement has been emphasized. We have seen that it is

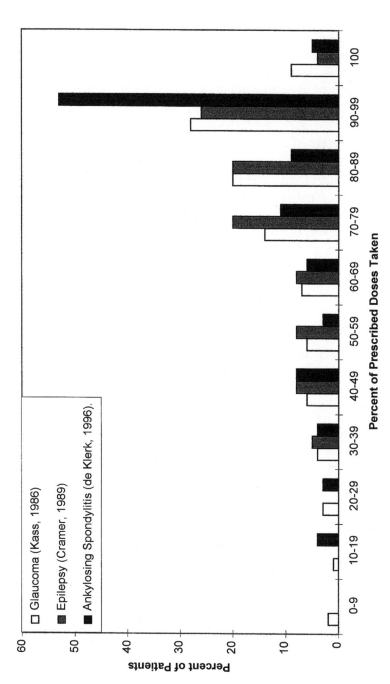

Figure 11.3. Frequency histogram of the percentages of prescribed doses taken by three groups of patients with different diseases.

possible to combine instruments and tailor them to specific research questions.

Three examples of studies utilizing the various methods to their advantage have been discussed, and several important aspects of the methods have been described. This overview can serve as a starting point for the development of new compliance-focused research questions.

## Acknowledgment

The author is indebted to John Urquhart for introducing him to the various aspects of patient compliance and for many cheerful discussions on the subject and useful comments on the content of this chapter. In addition, the author would like to thank Désirée van der Heijde and Sjef van der Linden for reviewing the chapter. This work was completed under a grant from the Dutch Rheumatism Foundation.

## References

Bandura, A. (1977) Analysis of self-efficacy theory of behavioral change. *Cognitive Therapy Research, 1*, 287–310.

CDP Group (1973). The Coronary Drug Project: Design, methods, and baseline results. *Circulation, 47 (Suppl 1)*, 1–179.

CDP Group (1974). Clofibrate and niacin in coronary heart disease. *Journal of Chronic Diseases, 27*, 267–285.

CDP (1980). Influence of adherence to treatment and response of cholesterol on mortality in the coronary drug project. *New England Journal of Medicine, 303*, 1038–1041.

Cox, D.R. (1998). Analyzing non-compliance in clinical trials. Invited discussion. *Statistics in Medicine*, 387–389.

Cramer, J.A., Mattson, R.H., Prevey, M.L., Scheyer, R.D., & Ouellette, V.L. (1989). How often is medication taken as prescribed? A novel assessment technique. *Journal of American Medial Association, 261*, 3273–3277.

Cramer, J., Vachon, L., Desforges, C., & Sussman, N.M. (1995). Dose frequency and dose interval compliance with multiple antiepileptic medications during a controlled clinical trial. *Epilepsia, 36*, 1111–1117.

de Geest, S. (1996). *Subclinical non-compliance with immunosuppresive therapy in heart transplant recipients: A cluster analytic study*. Doctoral thesis, Katholieke Universiteit Leuven, Leuven, Belgium.

de Geest, S. (1997). Personal communication with Dr. S. de Geest, Department of Public Health, University of Leuven, Belgium.

de Geest, S., Abraham, I., Gemoets, H., & Evers, G. (1994). Development of the long-term medication behaviour self-efficacy scale: Qualitative study for item development. *Journal of Advanced Nursing, 19*, 233–238.

de Klerk, E. (1997). Patient compliance in hypertension. *CardioTopics, 4*, 7–21.

de Klerk, E., & van der Linden, S.J. (1996). Compliance monitoring of NSAID drug therapy in ankylosing spondylitis: Experiences with an electronic monitoring device. *British Journal of Rheumatology, 35*, 60–65.

de Klerk, E., van der Heijde, D., & van der Linden, S. (1997a). Development of a measure for exploring variable patient compliance. *Arthritis and Rheumatism, 40*, S114.

de Klerk, E., van der Heijde, D., van der Linden, S., & Urquhart, J. (1997b). *A simple yet effective patient compliance simulation model.* Paper presented at the Modelling and Simulation of Clinical Trials and Drug Development Congress, Washington DC, USA.

de Klerk, E., van der Heijde, D., van der Tempel, H., & van der Linden, S. (1999). Development of a questionnaire to investigate patient compliance with antirheumatic drug therapy. *Journal of Rheumatology, 26*, 2635–2641.

Dolan-Mullen, P. (1997). Compliance becomes concordance. *British Medical Journal, 314*, 691–692.

Efron, B., & Feldman, D. (1991). Compliance as an explanatory variable in clinical trials. *Journal of the American Statistical Association, 86*, 9–26.

Feely, M., Cooke, J., Price, D., Singleton, S., Mehta, A., Bradford, L., & Calvert, R. (1987). Low-dose phenobarbitone as an indicator of compliance with drug therapy. *British Journal of Clinical Pharmacology, 24*, 77–83.

Feely, M., Price, D., Bodansky, H.J., & Tindall, H. (1989). Use of a pharmacologic indicator to assess compliance with drug therapy in patients with poorly-controlled type II diabetes. *British Journal of Clinical Pharmacology, 27*, 101P–102P.

Feinstein, A.R. (1990). On white-coat effects and the electronic monitoring of compliance. *Archives of Internal Medicine, 150*, 1377–1378.

Feinstein, A.R. (1991). Intent-to-treat policy for analyzing randomized trials. Statistical distortions and neglected clinical challenges. In: J.A. Cramer & B. Spilker (Eds.), *Patient compliance in medical practice and clinical trials* (pp. 359–370). New York: Raven Press Ltd.

Girard, P., Sheiner, L.B., Kastrissios, H., & Blaschke, T.F. (1996). Do we need full compliance data for population pharmacokinetic analysis? *Journal of Pharmacokinetics and Biopharmaceutics, 24*, 265–281.

Goetghebeur, E.J., & Shapiro, S.H. (1996). Analysing non-compliance in clinical trials: Ethical imperative or mission impossible? *Statistics in Medicine, 15*, 2813–2826.

Guillebaud, J. (1993). Any questions? *British Medical Journal, 307*, 617.

Harter, J.G., & Peck, C.C. (1991). Chronobiology. Suggestions for integrating it into drug development. *Annals of the New York Academy of Science, 618*, 563–571

Hasford, J. (1991). Biometric issues in measuring and analyzing partial compliance in clinical trials. In: J.A. Cramer & B. Spilker (Eds.), *Patient compliance in medical practice and clinical trials* (pp. 265–281). New York: Raven Press Ltd.

Hippocrates. (ca 400 BC). *Decorum.*

Joyce, C.R.B. (1962). Patient cooperation and the sensitivity of clinical trials. *Journal of Chronic Diseases, 15,* 1025–1036.

Kass, M.A., Gordon, M., Morley, R.E., Jr., Meltzer, D.W., & Goldberg, J.J. (1987). Compliance with topical timolol treatment. *American Journal of Ophthalmology 103,* 188–193.

Lasagna, L., & Hutt, P.B. (1991). Health care, research and regulatory impact of non-compliance. In: J.A. Cramer & B. Spilker (Eds.), *Patient compliance in medical practice and clinical trials* (pp. 393–403). New York: Raven Press Ltd.

LRCPPT (1984a). The Lipid Research Clinics Coronary Primary Prevention Trial results. I. Reduction in incidence of coronary heart disease. *Journal of the American Medical Association, 251,* 351–364.

LRCPPT (1984b). The Lipid Research Clinics Coronary Primary Prevention Trial results. II. The relationship of reduction in incidence of coronary heart disease to cholesterol lowering. *Journal of the American Medical Association, 251,* 365–374.

McGavock, H. (1996). *A review of the literature on drug adherence.* Queen's University, Belfast.

Moulding, T. (1962). Proposal for a time recording pill dispenser as a method for studying and supervising the self-administration of drugs. *American Review of Respiratory Disorders, 85,* 754–757.

Mushlin, A.I., & Appel, F.A. (1977). Diagnosing potential non-compliance. Physicians' ability in a behavioral dimension of medical care. *Archives of Internal Medicine, 137,* 318–321.

Peaker, S., Mehta, A.C., Kumar, S., & Feely, M. (1989). Measurement of low (sub-therapeutic) phenobarbitone levels in plasma by high-performance liquid chromatography: Application to patient compliance studies. *Journal of Chromatography, 497,* 308–312.

Pullar, T., Birtwell, A.J., Wiles, P.G., Hay, A., & Feely, M.P. (1988a). Use of a pharmacologic indicator to compare compliance with tablets prescribed to be taken once, twice, or three times daily. *Clinical Pharmacology and Therapeutics, 44,* 540–545.

Pullar, T., Kumar, S., Tindall, H., & Feely, M. (1989). Time to stop counting the tablets? *Clinical Pharmacology and Therapeutics, 46,* 163–168.

Pullar, T., Peaker, S., Martin, M.F., Bird, H.A., & Feely, M.P. (1988b). The use of a pharmacological indicator to investigate compliance in patients with a poor response to antirheumatic therapy. *British Journal of Rheumatology, 27,* 381–384.

Rubin, D.B. (1998). More powerful randomization-based p-values in double-blind trials with non-compliance. *Statistics in Medicine, 17,* 251–267.

Sackett, D.L., & Haynes, R.B. (1976). *Compliance with therapeutic regimens.* Baltimore, MD: Johns Hopkins University Press.

Svarstad, B.L. Chewning, B.A., Sleath, B.L. & Claesson, C. (1999), The brief medication questionnaire: A tool for screening patient adherence and barriers to adherence. *Patient Education & Counselling, 37,* 113–124.

Urquhart, J. (1997). The electronic medication event monitor – lessons for pharmacotherapy. *Clinical Pharmacokinetics, 32,* 345–356.

Urquhart, J., & Chevalley, C. (1988). Impact of unrecognized dosing errors on the cost and effectiveness of pharmaceuticals. *Drug Information Journal, 22,* 363–378.

van Wanghe, P., & Dequeker, J. (1982). Compliance and long-term effect of azathioprine in 65 rheumatoid arthritis cases. *Annals of Rheumatic Disorders, 41( Suppl 1),* 40–43.

Vanhove, G.F., Schapiro, J.M., Winters, M.A., Merigan, T.C., & Blaschke, T.F. (1996). Patient compliance and drug failure in protease inhibitor monotherapy. *Journal of the American Medical Association, 276,* 1955–1956.

Vrijens, B., & Goetghebeur, E. (1997). Comparing compliance patterns between randomized treatments. *Controlled Clinical Trials, 18,* 187–203.

Waterhouse, D.M., Calzone, K.A., Mele, C., & Brenner, D.E. (1993). Adherence to oral tamoxifen: A comparison of patient self-report, pill counts, and microelectronic monitoring. *Journal of Clinical Oncology, 11,* 1189–1197.

Weis, S.E., Slocum, P.C., Blais, F.X., King, B., Nunn, M., Matney, G.B., Gomez, E., & Foresman, B.H. (1994). The effect of directly observed therapy on the rates of drug resistance and relapse in tuberculosis. *New England Journal of Medicine, 330,* 1179–1184.

# 2 ASSESSMENT OF LIFE STYLE

Jan Snel and Jos Twisk

The assessment of lifestyle is an important issue in behavioral medicine and health psychology. First of all it is assumed that a "healthy" lifestyle is preventive for many chronic diseases, and so lifestyle is frequently used as an independent variable in (mainly epidemiological) studies. Secondly, lifestyle parameters are used as dependent variables in studies investigating its determinants of lifestyle or in studies evaluating prevention programs like the promotion of physical activity or quitting smoking. Another example of the importance of lifestyle parameters concerns their mediating role in studies relating personality characteristics or stressor exposure to health outcomes. Because in (epidemiological) research lifestyle generally includes physical activity, dietary intake, alcohol consumption, smoking, and caffeine consumption, this chapter will be focused on these lifestyle parameters.

## Activity and diet

Methods of measuring activity and dietary patterns have been described and are available in some excellent textbooks and review papers (Montoye et al., 1996; Willet, 1990). The aim of this chapter is not to give an extensive overview of all these methods but rather to mention the different methods briefly and then focus on some related methodological issues. Furthermore, the different methods will be discussed in light of the assessment of overall, general habitual physical activity and dietary intake, because these are the parameters of most interest.

### HABITUAL PHYSICAL ACTIVITY
Habitual physical activity has been recognized as an important component of lifestyle. Physical inactivity is not only related to chronic somatic diseases like coronary heart disease (Paffenbarger et al., 1986), diabetes mellitus (Helmrich et al., 1991), certain types of cancer (Lee et al., 1991), osteoporosis (Marcus et al., 1992), and chronic lung disease

(McClaren et al., 1995), but also to chronic mental diseases (King et al., 1989). The importance of habitual physical activity is not only reflected in the relative risk of physical inactivity, but also by the high prevalence of physical inactivity in Western society; the so-called population attributable risk (PAR) of physical inactivity for different chronic diseases is very high (Powel & Blair, 1994).

## ASSESSMENT OF HABITUAL PHYSICAL ACTIVITY

The methods used to measure physical activity can be divided into *direct* and *indirect* measurements. With the direct measurements one is trying to measure the absolute amount of habitual physical activity; examples are behavioral (activity) observation, the activity diary, the activity questionnaire and interview. With indirect measurements one is trying to measure an indicator of the amount of habitual physical activity; examples are job classification, mechanical devices, physiological measurements and the method of "doubly labeled" water.

*Direct measurements of activity*: Behavioral (activity) observation (on site or by video assessment) is in principle probably the most valid way to measure habitual physical activity in individual subjects (McKenzie, 1991). One of the problems is that this method is very time consuming for the researcher, because when one is trying to get an idea of the habitual activity of the individual the observation period must be quite long. Another important problem of activity observation is that the subjects are (mostly) aware of the fact that they are observed, which may influence their "normal" activity pattern. The method is particularly useful when only a few particular activities must be observed (e.g., in ergonomics).

Activity questionnaires are widely used to assess habitual physical activity of individuals. The method is easy to apply, self-administered, not expensive, and therefore suitable for large (epidemiological) studies. Although many questionnaires are available (e.g., the Baecke questionnaire of habitual physical activity, the Bouchard three-day physical activity record, the Yale physical activity survey, etc.) they all basically assess the same concept. The questionnaires only differ in length, their focus on specific age groups, specific activities, specific countries, etc. An extensive review of available questionnaires was published by Kriska and Caspersen (1997).

The physical activity interview is more or less comparable to the activity questionnaire, but the interview is less widely used, because it is more time consuming for the researcher. However, more detailed information can be gathered with an interview than with a question-naire. Because for both interviews and questionnaires the subjects have to recall their habitual physical activity, self-report bias can be a problem. When using an interview technique, a new sort of bias, i.e., interviewer bias may be introduced. The only valid way to use an inter-view technique is for all subjects to be interviewed by the same person, which is almost impossible in large studies.

A final self-report methodology is the application of the activity diary, in which an individual reports his/her own activity periodically (Acheson et al., 1980). The reports can be very detailed or more gener-alized, and the time span over which activities must be recorded can range from several minutes to several days (or even longer periods). The major problem of using an activity diary is that it requires much effort from the participants, especially when one is interested in physi-cal activity over a longer period of time. With the activity diary, the subjects are more or less forced to think about their own physical activity, which can possibly influence their activity pattern. Furthermore, like all methods in which subjects report their own activ-ities, the diary method can be influenced by self-report bias.

*Indirect measurements of activity*: One of the most simple forms of measuring habitual physical activity indirectly is by job classification (Powel et al., 1987). It is obvious that this method is very limited and will only give a very rough estimation of habitual physical activity.

Other examples of indirect measurements of physical activity are the movement assessment devices. Probably the first device used was the pedometer (Kemper & Verschuur, 1977), which counts steps. Later, devices were invented with which not only steps, but also more general movements of the body could be measured. The latest innova-tion in this field is the three dimensional accelerometer (e.g., caltrac). The major advantage of these methods is that they are not influenced by self-report bias. However, with these methods the subjects are aware of the fact that they are measured, which can influence their activity pattern. Furthermore, if one is interested in intensities of the performed activities, these devices must be used in addition to other methods.

Sometimes heart rate monitoring is used to get an indication of habitual physical activity (Leger & Thivierge, 1988). Heart rate can be registered with different time intervals and can be stored over a longer period of time. Besides the problem that subjects are aware of the fact that they are measured, the fact that heart rate only gives an raw indication of habitual physical activity is also a problem. Increases in heart rate due to causes other than an increase in physical activity are also registered. Like the movement assessment devices, the heart rate monitors are only suitable for measuring habitual physical activity in combination with other methods.

Another indirect method to assess habitual physical activity is the measurement of physical fitness; i.e., maximal oxygen uptake (Saris, 1982). However, like most of the indirect measurements, maximal oxygen uptake gives only a raw indication of habitual physical activity; in fact it measures a different concept. It is therefore remarkable that it is widely used as an indicator of habitual physical activity, especially because maximal oxygen uptake is difficult to measure and very time consuming; i.e., not suitable in large studies. To illustrate the difficulties in using indirect measures to estimate habitual physical activity, in the Amsterdam Growth and Health Study (AGHS), maximal oxygen uptake was measured in combination with habitual physical activity assessed by a structured interview. The correlation coefficient between habitual physical activity and maximal oxygen uptake was lower than 0.15 (Van Mechelen et al., 1997).

Finally, a relatively new approach for measuring physical activity is the method of "doubly labeled" water (Schoeller, 1983). The idea behind the method is as follows: A known quantity of water in which both hydrogen and oxygen are "labeled" is consumed by the subjects under study. The labeled hydrogen and oxygen will leave the body as water (e.g., in urine, sweat, etc.) and as carbon dioxide. From the difference between the elimination rates of the two "isotopes" and the respiratory quotient, the uptake of oxygen (i.e., energy expenditure) for a particular time period can be calculated. Although the idea is quite simple, the technique is rather difficult to accomplish and expensive, so to date it is impossible to use in large studies. However, it can be used to validate other less precise methods (Seale et al., 1993). One of the problems is that this method is limited to the estimation of energy expenditure, which is only a rough estimation of habitual physical activity which is not always the variable unit in which one is interested.

## HABITUAL DIETARY INTAKE

Diet is not only a basic need for human beings in order to grow and develop, it is also associated with health and disease. Several dietary parameters are recognized as determinants of chronic diseases: the intake of fat (especially saturated fat) and cholesterol are related to coronary heart disease (Grundy & Denke, 1990); the intake of calcium is associated with osteoporosis (Cumming, 1990); several nutrients are related to different cancers (Willet et al., 1987); and the intake of retinol and unsaturated fatty acids to chronic lung disease (Morabia et al., 1990). The importance of dietary factors in the development of chronic diseases is not fully understood and is mostly based on indirect evidence. For instance, the fact that the lowest incidence of cardiovascular disease is observed in Japan, although the smoking prevalence is very high, is often attributed to differences in diet between Japan and other developed countries (Wright et al., 1994).

## ASSESSMENT OF HABITUAL DIETARY INTAKE

The methods to assess habitual dietary intake can also be divided into direct and indirect methods. The direct methods include the following approaches: (1) quantitative daily consumption recall methods (i.e., the 24-hour recall and the dietary diary); (2) behavioral (dietary) observation; and (3) dietary history methods (i.e., food frequency questionnaire and the cross-check dietary history). An indirect method to assess habitual dietary intake is the use of biological markers. One should take into account that no one method suits all purposes, and that a combination of different methods probably gives the most valid estimate of habitual dietary intake. Measuring habitual dietary intake deals with measurement of certain foods. Most researchers are not only interested in foods or food groups, but also in the habitual intake of macro- and micro-nutrients. So a transformation is needed in which foods are transformed into nutrients. For the macro-nutrients like carbohydrates, protein and fat this transformation does not introduce much error. However for micro-nutrients like sodium, potassium, etc., the validity of this transformation is often doubtful, even though special computer programs are available for this transformation.

*Direct dietary measurements: (1) Quantitative recall methods.* With the quantitative daily consumption recall methods, subjects are asked to recall or report their exact dietary intake of one or more days (Block, 1982). The 24-hour recall is probably the best described quantitative method to assess dietary intake. The purpose is to recall all foods and beverages consumed in the past 24 hours, including cooking methods, brand names, supplements, and other details. Furthermore, food models are used to document or estimate portion sizes. However, research suggests that individuals have great difficulty in estimating portion sizes, even when food models are used (Guthrie, 1984). It is further doubtful whether one single 24-hour recall accurately characterizes an individual's habitual dietary intake. Because the number of dietary products in Western countries has increased enormously, day-to-day variation can be a huge problem in the assessment of habitual dietary intake. Given this large day-to-day variation, the consensus is that multiple 24-hour recalls (in nutritional epidemiology also known as multiple-day food records) are best suited for most nutrition monitoring studies. However, infrequent or seasonal consumption of foods, such as fresh fruits and vegetables, may be difficult to assess even using multiple 24-hour recalls.

The dietary diary is used to recall all foods consumed over a certain amount of time. To get a more objective estimate of the amount of the different foods consumed, the participants using a dietary diary are often asked to weigh the consumed foods. This method is very demanding for the participants (sometimes they even need a training period) and is mostly limited to a short period of time. The shorter the time period, the more the estimation of habitual dietary intake is biased by day-to-day variation. Both quantitative recall methods are influenced by self-report bias.

*(2) Dietary observation.* With a dietary observation method (which can be limited to a one day observation or can take several days) the same information is collected as with the quantitative daily consumption recall methods; but in the dietary observation method the information is gathered by the researcher, so reducing the influence of self-report bias. Like the activity observation, however, the method is very time consuming for the researcher and dietary intake can be influenced by the fact that the participants are aware that they are observed. Furthermore, the method is biased by, day-to-day dietary variation; a problem which is reduced the longer the observation period will last.

*(3) Dietary history methods.* The purpose of food frequency questionnaires (FFQ) is to obtain information on habitual dietary intake over an extended period (for example the last three months or the last year) (Hankin, 1992). FFQs are used to obtain qualitative, descriptive information about habitual food consumption patterns. They use a list of food and frequency-of-use response categories from which the intakes are supposed to represent usual intakes over an extended period of time. An FFQ can be self- or interviewer administered.

With the cross-check dietary history method, subjects are asked by the interviewer to estimate their "average daily consumption" over a period of one or more months before the interview. As with the FFQ, the bias caused by day-to-day variation is reduced, but it seems to be very difficult to estimate the "average daily consumption". In large (epidemiological) studies it is often not feasible to use extensive dietary survey methods. Therefore short FFQs are mostly used to assess the food intake, with the limitation that the method is rather crude and inexact. Both dietary history methods can be very extensive to cover one's complete daily food intake but also short in order to measure the intake of specific foods or food groups (e.g., the intake of calcium in relation to osteoporosis). One of the problems with these methods is the difficulty in making the distinction between frequency and quantity. In general two approaches can be used: (1) recall of the quantity separate from the frequency (which is the usual approach); and (2) recall of the frequency of a given quantity. It is obvious that the accuracy of the estimate of the subjects' "average daily consumption" diminishes the longer the reference period. It is also not clear whether people really use the reference period they are asked to use in formulating their answers. Comparable to the assessment of physical activity all methods using an interview technique are potentially vulnerable to interviewer bias.

*Indirect dietary measurements.* An indirect way to assess dietary intake is the use of biological markers (Nierenberg & Nann, 1992). The motivation for looking at biological markers results from the search for objectivity. It is further enhanced by the attractiveness of technology. However, when using biological markers is often questionable if biological concentration is a valid indicator for nutritional intake. Nierenberg et al. (1997) investigated the intake of beta carotene in relation to blood levels of beta carotene. They found that a doubling of the intake was reflected in an increase of just 29% in blood levels. Another problem is the time integration of diet effects; how long are dietary factors traceable as biological markers? This depends partly on where the biological markers are assayed. For urine it varies from a few hours to a few days; for blood from a few days to a few weeks; for adipose tissue more than a year; for hair from a month to a year and for nails the biological marker will be present for more than three years. The major limitation of this method is the fact that the concentration of a certain marker is not only determined by the intake of the nutrients, but by many other (often unknown) factors. In conclusion, although biomarkers can be used as an objective indicator for the dietary intake of particular nutrients, they are highly biased and not necessarily a valid indicator for habitual dietary intake.

## General comments regarding diet and activity assessment

The choice of a certain method to measure physical activity or dietary intake depends to a great extent on the design of the study. There are roughly two kind of studies (observational and experimental) where the observational can be divided into cohort studies and case control studies. The idea behind case control studies is that determinants of a certain disease are measured after the disease has become manifest. This implicates that case-control studies are by definition retrospective and this limits the choice to a questionnaire/interview technique. Another problem with case control studies is that the subjects are ill at the moment their habitual physical activity or dietary intake (in the period before they were ill) is measured. However, it is possible that the disease has a strong influence on the activity and/or dietary pattern of the patient and that this "altered" pattern influences the retrospective recall. Another problem with retrospective recall is that the amount of activity or the intake of certain foods seems to be a poor indication of the real habitual activity or dietary intake over the particular time-period of interest; it is mostly an overestimation (Welten et al., 1996). For observational cohort studies a distinction must be made between retrospective cohort studies, which have the same problems as case control studies, and cross-sectional and prospective cohort studies. With the latter, one is not limited to questionnaire/interview techniques to measure habitual physical activity and habitual dietary intake, but all possible methods can be used. In experimental studies often activity or dietary interventions are given, implying that the assessment of physical activity and/or dietary intake is not the main point of interest. In observational and experimental studies in which physical activity and/or dietary intake are outcome variables in principle all methods can be used.

The choice of the most appropriate method to assess habitual physical activity or dietary intake is further influenced by the age and number of subjects.

Table 12.1 gives an overview of the different methods with the suitability for different age groups, the possibility to use the methods in

Table 12.1. Different methods for the assessment of daily physical activity and dietary intake

| | Age groups** | | | | | Large studies | Costs |
|---|---|---|---|---|---|---|---|
| | I | C | T | A | E | | |
| *Activity measurements* | | | | | | | |
| Job classification | – | – | – | ++ | + | ++ | low |
| Diary | – | – | + | ++ | ++ | ++ | moderate |
| Observation | + | ++ | ++ | ++ | ++ | + | high |
| Activity recall questionnaire/interview | – | + | ++ | ++ | ++ | ++ | moderate |
| Cardiorespiratory fitness | – | + | ++ | ++ | + | ++ | high |
| Doubly labeled water | + | ++ | ++ | ++ | ++ | + | high |
| Accelerometers/heart rate monitors | + | ++ | ++ | ++ | ++ | + | high |
| *Dietary measurements* | | | | | | | |
| 24-hours recall | – | + | ++ | ++ | ++ | ++ | low |
| Diary | – | – | + | ++ | ++ | ++ | moderate |
| Observation | + | ++ | ++ | ++ | ++ | + | high |
| Food frequency questionnaire | – | + | ++ | ++ | ++ | ++ | moderate |
| Cross-check dietary history | – | + | ++ | ++ | ++ | ++ | moderate |
| Biological markers | + | ++ | ++ | ++ | ++ | + | high |

Key:* ++ = highly suitable; + = suitable; – = not suitable

** I = infants; C = children; T = teenagers; A = adults; E = the elderly.

large studies, and the costs related to the different methods. Last but certainly not least, the choice for a particular method has to be related to the research question of the study. This looks very obvious, but it is often neglected in studies investigating habitual physical activity and habitual dietary intake.

In the discussion of the different methods to assess habitual physical activity and dietary intake, attention is given to possible sources of bias, because this may have important implications for the estimation of relationships between lifestyle parameters and health outcomes. The magnitude of the bias (i.e., measurement error) is in general non-differential; i.e., not related to the health outcome. This non-differential misclassification will lead to "bias towards the null"; i.e., relationships ought to be underestimated. This phenomenon exists both for under-reporting and over-reporting.

One of the problems in the assessment of habitual physical activity and/or dietary intake is that with the measurement of the recent activity, researchers want to obtain insight into past activity (or habitual physical activity). The idea behind this is that the present level of physical activity or dietary intake is a good representation of past activity or diet. However, this only holds when activity and dietary intake are relatively stable over time (this refers not to day-to-day variation, but to variation over a longer period). In epidemiology the long-term relative stability of a certain parameter over time is called tracking. In the AGHS, tracking of both physical activity and dietary intake has been investigated over a period of more than 15 years covering adolescence and young adulthood. The results showed low tracking for both physical activity and dietary intake (Twisk et al., 1997), implying that present activity and dietary patterns are poor estimates of past activity and dietary patterns. This poor long-term stability of both physical activity and dietary intake is only partly due to seasonal changes among others. For physical activity there are particular summer activities like tennis, gardening, etc., and specific winter activities like skiing, ice skating, etc., and regarding dietary intake a distinction can be made between typical winter and summer foods. In fact, the assessment of both habitual physical activity and dietary intake can be highly biased by these seasonal changes.

In physical activity research three parameters are of interest in the estimation of habitual physical activity: (1) the frequency of certain activities per week; (2) the duration of the activities in minutes; and (3) the intensity of the activities. A major problem with questionnaires/

interviews is that it is difficult to assess the intensity of the different activities carried out by a particular subject. Mostly this is done using standard tables in which a different kind of activity is related to a certain amount of energy expenditure, which can be seen as an indication for intensity. This not only introduces a new source of bias, it also has another problem: For example, playing soccer for 90 minutes can be done at a very different intensity by different players depending on the level, position, etc. Different levels of physical fitness can also have important implications for the translation of certain (sports) activities into energy expenditure. This is probably why questions like "did you sweat?", "were you very tired?," etc., are now added to the questionnaire or interview. The only method by which the intensity of different activities can be estimated objectively is using heart rate monitors. Therefore, a combination of different methods (for instance heart rate monitoring with an activity dietary) may be considered the most valid way to estimate the individual intensity of a particular physical activity.

In dietary research, portion sizes are used as a measure of "intensity". Although the between-subjects variability of portion sizes is remarkable, some researchers try to apply standard portion sizes in order to increase the reproducibility of the measurement. However the validity of the use of standard portions is highly questionable.

In the literature a lot of attention is devoted to the validity and reproducibility of the different methods to assess habitual physical activity or habitual dietary intake. One of the problems in investigating the reproducibility of these methods is the fact that the time-period between the two measurements must not be too short, because that can lead to some sort of "test-effect" resulting in an overestimation of the reproducibility. On the other hand, when the time period is too long the activity or dietary pattern is more likely to be changed, which leads to an underestimation of the reproducibility. Unfortunately, it is almost impossible to examine the validity of the methods to assess habitual physical activity and dietary intake because of the lack of a golden standard (although some people think one exists). The validity studies are always limited to a comparison between two or more methods which in theory measure the same phenomenon, although we are not sure whether they really do so. Validity studies are thus of limited value. Regarding habitual physical activity it has been argued that the method of doubly labeled water can be used as the golden standard (Bouten et al., 1996; Montoye et al., 1996). However, it is questionable if that is really true, and if it is true it only holds for energy expenditure, which is not the same as habitual physical activity.

In addition to the issue of validity and reproducibility in the literature regarding physical activity and dietary intake, much attention is given to the important relationship between physical activity or dietary intake and health or disease. However this does not cover the whole picture. In preventive medicine one of the most important issues should be to try to change physical inactivity and "unhealthy" dietary patterns. It is therefore surprising that less attention has been given to the assessment of the determinants of physical activity and dietary intake, because to start preventive strategies in order to change "unhealthy" behavior one should have insight into the determinants of that behavior (cf. Conner & Norman, 1966). The fact that both inactivity and "unhealthy" dietary patterns tend to cluster into some sort of "unhealthy" behavior pattern is also mostly not covered in the literature. These "unhealthy" behaviors interact with each other leading to a higher risk for chronic diseases than the sum of the risks of the "unhealthy" behaviors separately (Hulshof et al., 1992). Maybe researchers should focus more on these topics instead of trying to validate new (or old) methods of assessment.

It appears to be impossible to measure habitual physical activity or habitual dietary intake adequately. The best choice is to apply a combination of different methods. Results of studies using these lifestyle parameters should therefore be interpreted with caution.

## Alcohol, coffee and smoking

The major part of the alcohol consumption, coffee, and smoking research draws upon epidemiological data. The focus of this type of research lies on the measurement of the level of consumption and indicators of health problems related to consumption. There is a growing body of evidence supporting the positive effects of moderate alcohol intake, in particular on the risk of cardiovascular disease, and of caffeine on alertness and task performance (Lorist, 1995). Research on the genetic basis and biomarkers of alcoholism (Van der Stelt, 1997) and on neurocognitive effects of caffeine (Lorist, 1995; Snel and Lorist, 1998) has yielded more detailed information on their specific effects on behavior and brain activity. Most attention has been given to the measurement of consumption level for each product separately and to how differences in consumption are associated with health and psychosocial functioning. Nevertheless, the everyday practice of smoking, drinking coffee and taking alcohol in changeable combinations requires investigators to pay attention to their interactive effects.

However, studies which do not focus on the consequences but on possible behavioral and social determinants of use of these socially acceptable substances rarely restrict their focus to one of them alone: alcohol and nicotine consumption are highly correlated, average smokers consume more coffee than non-smokers, and smoking seems to increase the clearance of caffeine (Istvan & Matarazzo, 1984; Klatsky & Armstrong, 1992; Rehm et al., 1993; Shu et al., 1995). Caffeine consumption alone or together with alcohol intake does not appear to play a role in the link between smoking and coffee drinking (Pritchard et al., 1995). For this reason when evaluating the influence of one of these substances it is necessary to control for the consumption of the other substances, as has been done in the "social drinking" study of Zeef et al. (1998), who excluded social drinkers who also smoked. Lorist and Snel (1997) recruited only non-smoking coffee drinkers in their study on the effects of caffeine on human information processing.

Whether co-occurring intake of smoking and alcohol also occurs in young subjects from their teens through young adulthood was analyzed in the longitudinal AGHS for the age range 14 to 27 years (Twisk & Snel, 1999). For the 181 subjects it was found that those who used alcohol had a 2.98 times higher "risk" of smoking as well.

Further, the dichotomized life style factors drinking alcohol, smoking, inactivity and high energy intake were clustered and used as an *outcome* variable. For the age period from 16 to 27 years, a high score on this cluster (unhealthy lifestyle) was predicted by the personality factors rigidity and inadequacy; for the age period 21 to 27 years by dominance, inadequacy and low rigidity. Using this cluster as a *predictor*, the higher (unhealthy) this lifestyle score was, the higher the body mass index and obesity and the worse the aerobic condition.

To evaluate effects of separate and combined use reliably and validly, measurements of consumption are needed. Predominantly it is the absolute *per capita* consumption level that is used, while the pattern of consumption is hardly assessed in most research. To evaluate relationships of the *per capita* consumption or the pattern of consumption with health and social functioning, other factors like situation, context, age, sex and (sub)cultural settings should be considered as well.

## ALCOHOL CONSUMPTION
The 1999 mean world wide annual alcohol consumption *per capita* was 3.41 liters (World Drink Trends, 2000). In the European Union

this figure is 9.29 LPA (liters per annum), for Eastern Europe 7.19, for North America 6.66 and for Latin America 3.84.

When assessing absolute levels or patterns of use, other factors are also of importance. These factors are gender, age (i.e., binge drinking at a young age, especially during adolescence), personality, ethnicity (many Asian people have low levels of the enzyme acetaldehyde dehydrogenase to convert acetaldehyde into acetic acid and hence feel easily ill after drinking alcohol), genetics (positive or negative family history of excessive alcohol consumption), and socioeconomic status (Rehm et al., 1996). One should also realize that most drinkers do not stick to one type of beverage exclusively, but may change types of drink or use them in varying combinations depending on mood, setting, context, time of day and season, and availability.

Variability of consumption level and pattern is not only found on the individual level, but also across cultures. For example, young Dutchmen consume more beer, especially at a few specific occasions such as birthdays and celebrations and during the weekend, while older persons generally prefer wine or spirits. Men drink more alcohol than women. In addition, there is a temporal and seasonal rhythm of drinking. Beer and spirits are drunk more on a weekly base, while in general wine is taken daily.

## ASSESSMENT OF ALCOHOL CONSUMPTION

The usual parameters for measuring alcohol consumption are quantity and frequency. However, the measurement of specific patterns of consumption is also needed. To illustrate the latter, an average *per capita* consumption of 2 units per day may mean the regular use of 2 units a day or 14 units at one single occasion or during the weekend. Obviously, the effects on health and social functioning might be quite different. The measurement of *quantity* only, for example in order to classify moderate, regular and heavy drinkers is inadequate when not taking into account the pattern of consumption. Since it is the heavy drinker who experiences the adverse consequences most seriously, whereas the moderate drinker experiences the beneficial effects most, it is important to make these categorizations reliably. An additional problem of measurement of volume, based on the number of drinks is the concept of "drink" which may differ widely from country to country. The definition of a standard drink ranges from 6.0 gr. of alcohol in Austria for spirits, and for all types of alcohol-containing beverages 10 gr. in Australia to 19.75 gr. in Japan (ARISE, 1998).

Assessment of alcohol consumption may serve two goals: assessing acute alcohol consumption and alcohol use during longer periods (Weijers-Everhard, 1996). Acute alcohol use can be assessed as the Blood Alcohol Concentration or in a less invasive way with breath analyzers and in saliva or in urine.

To acquire an indication of the extent of alcohol use during long periods the following tests are used. Assessment of gamma-glutamyl-transferase (GGT) is a cheap method, that can be done in every laboratory. The sensitivity of this test is 30 to 50% in an ambulant population and between 60–70% in hospitalized patients. The specificity of this test depends on the presence of liver and gall-disorders and the use of anti-epileptica. Measurement of aspartaat-amino-transferase (ASAT) and alanine-aminotransferase (ALAT) form an indication of liver damage and less of alcohol abuse. An ASAT/ALAT ratio higher than 2.0 may indicate liver damage caused by alcohol. The assessment of the mean corpuscular volume (MCV) is highly specific (>90%) for long term alcohol use, its sensitivity lies between 20 and 50%. A useful test to discover high alcohol consumption is assessment of carbohydrate deficient transferrine (CDT). Although its sensitivity in alcohol-dependent patients is 81 to 100%, for heavy drinkers it is unclear. It is obvious that the use of these laboratory tests makes sense only if other information about the subject is also available. Needless to say, these methods are less easily applicable in large scale studies.

*Volume of drinking.* Self-reports of alcohol consumption depend on the subjects' willingness and motives to report. If the assumption of 50% underreporting is valid, this implies that the amounts of alcohol related to adverse health effects should be doubled, and that heavy drinkers who experience the most adverse effects in fact drink twice as much as reported. Conversely, it means that the amounts of alcohol indicative of protection for cardiovascular disease also should be doubled and that improvement of mood and social functioning should be based on higher consumption levels than the routinely recommended two to three units a day. On the other hand, the extent of underreporting, because of social unacceptability, fear of exposure and its possible consequences may differ considerably for moderate drinkers and alcoholics (Midanik & Harford, 1994). Conversely, overreporting may occur among young people to achieve higher status among their peers. Single and Wortley (1994) state that, in general, self-reported estimates are lower than alcohol consumption estimates derived from alcohol sales, demonstrating that underreporting is the rule. To increase the reliability of self-report consumption data, questions should be worded as unambiguously as possible and repeatedly formulated in other ways to check for response tendencies and socially desirable answers.

*Frequency of drinking.* Similar to the problems concerning the assessment of volume are the problems with self-reporting frequency of drinking. There are two ways to obtain information about frequency. The *summary method* asks for the number of occasions on which more than a given number of drinks was consumed within a certain time period, usually for the past year. The accuracy of reporting may decrease with the length of the interval due to weakness of memory or biased recall. In addition, it is a serious shortcoming that often no information is asked concerning the pattern of consumption. With the *recent-period summary* approach, the respondent is asked to summarize his drinking over a shorter period of time, for example the past 30 days. Study participants may be asked to recall the number of occasions at which more than a certain number of drinks were consumed. Using this method, inaccuracy might be less due to the shorter recall period, although this is not certain.

Although the accuracy and reliability of this method might be increased further by taking even shorter intervals, the shorter the interval the less representative the data may be for the subject's characteristic drinking behavior. One way to solve these problems is by extensively focusing on the most recent drinking occasions (Martinic, 1998). By asking questions relating to pattern, quantity, beverage type, length of drinking occasion, the time of drinking, drinking style, drinking companions, as well as assessment of the expectancies of drinking outcome (Wiers, 1998) and the degree of satisfaction or pleasure derived, it is possible to attain sufficient reliability and accuracy.

A more indirect method is to collect information concerning problems related to drinking. However, to be sure that the cause of such problems is drinking, detailed information should be gathered on the intensity of the problem, the self perception of the drinker and his expectations of the alcohol effects, drinking style in terms of quantity and frequency, type of beverage, when, where and with whom he is drinking, and his family's drinking history.

Moreover, in order to interpret such drinking-problem relationships in terms of the individual's health correctly, one should be aware that changes of *per capita* consumption over time might be socially induced, for example by changes in general lifestyle, in (sub)groups, or by attitude of the public health considerations or availability of alcohol. In addition, the use of at risk populations is questionable, especially when the aim is to extrapolate the findings to the general population. For example, in the general population moderate alcohol use may have beneficial effects and complete abstention may be a risk factor (Rimm et al., 1996). Information from patterns that do *not* result in problems may be more applicable to the general population than information gathered from clinical, alcoholic or heavily drinking samples. Martinic's (1998) conclusion that moderate consumers might be better controls than abstainers for measuring alcohol problems, is worth considering.

In conclusion, for the assessment of alcohol consumption to be reliable and valid, not only the measurement of quantity, frequency, and the pattern of use should be performed, but also information on the individual and the situational and sociocultural context in which drinking takes place.

*Coffee consumption.* According to the United States Department of Agriculture (USDA) the world coffee consumption in the harvest year 1998/1999 was 106.0 million bags of 60 kg each. Of these 106.0 million bags, 26.1 million bags were consumed in the producing countries and 79.9 million bags in the coffee importing countries (VNKT, 1999). In 1999 the Dutch *per capita* roasted coffee consumption was 7.4 kg or 154 litres, a daily average of 3.5 cups of coffee. Using as Burg (1975) proposes a standard dose of 85 mg caffeine per cup (Dutch standard size: 125 ml or 4 ounces), for a person weighing 75 kg, it means a daily intake of 4.0 mg/kg BW. In comparison, the estimated intake from all caffeine-containing drinks and foods for the average US consumer is 4.0 mg/kg BW (of which 2.7 mg/kg BW from coffee and tea, Barone & Roberts, 1984), and for the UK citizen less than 3 mg (Barone & Grice, 1994). These data illustrate that to answer questions on the relation between caffeine intake and health, questionnaires on coffee consumption should also ask for other caffeine-containing products as well, including soft drinks, tea, chocolate and certain medications.

The national consumption of coffee is a poor indicator of consumption *per capita* and this in turn is a poor indicator of the pattern of consumption, not to say of the exact caffeine intake. Although there is a vast amount of literature on the effects of coffee on health, estimates of the total caffeine intake based on caffeine content of all consumed caffeine-containing food, beverages and medicines have to our knowledge not been reported. In general, validity of caffeine intake should be determined by the correspondence of information gathered by asking people about their caffeine consumption from all sources and some independent assessments of the true state of caffeine intake, for examples from the coffee and soft drinks purchased in one month and/or from blood or salivary caffeine levels. James et al. (1989) found a correlation of 0.31 between self-reported caffeine use and salivary caffeine, explaining a meager 10% variance.

Factors in the physical nature of coffee that affect the validity of caffeine estimates are plant variety (caffeine content may range from 0.8% to 1.8% in freshly ground roasted coffee beans), cultivation methods, the coffee "grind" used for brewing, method and length of brewing, the amount used for brewing and cup size.

There are also such factors as sensitivity to and metabolic rate of caffeine absorption: (half-life ranging from 2 to 8 hours), personality, and demographic characteristics including gender and age (Knibbe & De Haan, 1998), situational context and the co-occurring use of other substances like alcohol and nicotine. Notwithstanding these difficulties, several "standard" values have been published (Lieberman, 1992) for the principal dietary sources of caffeine, ranging for a cup of 142 ml (5 ounces) from 2 mg for decaffeinated instant coffee to 90–150 mg in coffee brewed with the drip method and from 64 to 124 mg for percolated coffee. For tea the content may range from 9 mg (1 minute brew) to 50 mg (5 minute brew) and from 12 to 36 mg in instant or iced tea. Burg (1975) proposed as a standard average for a cup of brewed coffee: 85 mg, 60 mg for instant coffee and 3 mg for decaffeinated coffee. Similar "standards" have been proposed more recently in 1984 and 1987 (James, 1991). The range of daily consumption may vary from 1 to 17 cups (Bättig, 1991) with an average of about 3 to 4 cups. In Bättig's study among Swiss women aged 20–40 years, coffee is consumed over the whole day with a peak consumption at breakfast and morning break and a relatively low consumption with dinner, during the morning without a defined break and for wake up. It is difficult to say whether this distribution of consumption over the day can be generalized to other populations.

## ASSESSMENT OF CAFFEINE CONSUMPTION

Extensive descriptions of the methods applied to measure coffee consumption are scarce. The literature generally reports on average consumption without information on the specific method used, although there are some notable exceptions. For example, Bättig (1991) asked for coffee consumption in two different ways and correlated the obtained consumption data. Overall questions asked for usual consumption of regular coffee, decaffeinated coffee, and tea. In addition, the subjects filled out a detailed form about their consumption at different times of the day and the occasions at which they did not consume coffee or consumed more than usually. These two methods correlated 0.92 for the number of cups of coffee per day: 0.92 for the caffeine-containing cups and 0.77 for the decaffeinated cups. The actual and usual coffee consumption correlated 0.55.

Another approach was made by Barr et al., (1981), who examined the test-retest reliability of self-reported caffeine intake with an interval of one week and found values ranging from 0.86 to 0.94 for total caffeine intake. Further support for the reliability of self reported caffeine intake is offered by Schreiber et al., (1988) who followed up coffee drinking respondents three months later. Overall there was a high level of consistency of the subjects' reports on the number of cups drunk and their volume, the type of beverage and the brewing method. They also pointed to causes of imprecision in the reporting such as changes in type of beverage and other brewing methods but also to seasonal variations and true changes in habits over time.

More sophisticated methods concern computer programmed estimates of systemic caffeine concentrations based on individual caffeine-intake data, pharmokinetics of caffeine and the caffeine content of foods and beverages for a specific individual (Pfeifer & Notari, 1988). The weakness of this approach is the invalid assumption of "standard" caffeine contents for the variety of food and beverages that individuals consume. The quantitative measurement of serum and salivary caffeine content following an oral caffeine load can be done with the so-called high performance liquid chromatography assay (Setchell et al., 1987). This method is precise and sensitive enough (signal-noise ratio 2.5) to detect 0.005 $\mu$g caffeine/ml in saliva or serum. The agreement between saliva and serum values is 0.98.

*Coffee consumption as part of dietary intake.* When coffee consumption is considered as a part of diet, the methods used are as described before. Examples are Ellison et al.'s (1994) study on caffeine intake in children in which a detailed 3-day food diary is used. The same method was used in the 1977 Market Facts Survey for seven days. Other methods are part of dietary intake related methods, such as the 24-hour recall method (USDA 1965 survey of food intake, in Barone & Roberts, 1984). A similar method is a telephone survey regarding coffee consumption "yesterday". This method is used in the so-called "winter coffee drinking study", conducted annually by the International Coffee Organisation, and in food frequency methods (the MRCA national household menu census in 1972–73 in Barone & Roberts, 1984). With these methods not only the amount of consumed coffee or caffeine-containing beverages and nutritional products is asked for, but sometimes also where coffee is consumed, the type of coffee used, the brewing method and at which times of the day coffee consumption takes place. For all these methods it remains necessary to convert the amount of coffee drunk to estimates of caffeine taken by the respondent.

*Over- or underreporting of coffee consumption.* Reliability of the estimates of caffeine intake also depends on possible biases. One source of error might be the incompleteness of reporting of nutritional products other than coffee which contain caffeine. This could sufficiently be met by using the widely accepted dietary intake measures as referred to above. However, similar to the issue of over- and underreporting of alcohol consumption, the ambivalent appreciation of coffee, attributing negative health consequences to coffee drinking next to the pleasure of drinking coffee might induce underreporting. Indeed, Knibbe and De Haan (1998) found in 1240 men and women, aged 16 to 70 years, that the higher the consumption level, the more negative health consequences were attributed to coffee. They also collected questionnaire and diary estimates of coffee consumption for seven days. It appeared that questionnaire estimates (37.1 cups/week) were about 0.8 cup/day higher than the diary estimates (31.5 cups/week) and this was true at all levels of coffee consumption. Whether this difference reflects over-reporting (questionnaire estimate) or underreporting (diary estimate) is not clear. It is also unknown whether such difference is consistently present in other studies. In the only comparable study (Bättig, 1991) the opposite was found. The questionnaire on coffee consumption revealed 4.7 cups/day, while the detailed diary form to be filled out for one day found an daily average of 4.88 cups, a slight but significant difference of 0.2 cups/day. It is difficult to interpret these findings, because it is uncertain whether it concerns under- or overreporting of coffee consumption. Similarly to procedures used in studies on smoking, validity of self reported coffee consumption could possibly be increased by telling the respondents that a laboratory assessment of their salivary caffeine contents will also be made. As already indicated, estimates of caffeine contents from these self report data are inaccurate, at least partially due to the lack of information on consumption of caffeine containing products other than coffee. The unknown exact caffeine content of these products and their methods of production, the doubtful reliability and validity and the incompleteness of monitoring total caffeine consumption emphasize the need for more adequate methods to assess caffeine intake. For this reason information on caffeine-containing products other than coffee and the quantitative measurement of caffeine in saliva could be used to improve the estimates of caffeine intake.

SMOKING

In 1997, the percentage of the population in the USA older than 18 years that smoked was about 25%, in the Netherlands 33%; and in Eastern Europe 50%. According to the Centers for Disease Control, of the 46 million US smokers, 41.5% smoke less than 15 cigarettes a day, 41% smoke between 15 and 24 cigarettes a day, and 17.5% smoke more than 25 cigarettes a day; a rough average of 18 cigarettes daily (Hajari, 1997). In Japan, the 1998 consumption of cigarettes was 2,403 cigarettes for every Japanese, or 6.6 cigarettes daily. According to the Central Bureau for Statistics in The Netherlands (2001), 11% of smokers smoke more than 20 cigarettes a day. In 2000, the daily consumption of cigarettes, per smoker was 20.1 (STIVORO, 2001), per capita daily 6.2 cigarettes.

Cigarette smoking can be viewed as a series of discrete episodes of self-regulatory behavior with the aim to control one's physiological and mental state. The maintenance of a characteristic level of nicotine in a smoker's body is referred to as nicotine regulation. This view implies that a smoker depends for his smoking more on "internal" factors than on non-subject, "external" factors such as the family context, social setting, situation, educational level, age and gender. "Internal" or subject-bound variables are for example personality (O'Connor, 1989), gender and age and in particular style of smoking. The style of a smoker's puff, duration, volume and pattern appears to be consistently stable over time (O'Connor, 1989). It may also explain the so-called paradoxical effects of smoking, the "nicotine paradox", that stimulating (see Snel & Lorist, part 1, 1998) as well as relaxing effects of tobacco consumption have been found (Perkins et al., 1992). To be reliable and valid, an assessment of smoking cannot restrict itself to asking subjects to report the amount of tobacco products smoked, type or brand and the frequency of smoking, but should also involve a measurement of the subject's typical smoking style.

## ASSESSMENT OF SMOKING BEHAVIOR

Self-reports of smoking have the same advantages and disadvantages as discussed for alcohol and coffee. Overreporting by young people as a means to achieve higher status might be possible, but underreporting due to the increasing social unacceptability of smoking, especially of large amounts of smoking (chain smoking) and in the vicinity of other people, may also occur. Since there are large cultural differences of acceptance of smoking (from the least tolerant in the USA via the European Community to the most tolerant in Japan) methods to assess smoking behavior reliably should take these into account. Gathering data on the absolute amount of tobacco consumed in a relatively short time for epidemiological research is a quick, easy and practical method. The disadvantages of such an approach are obvious. Such data lack information on the extent of under- or overreporting, on the constituents of smoke inhaled and on smoking style. If no information is available on the brand used, only crude estimates of the nicotine amount the subjects are exposed to can be made. The actual content of nicotine in tobacco may vary from 0.2 to 5%, in general lying between 1 and 2% for more readily absorbable smoking tobaccos as found in cigars, pipe tobaccos and smokeless tobaccos. Also the tar content may vary considerably per cigarette from between 0.5 to 35 mg (Goodman et al., 1990). However, even if such an estimate of the smoke components can be made, knowledge concerning the characteristic smoking style of each subject is still necessary to reach valid estimates of the inhaled components of tobacco. A proposal to solve the problem of how to estimate nicotine content is given by DeGrandpere et al. (1992). First, nicotine can be estimated from the product of the number of cigarettes smoked and the nicotine yield of the specific brand smoked. A second measure can be derived from puff measures: puff volume, total number of puffs and nicotine yield, provided the type of cigarettes smoked is known. Third, nicotine intake can be estimated from blood nicotine levels. Daily nicotine intake and cotinine, the primary metabolite of nicotine, are far more accurately characterized by measuring blood or salivary cotinine concentrations than by nicotine estimates derived from self-reported number, type of cigarettes consumed and smoking style. However, the daily number of cigarettes smoked and cigarette nicotine delivery (half-life 2 hours; Goodman et al., 1990) correlate not significantly with cotinine concentrations (half life 20–30 hour; Pomerleau and Pomerleau, 1987). Moreover, laboratory measurements of nicotine and cotinine are only possible in small-scale studies with a limited number of subjects, sufficient financial resources, adequate laboratory equipment and manpower, and for these practical reasons are less useful in large scale epidemiological research.

## VALIDITY AND RELIABILITY

In spite of the growing interest in the relationship between smoking and health, methods to assess smoking are still surprisingly simple, hardly standardized and information about their reliability or validity is lacking. Mostly, data on smoking are collected by personal interview, or by telephone, and with self-report questionnaires. Questions always concern the number of cigarettes smoked daily and/or during the weekend. Internationally, there is informal agreement that the amount of smoking asked for should cover the last 24 hours, the last seven days and the last year. Sometimes questions also focus on smoking history, quitting of smoking and attempts to do so, the age at which the first cigarette was smoked and the brand of tobacco product(s). To enhance the validity of self-reports, a proven method is to inform the subjects that for a part of them, self-reported smoking may be validated through a saliva test (Murray et al., 1993). When smoking is seen as a habit with implications for the subjects' nutrition, it can be assessed as a part of the applied dietary intake methods (see above).

The collected data can be used to classify the respondents into lifetime non-smoker, non-smoking smoker, quitted smoking temporarily, non-smoking ex-smoker, smoker, smoking (relapsed) ex-smoker. Parallel to drinking types, another classification is into non-smokers, light, moderate or heavy smokers. These categorizations are to the taste of the researcher or tuned to the aim of the study, since there are to date no internationally accepted criteria for classifying smokers.

## SMOKING DEPENDENCE, TOLERANCE AND SENSITIVITY

An alternative, more indirect, approach to relate smoking behavior to health is assessing the extent of nicotine dependence. Unfortunately, there is no adequately valid measure for psychological dependence on smoking and nicotine (Gilbert, 1995). Different measures of proposed markers of dependence generally have low intercorrelations and suffer from a poor predictive validity. Gilbert (1995) blames this on the failure to incorporate situational and personality factors. If that is true, the severity of the abstinence response and success of stopping smoking can be predicted from the assessment of nicotine intake history, abstinence, tolerance, dependence and sensitivity.

The most frequently used instrument to measure tolerance and dependence is the Fagerström Tolerance Questionnaire (FTQ; Fagerström, 1987). Unfortunately, the FTQ has a poor internal consistency, does not reliably assess a single construct and correlates significantly positively with neuroticism and depression and with reasons for smoking. In the few studies in which the FTQ correlated significantly with physiological responses to smoking and with relapse, the association could be explained by personality and reasons for smoking. Studies applying standard challenge doses of nicotine also failed to find significant associations with FTQ-scores and cardiovascular or other responses (Gilbert et al., 1994).

The Fagerström Test for Nicotine Dependence (FTND), the improved version of the FTQ, has slightly improved psychometric properties (Heatherton et al., 1991) but still has a poor ability to predict smoking and again there is a link to neuroticism. Factor analysis showed two factors (morning smoking and cigarette consumption) while the Nicotine Dependence Scale of Covey et al., (1994) has three factors, explaining 57% of the variance and correlating 0.34 with the FTND.

Most studies assessing responses to quantified doses of tobacco smoke have failed to find significant associations between nicotine-induced physiological changes and the FTQ, but have found links with neuroticism and depression (Gilbert et al., 1994), both personality factors related to relapse and nicotine abstinence responses.

Apparently, nicotine dependence is a multidimensional construct that is not well covered by the FTQ and the FTND. Thus, to get some indication of nicotine dependence the best method is to use both questionnaires together, supplemented with data on situational and contextual aspects, personality and sensitivity for an adequate characterization of nicotine dependence. The best approach to our knowledge is the Situational x Trait Adaptive Response model (Gilbert, 1995; Gilbert & Gilbert, 1998).

In sum, in spite of a lack of reliable, validated and standardized methods to assess smoking, the available literature indicates roughly two methods. Direct measurements could be done by asking for amount and frequency of smoking, types of tobacco products and smoking style to estimate the inhaled nicotine content. Indirect measurements concern assessment of dependence, tolerance and sensitivity to smoking, possible supplemented with data on systemic nicotine and cotinine concentrations. Assessment of nicotine tolerance and sensitivity could be best done by using a quantified smoke and nicotine delivery system (Gilbert et al., 1989).

# Conclusion

To summarize, the currently available methods to assess smoking, alcohol consumption and coffee consumption suffer from serious methodological flaws. They are highly susceptible to social ideas related to acceptability of the consumption of the involved substances and therefore either over- or underreporting might be a serious problem. In addition, these substances are quite often consumed in variable patterns and changeable combinations. Furthermore the assessment of these parameters should be supplemented with information of the physiological and behavioral characteristics of the individual and with the situational and sociocultural context in which the consumption occurs. The methods used to date are of doubtful usefulness in epidemiological research with the aim of studying consumption related effects on health of the whole population, not to say at the individual level. More advanced methods to assesses the intake of these generally accepted substances, which take account of the before mentioned comments, will enable more reliable and valid conclusions on the consumption of alcohol, coffee and smoking and their relation with health.

# References

Acheson, K.J., Campbell, I.T., Edholm, O.G., Miller, D.S., & Stoch, M.J. (1980). The measurement of daily energy expenditure: An evaluation of some techniques. *American Journal of Clinical Nutrition, 33*, 1155–1164.

ARISE (1998). *Dietary disarray—A comparison of international comparisons of recommended amounts of nutritional products.* Internal report, Warburton D.M., University of Reading, UK.

Barone, J.C., & Roberts, H. (1984). Human consumption of caffeine. In: P.B. Dews (Ed.), *Caffeine: Perspectives from recent research* (pp. 59–73). Berlin: Springer Verlag.

Barone, J.J., & Grice, H.C. (1994). Meeting Report, Seventh International Caffeine workshop, Santorini, Greece, 13–17 June 1993, *Food Chemistry and Toxicity, 32*, 65–77.

Barr, H.M., Streissguth, P., Martin, D.C., & Horst, T.E. (1981). Methodological issues in assessment of caffeine intake: A method for quantifying consumption and a test-retest reliability study. In: L.F. Soyka & G.P. Redmond (Eds.), *Drug metabolism in the immature human* (pp. 265–280). New York: Raven Press.

Bättig, K. (1991). *Cross-sectional study: Coffee consumption, life-style, personality and cardiovascular reactivity* (pp. 1–27). Internal Report. Zürich: ETH-Zentrum.

Block, G. (1982). A review of validations of dietary assessment methods. *American Journal of Epidemiology, 115*, 492–505.

Bouten, C.V.C., Verboeket-van de Venne, W.P.H.G., Westerterp, K.R., Verduin, M., & Janssen, J.D. (1996). Daily physical activity assessment: Comparison between movement registration and doubly labeled water. *Journal of Applied Physiology, 81*, 1019–1026.

Burg, A.W. (1975). Effects of caffeine on the human system. *Tea and Coffee Trade Journal, 147*, 40–42.

Central Bureau of Statistics. (2001). The Hague, The Netherlands: www.cbs.nl/ln/diensten/persberichten/2001.

Conner, M., & Norman, P. (1996). *Predicting health behavior*. Buckinghamshire, UK: Open University Press.

Covey, L.S., Glassman, A.H., & Stetner, F. (1994). The Nicotine Dependence scale: A measure based on psychiatric criteria. *Annals of Behavioral Medicine, 16S*, 60.

Cumming, R.G. (1990). Calcium intake and bone mass: A quantitative review of the evidence. *Calcified Tissue International, 47*, 194–201.

DeGrandpere, R.J., Bickel, W.K., Hughes, J.R., & Higgins, S.T. (1992). Behavioral economics of drug self-administration. *Psychopharmacology, 108*, 1–10.

Ellison, R.C., Singer, M.R., Moore, L.L., Nguyen, U-S., Marmor, J.K, & Pawlik, E.J. (1994). *Caffeine intake and salivary levels in children*. Proceedings of the Seventh International Caffeine workshop, Santorini, Greece, 1994. Washington: ILSI (International Life Sciences Institute).

Fagerström, K.O. (1987). Measuring degree of physical dependence to tobacco smoking with reference to individualization of treatment. *Addictive Behaviors, 3*, 235–241.

Gilbert, D.G. (1995). *Smoking—individual differences, psychopathology and emotion*. London: Taylor & Francis.

Gilbert D.G., & Gilbert, B.O. (1998). Nicotine and the Situation by Trait Adaptive Response (STAR) model: Emotional states and information processing. In: J. Snel & M.M. Lorist (Eds.), *Nicotine, caffeine and social drinking—Behaviour and brain function* (pp. 131–149). Reading, UK: Harwood Academic Publishers.

Gilbert, D.G., Jensen, R.A., & Meliska, C.J. (1989). A system for administering quantified doses of tobacco smoke to human subjects: Plasma nicotine and filter pad validation. *Pharmacology, Biochemistry and Behaviour, 31*, 905–908.

Gilbert, D.G., Meliska, C.J., Welser, R., & Estes, S.L. (1994). Depression, personality, and gender influence EEG, cortisol, beta-endorphin, heart rate, and subjective responses to smoking multiple cigarettes. *Personality and Individual Differences, 16*, 247–264.

Goodman, A., Gilman, Th., Rall, W., Nies, A.S., & Taylor, P. (Eds.) (1990). *Goodman and Gilman's The pharmacological basis of therapeutics* (8th ed., pp. 545–549). New York: Pergamon Press.

Grundy, S.M., & Denke, M.A. (1990). Dietary influences on serum lipids and lipoproteins. *Journal of Lipid Research, 30,* 1149–1172.

Guthrie, H.A. (1984). Selection and quantification of typical food portions by young adults. *Journal of the American Dietary Association, 78,* 377–386.

Hajari, N. (1997). Where there's smoke. *Time, September,* 56–58.

Hankin, J.H. (1992). Dietary intake methodology. In: E.R. Monson (Ed.), *Research: Successful approach* (pp. 173–194). Chicago: American Dietetic Association.

Heatherton, T.F., Koslowski, L.T., Frecker, R.C., & Fagerström, K.O. (1991). The Fagerström Test for Nicotine Dependence: A revision of the Fagerström Tolerance Questonnaire. *British Journal of Addiction, 86,* 1119–1127.

Helmrich, S.P., Ragland, D.R., Leung, R.W., & Paffenbarger, R.S. (1991). Physical activity and reduced occurrence of non-insulin-dependent diabetes mellitus. *New England Journal of Medicine, 325,* 147–152.

Hulshof, K.F.A.M., Wedel, M., Löwik, M.R.H., Kok, F.J., Kistenmaker, C., Hermus, R.J.J., Hoor, F. ten, & Ockhuizen T. (1992). Clustering of dietary variables and other lifestyle factors. *Journal of Epidemiology and Community Health, 46,* 417–424.

Istvan, J., & Matarazzo, J.D. (1984). Tobacco, alcohol, and caffeine use: A review of their interrelationships. *Psychological Bulletin, 95,* 301–326.

James, J.E. (1991). *Caffeine and health.* London: Academic Press.

James, J.E., Bruce, M.S., Lader, M.H., & Scott, N.R. (1989). Self-report reliability and symptomatology of habitual caffeine consumption. *British Journal of Clinical Pharmacology, 27,* 507–514.

Kemper, H.C.G., & Verschuur, R. (1977). Validity and reliability of pedometers in habitual physical activity research. *European Journal of Applied Physiology, 37,* 71–82.

King, A.C., Taylor, C.B., Haskell, W.L., & DeBusk, R.F. (1989). Influence of regular aerobic exercise on psychological health. *Health Psychology, 8,* 305–324.

Klatsky, A.L., & Armstrong, M.A. (1992). Alcohol, smoking, coffee and cirrhosis. *American Journal of Epidemiology, 136,* 1248–1257.

Knibbe, R.A., & De Haan, Y.T. (1998). Coffee consumption and subjective health: Interrelations with tobacco and alcohol. In: J. Snel & M.M. Lorist (Eds.), *Nicotine, caffeine and social drinking—Behaviour and brain function* (pp. 229–243). Reading, UK: Harwood Academic Publishers.

Kriska, A.M., & Caspersen, C.J. (Eds.) (1997). A collection of physical activity questionnaires for health-related research. *Medicine and Science in Sports and Exercise, 29(Suppl),* S3-S204.

Lee, I., Paffenbarger, R.S., & Hsieh, C. (1991). Physical activity and risk of developing colorectal cancer among college alumni. *Journal of the National Cancer Institute, 83,* 1324–1329.

Leger, L., & Thivierge, M. (1988). Heart rate monitors: Validity, stability and functionality. *The Physician and Sports Medicine, 16*, 143–151.

Lieberman, H.R. (1992). Caffeine. In: A.P. Smith & D.M. Jones (Eds.) *Handbook of human performance* (Vol. 2, pp. 49–72). London: Academic Press.

Lorist, M.M. (1995). *Caffeine and human information processing.* Ph.D. thesis, Faculty of Psychology, University of Amsterdam, The Netherlands.

Lorist, M.M., & Snel, J. (1997). Caffeine effects on perceptual and motor processes. *Electroencephalography and Clinical Neurophysiology, 102*, 401–413.

Marcus, R., Drinkwater, B., Dalsky, G., Dufek, J., Raab, D., Slemenda, C., & Snow–Harter, C. (1992). Osteoporosis and exercise in women. *Medicine and Science in Sports and Exercise, 24(suppl)*, S301-S307.

Martinic, M. (1998). The implications for measurement and research. In: M. Grant & J. Litvak (Eds.), *Consumption patterns and their consequences* (pp. 221–241). London: Taylor & Francis.

McClaren, S.R., Babcock, M.A., Pegelow, D.F., Reddan, W.G., & Dempsey, J.A. (1995). Longitudinal effects on aging on lung function at rest and exercise in healthy active fit elderly adults. *Journal of Applied Physiology, 78*, 1957–1968.

McKenzie, T.L. (1991). Observational measures of children's physical activity. *Journal of School Health, 61*, 224–227.

Midanik, L.T., & Harford, T.C. (1994). Alcohol consumption measurement, introduction to workshop. *Addiction, 86*, 43–47.

Montoye, H.J., Kemper, H.C.G., Saris, W.H.M., & Washburn, R.A. (Eds.) (1996). *Measuring physical activity and energy expenditure.* Champaign, Ill.: Human Kinetics.

Morabia, A., Menkes, M.J.S., Comstock, G.W., & Tockman, M.S (1990). Serum retinol and airway obstruction. *American Journal of Epidemiology, 132*, 77–82.

Murray, R.P., Connett, J.E., Lauger, C.G., & Voelker, H.T. (1993). Error in smoking measures, effects of intervention on relations of cotinine and carbon monoxide to self-reported smoking. *American Journal of Public Health, 83*, 1251–1257.

Nierenberg, D.W., & Nann, S.L. (1992). A method of determining concentrations of retinol, tocopherol, and five cartenoids in human plasma and tissue samples. *American Journal of Clinical Nutrition, 56*, 417–426.

Nierenberg, D.W., Dain, B.J., Mott, L.A., Baron, J.A., & Greenberg, E.R. (1997). Effects of 4-years of oral supplementation with beta-carotene on serum concentrations of retinol, tocopherol, and five cartenoids. *American Journal of Clinical Nutrition, 66*, 315–319.

O'Connor K. (1989). A motor psychophysiological model of smoking and personality. *Personality and Individual Differences, 10*, 889–901.

Paffenbarger, R.S., Hyde, R.T., Wing, A.L., & Hsieh C-C. (1986). Physical activity, all cause mortality, and longevity of college alumni. *New England Journal of Medicine, 324,* 605–613.

Perkins, K.A., Grobe, J.E., Fonte, C., & Breus, M. (1992). Paradoxical effect of smoking on subjective stress versus cardiovascular arousal in males and females. *Pharmacology, Biochemistry and Behavior, 42,* 301–311.

Pfeifer, R.W., & Notari, R.E. (1988). Predicting caffeine plasma concentrations resulting from consumption of food or beverages: A simple method and its origin. *Drug Intelligence and Clinical Pharmacy, 22,* 953–959.

Pomerleau, C.S., & Pomerleau, O.F. (1987). The effect of a psychological stressor on cigarette smoking and subsequent behavioral and physiological responses. *Psychophysiology, 24,* 278–285.

Powel, K.E., & Blair, S.N. (1994). The public health burden of sedentary living habits, theoretical but realistic estimates. *Medicine and Science in Sports and Exercise, 26,* 851–856.

Powel, K.E., Thompson, P.D., Caspersen, C.J., & Kendrick, J.S. (1987). Physical activity and the incidence of coronary heart disease. *Annual Review of Public Health, 8,* 253–387.

Pritchard, W.S., Robinson, J.H., Donald DeBethizy, J., Davis, R.A., & Stiles, M.F. (1995). Caffeine and smoking: Subjective, performance, and psychophysiological effects. *Psychophysiology, 32,* 19–27.

Rehm, J., Fichter, M.M., & Elton, M. (1993). Effects on mortality of alcohol consumption, smoking, physical activity and close personal relationships. *Addiction, 88,* 101–112.

Rehm, J., Ashley, M.J., Room, R., Single, E., et al. (1996). On the emerging paradigm of drinking patterns and their social and health consequences. *Addiction, 91,* 1615–1621.

Rimm, E.B., Klatsky, A., Grobbee, D., & Stampfer, M.J. (1996). Review of moderate consumption and reduced risk of coronary heart disease: Is the effect due to wine, beer, or spirits? *British Medical Journal, 312,* 731–736.

Saris, W.H.M. (1982). *Aerobic power and daily physical activity in children.* PhD Thesis, University of Nijmegen, Meppel, The Netherlands: Krips-Repro.

Schoeller, D.A. (1983). Energy expenditure from doubly labelled water. Some fundamental considerations in humans. *American Journal of Clinical Nutrition 38,* 999–1005.

Schreiber, G.B., Maffeo, C.E., Robins, M., Masters, M.N., & Bond, A.P. (1988). Measurement of coffee and caffeine intake: Implications for epidemiological research. *Preventive Medicine, 17,* 280–294.

Seale, J.L., Conway, J.M., & Canary, J.J. (1993). Seven day validation of doubly labelled water method using indirect room calorimetry. *Journal of Applied Physiology, 74,* 402–409.

Setchell, K.D.R., Welsh, B.M., Klooster, M.J., & Balistreri, W.F. (1987). Rapid high-performance liquid chromotography assay for salivary and serum caffeine following an oral load as indicator of liver function. *Journal of Chromatograhy 385*, 267–274.

Shu, X.O., Hatch, M.C., Mills, J., Clemens, J., & Susser M. (1995). Maternal smoking, alcohol drinking, caffeine consumption, and fetal growth, results from a prospective study. *Epidemiology, 6*, 115–120.

Single, E., & Wortley, S. (1994). Drinking in various settings, findings from a national survey in Canada. *Journal of Studies on Alcohol, 57*, 77–84.

Snel, J., & Lorist, M.M. (Eds.) (1998). *Nicotine, caffeine and social drinking—Behaviour and brain function*, Reading, UK: Harwood Academic Publishers.

STIVORO (2001). *Annual report 2000*. The Hague, The Netherlands.

Twisk, J.W.R., Kemper, H.C.G., Mechelen, W. van, & Post, G.B. (1997). Tracking of risk factors for coronary heart disease over a 14-year period. A comparison between lifestyle and biological risk factors with data from the Amsterdam Growth and Health Study. *American Journal of Epidemiology, 145*, 888–898.

Twisk, J.W.R., & Snell, J. (1999). Co-occuring intake of smoking and alcohol use from adolescence through young adulthood. Internal Report, AGGO-project, Vrÿe Universiteit, Amsterdam, The Netherlands.

Van Mechelen, W., Kemper, H.C.G., Twisk, J.W.R., Lenthe, F.J. van, & Post, G.B. (1997). Longitudinal relationship between resting heart rate, maximal oxygen uptake and activity. In: N. Armstrong, B.J. Kirby, & J.R. Welsman (Eds.), *Children and exercise XIX*. London: E&FN Spon.

Van der Stelt, O. (1997). *Children of alcoholics, attention, information processing, and event-related brain potentials*, Ph.D. Thesis, Faculty of Psychology, University of Amsterdam, The Netherlands.

VNKT (2000). *Annual report 1999, Vereniging Nederlandse Koffiebranders en Theepakkers*. Amsterdam.

Weijers-Everhard, J. (1996). Laboratoriumdiagnostiek. In: M.J.A.J.M. Hoes & P.J. Geerlings (Eds.), *Informatorium Alcoholisme*. Leusden, The Netherlands: NZP Medical Publishing.

Welten, D.C., Kemper, H.C.G., Post, G.B., & Staveren, W.A. van (1996). Relative validity of 16-year recall of calcium intake by a dairy questionnaire in young Dutch adults. *Journal of Nutrition, 126*, 2843–2850.

Wiers, R. (1998). *Bad expectancies? Cognitive and neuropsychological indicators of enhanced risk for alcoholism*. Ph.D. Thesis, Faculty of Psychology, University of Amsterdam, The Netherlands.

Willet W. (2000). *Nutritional epidemiology*. New York/Oxford: Oxford University Press.

Willet, W.C., Stampfer, M.J., Colditz, G.A., Rosner, B.A., Hennekens, C.H., & Speizer, F.E. (1987). Dietary fat and the risk of breast cancer. *New England Journal of Medicine, 316*, 22–28.

World Drink Trends (2000). *Productschap voor gedistilleerde dranken*, in association with NTC Publications Ltd., Oxfordshire, UK, ISBN 1-84116-075-X.

Wright, J.D., Ervin, B., & Briefel, R.R. (Eds.) (1994). *Consensus workshop on dietary assessment, nutrition monitoring and tracking the year 2000 objectives*. Hyattsville, MD: National Centre for Health Statistics.

Zeef, E., Snel, J., & Maritz, B.. (1988). Selective attention and event related potentials in young and old social drinkers. In: J. Snel, & M.M. Lorist (Eds.), *Nicotine, caffeine and social drinking: Behaviour and brain function* (pp. 301–313). Reading, UK: Harwood Academic Publishers.

# 3 MULTIDIMENSIONAL ASSESSMENT OF PAIN

Johan W.S. Vlaeyen and Geert Crombez

Pain is a universal condition. There is, however, very little known about its mechanisms and influencing factors. From a biomedical perspective, pain has been considered almost synonymous with tissue damage. The French philosopher René Descartes was one of the first to present a mechanical pain model. In this model there are direct and unique pain pathways from the peripheral nervous system to the brain, in the same way the bell in a church tower rings when the rope attached to it is pulled. For Descartes, pain was a reflex of the mind upon nociceptive stimulation of the body. Pain was treated as a symptom, isomorphically related to the severity of the underlying pathology of the organism. According to this perspective, pain treatment consists of two acts: localization of the underlying pathology and removal of the pathology with appropriate remedy or cure. In the absence of bodily damage, the mind was assumed to be at fault, and a psychic pathology was inferred. This model has been extremely influential. Even today, most medical pain treatments are based on these assumptions.

The limitations of the biomedical model became apparent during the late 1970s. In a nice example of a Kuhnian shift of paradigm, the gate-control theory of Melzack and Wall (1965) adequately dealt with the shortcomings of the biomedical model. The gate-control theory has also figuratively opened the gate for research on the role of psychological variables moderating and mediating pain. This theory clearly stated that cortical processing was involved in the integration of both sensory-discriminative and affective-motivational aspects of pain. Taking this one stage further, pain was not only the result of information ascending from the periphery, but was profoundly moderated by descending pathways. According to the gate-control theory, the balance between sensory and central inputs determines the presence or absence of pain.

About a decade after the publication of the gate-control theory, Fordyce (1976) published his influential book *Behavioral methods for chronic pain and illness*. His work stemmed from the obvious shortcomings of the attempts of traditional health care to resolve chronic pain problems. Fordyce was the first to apply the principles of operant conditioning (Skinner, 1953) to problems of chronic pain. Central was the idea that "pain behavior", which refers to observable signs of pain and suffering, should be the focus of treatment. There are at least two assumptions to this approach: (1) the factors that maintain the pain problem can be different from those that have initiated it. Pain behaviors may be subject to a graded shift from structural/mechanical to environmental control; and (2) biomedical findings do not eliminate the possibility that psychological or social factors contribute to the level of pain disability.

After the so-called "cognitive revolution" in behavioral science, Turk et al. (1983) emphasized the role of attributions, efficacy expectations, personal control and problem-solving within a cognitive-behavioral perspective on chronic pain. The assumptions of this approach are the following: (1) individuals actively process information regarding internal stimuli and external events; (2) thoughts and beliefs may alter behavior by their direct influence on emotional and physiological responses; and (3) individuals can become active participants in their treatment if they learn skills to deal with their problems (Turk & Rudy, 1989). In the remainder of this chapter, multidimensional assessment of pain will be discussed from this cognitive-behavioral perspective.

## Triple response mode in chronic pain

The International Association for the Study of Pain (1986) has defined pain as "a sensory and emotional experience associated with actual or potential tissue damage, or described in terms of such damage". This definition radically breaks with the biomedical model in which pain and tissue damage are almost synonymous. Tissue damage is not even a necessary condition for pain. Pain is also considered an emotional experience. In line with this idea, we will further elaborate the view that pain, just like an emotion, is a multidimensional experience. In particular, the three-systems model of emotions will be applied to the experience of pain. According to this model, emotions are always subjective and never observable in themselves. They can only be inferred by their effects at an observable level. Likewise, (chronic) pain can best be approached as a hypothetical construct that can be inferred by at least three partially independent response systems: (1) psycho-physiological reactivity; (2) beliefs about pain and pain control; and (3) overt pain behaviors (Vlaeyen et al., 1989).

## PSYCHOPHYSIOLOGICAL REACTIVITY

Like any emotional experience, pain may variably affect several bodily systems including the muscular, cardiovascular, respiratory and electro-dermal system (see Flor et al., 1992b for an extensive review). Although some of the psychophysiological responses during pain may be biologically hardwired and relatively specific to pain, psychophysio-logical reactivity to pain is specific for particular groups of subjects (response stereotypy) and is extremely sensitive to the environmental characteristics in which pain emerges. Therefore, psychophysiological reactivity to pain does not reflect a fixed set of unique and highly corre-lated responses, but refers to the selection of responses that allows an individual to prepare behavior that is tuned to its ecological environ-ment (Crombez et al., 1997b). From a functional perspective, psy-chophysiological reactivity may be best understood as a readiness or preparation to escape from a feeling of bodily harm (Sokolov, 1963). In other words, psychophysiological reactivity is there for a reason.

It has further become clear that psychophysiology is not a murky window to the mind; it does not allow a privileged look inside (Öhman, 1987). Questions about psychophysiological reactivity to pain have to be framed within a psychological model that provides answers to the following questions: when and how do we perceive pain? and when and how do we respond to pain? In such a model, key concepts are attention, attribution, expectations, coping and behavior.

## ATTENTION, ATTRIBUTIONS AND EXPECTATIONS

Pain seems designed to capture attention. Amongst many other com-peting demands in the environment, pain is quickly selected as the focus of attention. Once selected it is often difficult to disengage from. When pain demands the attention of the individual, three kinds of appraisal processes are hypothesized to occur (Lazarus et al., 1970): primary, secondary and tertiary (re)appraisals. Primary appraisals concern the immediate meaning of the invading stimulus: Am I OK or in trouble? Beecher (1959) was one of the first to highlight the effects of the meaning attached to pain. In one of his classic studies he investi-gated the differences in pain responses between a group of male civilian patients undergoing major surgery and a group of soldiers with compa-rable wounds. He found that four-fifths of the civilians requested anal-gesics whereas only one-third of the soldiers wanted medication. His explanation for this discrepancy was that for the soldiers, the painful wound meant an escape from the battlefield. In contrast, the surgery was a calamitous event for the civilian. A typical example of an extremely negative appraisal of pain in clinical practice is catastrophizing about pain. Pain is then appraised as extremely threatening and as having catastrophic consequences. It is well documented that pain catastrophizing is related to higher pain reports. In the experimental study by Spanos et al. (1978), for example, subjects who display catastrophizing attributions report higher pain levels to a cold pressor task than non-catastrophizing subjects.

After the interpretation of the stimulus, the individual will try to reduce his suffering. This process of evaluating an encounter with respect to coping resources and options is referred to as secondary appraisal. It concerns the question: What can I do about the pain? Not all coping strategies are beneficial. Patients with chronic low back pain who report ignoring or reinterpreting pain sensations, praying and hoping, and using attention diversion report greater pain levels and are more functionally disabled (Spinhoven et al., 1989). It is also very likely that different coping strategies may be relevant for different pain problems. In addition, there will be occasions when the required skills are not mastered or when some deficit will prevent the effective use of the resource. A pain patient may, for example, believe that exercise in general is a healthy thing to do, but not in his particular case because of the emerging pain increase.

This leads us to the third appraisal process which is referred to as efficacy expectations (Bandura, 1977) or the conviction that one is able to influence pain (perceived pain control). Patients who perceive themselves as having little control over their pain are likely to be more depressed and disabled. For example, patients with rheumatoid arthritis who believe that they can control their pain and who don't catastrophize are less distressed, and report better physical and psychological functioning (Parker et al., 1989). In studies with experimental pain, perceived control is also shown to increase pain tolerance levels (Arntz & Schmidt, 1989).

## OVERT PAIN BEHAVIORS

The overt-motoric responses cover a wide range of gross motor behaviors, referred to in the pain literature as pain behaviors. Fordyce (1976) particularly demonstrated the clinical and theoretical relevance of observable pain behaviors. The pain behavior construct should be considered multidimensional. Turk et al. (1985) employed multidimensional scaling and hierarchical clustering techniques to identify the latent structure of pain behaviors. They found that pain behavior could be characterized by two dimensions: "audible-visible" and "affective-behavioral". Four clusters of different pain behaviors were identified: distorted ambulation or posture; negative affect; facial/audible expressions of distress; and avoidance of activity. Similar results were found by Vlaeyen et al. (1987) who presented 78 behavior items to a group of independent behavioral scientists. Nurses working in the clinical setting of a pain rehabilitation department collected the behavior items. Multidimensional scaling resulted in three dimensions: "withdrawal-approach", "high arousal-low arousal" and "visible-audible". A hierarchical cluster analysis revealed nine clusters of behavior items, including behaviors related to affective distress such as nervousness and depression. The importance of assessing pain behaviors lies in the fact that they elicit reinforcing responses from the social environment, which can further worsen the pain problem. For example, Lousberg et al. (1992) reported that chronic low back pain patients with solicitous spouses reported more pain during a treadmill test than patients with nonsolicitous spouses.

## Measurement of pain

### SELF-REPORT METHODS
One of the early attempts to measure pain concerned the quantification of the experienced pain intensity. From a biomedical perspective, pain intensity is thought of as a direct and valid expression of some underlying pathology, and is therefore an essential part of the medical examination. If pain is viewed as a construct, however, such as anxiety or depression, it must be realized that the relationship between the pain report and the pain construct is not absolute or isomorphic. Because of the multidimensionality of pain, no single measure can adequately assess the whole construct. This points to a fundamental limitation of pain assessment. Jensen and Karoly (1992) distinguish three aspects of pain: pain location (where does it hurt?); pain intensity (how much does it hurt?); and pain affect (how does it hurt?).

### PAIN LOCATION
The instrument most commonly used to assess the sensory distribution of pain is the pain drawing. Patients are asked to indicate the location of their pain on a line drawing of a human body, which is divided in several regions (Margolis et al., 1986). A score can be calculated by summing the number of regions that are indicated. In the case where

pain is felt at different locations, symbols are used to combine quality or intensity of pain with these locations (Parker et al., 1995).

PAIN INTENSITY

There are three frequently used instruments to quantify pain intensity: Visual Analog Scale (VAS), Numerical Rating Scale (NRS), and Verbal Rating Scale (VRS). The VAS is usually presented as a 10 cm long horizontal line, whose ends are labeled as the extremes of pain such as "no pain at all" and "worst pain ever experienced". The patient is then requested to place a small vertical line according to the intensity of the pain experienced. The distance in millimeters between the left extreme and the vertical line is the pain intensity score. Advantages of the VAS are that they are strongly related to other measures of pain intensity and that they are sensitive to treatment effects as a result of the high number of response categories. One reported disadvantage is that, despite their simplicity, the patient needs careful instructions (Jensen et al., 1989). The NRS has similar qualities, but has the advantage of being more easily understood by patients. Patients are asked to assign a number, e.g., ranging from 0 to 100, to their pain, again with both extremes labeled as in a VAS. The main difference between VAS, NRS and VRS is that in the latter adjectives instead of number are used to describe the different levels of pain. The pain intensity score is the number assigned to the adjective chosen by the patient. An example of a 5-point scale would be: None, mild, moderate, severe, very severe. The obvious disadvantages of a VRS is that patients have to be familiar with the list of adjectives before they can make a choice, with the possibility that s/he cannot find the adjective that accurately describes the perceived pain intensity.

PAIN AFFECT

Pain affect is the emotional component of pain, defined as the degree of change in action readiness caused by the sensation of pain. By definition, pain affect is more complex than pain intensity and pain location as it is found to be multidimensional. There is less consensus about how to measure the emotional aspect of the pain experience. Although verbal rating scales and visual analog scales have been suggested (Price & Harkins, 1992), the most commonly used instrument to quantify the affective dimension of pain is the McGill Pain Questionnaire (MPQ; Melzack, 1975). The MPQ consists of a list of 20 classes of pain words such as sharp, flickering, jumping, etc. Each class belongs to one of four dimensions: sensory, affective, evaluative and miscellaneous. Each subclass contains two to five words that belong to the same dimension but differ in intensity. The words in each subclass are ranked in the order of increasing intensity. The patient is requested to choose only those words that describe his or her feelings and sensations at that moment. Two major indices are obtained: (1) The Pain Rating Index (PRI) which is the sum of the rank values of the chosen words. For each of the dimensions, separate PRIs can be calculated; and (2) The Number of Words Chosen (NWC). The MPQ also contains a verbal rating scale to quantify pain intensity. Pain affect can best be measured with the affective subscale of the MPQ. Examples of affective pain words are: "exhausting", "sickening", "terrifying", "killing". In 1987, a short form (SF-MPQ) consisting of only 15 pain words was developed for use in research settings when the time to obtain information from patients is limited (Melzack, 1987).

## PSYCHOPHYSIOLOGICAL APPROACHES

There are no absolute physiological correlates of pain. For that reason, receptors that are specialized in the translation of information about tissue damage are called nociceptors and not "pain" receptors. Also no specific "pain" nerves or "pain" centra in the brain have been identified. Often the assessment of (psycho)physiological correlates of pain is limited to a laboratory setup in which one has perfect control over the pain eliciting stimulus. Sokolov (1963) identified three dynamic reflex systems in the autonomic nervous system: the orienting system, the adaptive system and the defensive system. According to this author the defensive system is activated by aversive and/or painful stimuli. Whereas the function of the orienting system is to optimize the reception and transmission of incoming information, the primary function of the defensive system is to limit the impact of aversive/painful events.

Experimental pain is associated with: (1) large electrodermal responses that are difficult to extinguish completely with repeated presentations (Hardy et al., 1967); (2) a late acceleration component in heart rate that emerges about 20 sec. after stimulus onset (Graham, 1979); (3) peripheral and central vasoconstriction (Graham, 1979); (4) a pupil dilation response (Chapman et al., 1997); (5) a typical facial expression of pain which consists of lowering of the eyebrow and tightening of the eyelids (Crombez et al., 1997a), and (6) an EEG event-related response that is specific for somatosensory information (Zaslansky et al., 1996). Except for the latter, most of these responses are also observed when being exposed to non-painful threatening events, which may indicate that they are part of a more general defensive system. Due to the non-specific nature of the psychophysiological responses to pain, the relation of these measures to the pain construct is often ambiguous. Interpretation may be further confounded because there may occur a shift from an active to a more passive defensive mode along with the chronicification of the pain problem.

An interesting new development is the registration of the attentional component of an event-related potential, i.e., the P300 in the EEG. The P300 component is easily elicited in an oddball task in which subjects have to attend to rare discrete events (e.g., a few high pitch tones among a large series of low pitch tones). It has been demonstrated that the amplitude of the P300 to the rare events depends upon the availability of spare attentional resources. Because pain demands attention and depletes attentional resources, it may be expected that the P300 component to the rare events is diminished during pain. This is exactly what is observed using a tonic pain procedure (Lorenz & Bromm, 1997). In line with this is the finding that morphine, a traditional painkiller, enlarges the P300 in chronic pain patients, suggesting that this substance diminishes the attentional demand by pain.

Some psychophysiological responses are assumed to play a significant role in the initiation or maintenance of the chronic pain problem. A leading thesis is that of response stereotypy, i.e., the preference of (groups of) individuals to respond to a wide variety of stressors with the same pattern of physiological responses. There is some evidence in favor of response stereotypy in chronic pain patients. Patients with chronic pain in the temporomandibular region (cheek region) respond to personal stressors with high EMG activity in the masseter muscle (involved in chewing). In patients with chronic back pain, the paraspinal muscles (m. erector spinae muscles) are most responsive to personal stressors (Flor et al., 1992a). Migraine patients show a specific functional abnormality in one of the major head arteries in response to stressors (Rojahn & Gerhards, 1986). Despite this evidence, the function of response stereotypy in the initiation or maintenance of chronic pain is still unclear and poorly researched.

## OBSERVATIONAL MEASURES

Under the influence of Fordyce's theory of operant conditioning of pain behaviors (Fordyce, 1976), a great deal of clinical research has dealt with the role of environmental contingencies in the maintenance of chronic pain and with the modification of overt expressions of pain and suffering. In order to assess the effects of behavioral interventions, observational instruments have been developed to quantify the non-verbal signs of pain suffering. In addition, behavioral observation assessment strategies are needed for adults and children who lack the ability to articulate their pain experience. Generally, there are three domains in which observation methods have been developed: (1) facial expressions; (2) guarded and protective movements; and (3) reduced daily activity levels. One of the most sensitive non-verbal correlates of pain is facial activity. A number of studies have indicated that acute pain is associated with a distinct pattern of facial actions, including brow lowering, narrowing of the eye orbit as a result of tightening the eyelids and raising cheeks (e.g., Craig et al., 1991). Validity of facial action assessment has been demonstrated. For example, LeReche and Dworkin (1988) found positive correlations between self-report measurements of pain and various characteristics of facial expression.

For the assessment of guarded and protective movements, a number of observation methods have been developed. Keefe and Block (1982) developed an observation method for chronic low back pain designed to measure motor pain behaviors that occur during simple daily activities. Patients are videotaped during these activities and the tapes are subsequently scored by trained observers. The categories include guarding, bracing, rubbing painful areas, facial grimacing, and sighing. A similar method was developed by Follick et al. (1985) differentiating 16 categories. These observation systems have also been expanded for use with other pain patient populations such as rheumatoid arthritis (McDaniel et al., 1986) and cancer (Ahles et al., 1990). The disadvantage of these counting methods is that they are quite complex and difficult to use in a clinical context.

Alternative and more global observation scales are developed such as the UAB Pain Behavior Scale (Richards et al., 1982). This instrument lists 10 pain behavior categories rated on a 3-point scale of increasing frequency. A slightly modified version with only eight categories and during which patients are requested to perform standardized tasks is developed by Feuerstein et al. (1985). More recently, the Checklist for Interpersonal Pain Behavior (CHIP; Vlaeyen et al., 1990) was designed for use by nurses in clinical settings and by the spouses of pain patients. As well as categories concerning protective behaviors and guarded movement, the CHIP includes behavior categories related to depression and nervousness. Both the CHIP and UAB scale have been found to be responsive to behavioral treatment, and not be influenced by observer biases (Kole-Snijders et al., 1999). There are also observational instruments specially developed for the assessment of pain in children. One of these instruments is the Children's Hospital of Eastern Ontario Pain Scale (CHEOPS; McGrath et al., 1985) which includes six behaviors (crying, facial expression, verbal expression, torso position, touch behavior, and leg position).

Daily physical activity assessment can be done with self-report diaries (e.g., Fordyce, 1976) or by automated movement registration with body-fixed accelerometers (Bussman et al., 1998). The use of diaries, in which patients are requested to write down what kind of activity (e.g., sitting, lying, standing) they are engaged during a given period of time is time consuming, requires the full compliance of the patient, and may interfere with daily activity patterns. The method has now been replaced by the more sophisticated triaxial accelerometers. These are small portable devices with minimal interference, and which usually have a data-unit for on-line processing of output over 1-minute intervals. Moreover, these accelerometers have been shown to correlate highly with robust measurements of energy expenditure (Bouten et al., 1996).

## Measurement of functional limitations due to pain

One of the main goals of behavioral treatments of chronic pain is the restoration of functional abilities, rather than the reduction of pain. The need for measuring the functional capacity of chronic pain sufferers has led to the development of many scales and indexes. It is certainly beyond the scope of this chapter to review all of the existing instruments, and we will restrict the discussion to the most frequently used self-report instruments.

One of the earliest and most widely used, but general health instruments is the Sickness Impact Profile (SIP; Bergner et al., 1981) which covers the physical, social, and emotional aspects of health. Because the SIP was developed for people with chronic disabilities in general, and not specifically for a chronic pain population, modified versions have been developed such as the Roland Disability Questionnaire (RDQ; Roland & Morris, 1983) for back pain. Similar instruments have been developed for different diagnostic groups, such as The Fibromyalgia Impact Questionnaire (FIQ; Burckhardt et al., 1991) and the Arthritis Impact Measurement Scales (Meenan et al., 1980).

A short and easy to use instrument is the Disability Rating Index (DRI; Salén et al., 1994), which covers 12 items ranging from relatively basic activities of daily life such as dressing and climbing stairs to more vigorous activities such as lifting heavy objects and participating in sports. The DRI has been designed for application in clinical settings, and the questions are arranged in increasing order of physical demand, which also permits the health personnel to interpret the consistency of the answers. A general index is achieved by calculating the responses in terms of the percentages of the highest possible rating.

One of the most comprehensive instruments to quantify the daily life problems of chronic pain patients, irrespective of their diagnosis, is the Multidimensional Pain Inventory (MPI; Kerns et al., 1985). This questionnaire consists of 61 items and has three parts, of which the first measures the severity of the pain problem, the experienced support by family members, functional limitations, pain control, and emotional distress. The second part is designed for the quantification of the spouse's reactions to the pain including solicitous, diverting and punishing responses. Part three focuses on the functional limitations. The patient rates his participation in four categories of daily activities inside and outside the house, as well as social activities. A special feature of the MPI is that a pain profile can be made based on the scores of the individual scales. Cluster analyses consistently revealed three patient profiles: (1) "dysfunctional" patients, who have severe pain, limited control over pain and engaging in little activity. The pain interferes with their daily lives and they are distressed; (2) the "interpersonally distressed" patients who experience very little support from their social environment; and (3) the "adaptive coper" patients who are characterized by a profile which is opposite to the dysfunctional patients. The MPI typology appears to be quite robust and has been found in patients with benign pain such as fibromyalgia (Turk & Okifuji, 1996), as well as in cancer pain patients (Turk et al., 1998).

Although the objective of these instruments is to achieve a quantitative measure of the patient's level of functional capacity, the scores are also, as with any self-report instrument, influenced by the patients' attitude and personal opinions about their actual functioning. Therefore, it may be wise to complement the assessment with observational measures including some kind of physical performance.

## Quantification of biomedical findings in chronic pain

Although it is seldom carried out, the quantification of the biomedical findings is an essential part of the assessment of pain from a biopsychosocial perspective. In medicine, and chronic pain in particular, there is wide variability among clinicians in interpreting biomedical data that is based on the interview, physical examination and diagnostic tests such as X-rays, CT scans and clinical biology tests. Recently, an empirically derived index of organic pathology in patients with chronic pain has been developed. The Medical Examination and Diagnostic Information Coding System (MEDICS; Rudy et al., 1990) provides a list of 17 diagnostics tests (such as electromyography, contrast radiography, blood count) at which the clinician or researcher can indicate whether the test has been carried out, and whether the test has led to positive or negative findings. These indications can be used to calculate a weighted total score which is considered an index of the organic pathology and impairments found. MEDICS is a valuable tool for the quantification of the result of the endless list of diagnostic procedures often applied with chronic pain patients.

## Pain-related beliefs

In order to examine the ways individuals with pain think about their pain (appraisals) and about possible ways of dealing with pain and its consequences (efficacy expectations), several questionnaires have been developed. As most of these instruments show considerable overlap, only the most frequently used will be described here. For excellent reviews, the reader is referred to Jensen et al. (1991) and DeGood and Shutty (1992).

Four types of non-adaptive appraisals (catastrophizing, overgeneralization, personalization, and selective abstraction) can be examined with the Cognitive Error Questionnaire (CEQ; Lefebvre, 1981) using 24 short vignettes reflecting one of the four cognitive errors. The patient is then asked to rate how similar the cognition is to the thought they would have in a similar situation. Two forms of the CEQ are available, one for general life experiences and one for problems experienced by chronic low back pain patients. Pain-specific measures are found to be more valid in that they appear to be better predictors of functional ability and responsiveness to pain treatment programs.

The Survey of Pain Attitudes (SOPA; Jensen et al., 1989) is a 35-item self-report scale aimed at measuring the belief that a patient can gain control over his pain (control), the extent to which the patient experiences support from the family members (solicitude), the belief that physical exercise can cause reinjury (harm), reliance on health care (medical cure), the patient's view on his/her own disability (disability), reliance on medication (medication), and the belief that stress and emotions influence the pain experience (emotion). Several scales of the SOPA have been found to be predictive of the adjustment at seven years after an inpatient rehabilitation program (Jensen & Karoly, 1991).

A comparable instrument is the Pain Cognition List (PCL; Vlaeyen et al., 1990), which focuses on the patient's belief that pain has a great impact on daily life (pain impact), the exaggerated negative view on pain and its consequences (catastrophizing), the belief that pain can be controlled (outcome efficacy), the belief that the pain problem will remain the same, regardless of any efforts to deal with it (acquiescence), and the reliance on health care (reliance). The first two PCL scales have been shown to differentiate between individuals with chronic pain who consult a pain clinic (consumers) and those who carry on with their lives without utilizing health care facilities (non-consumers) (Reitsma & Meijler, 1997). A short and methodologically strong instrument to measure catastrophizing beliefs is the Pain Catastrophizing Scale (Crombez et al., 1998; Sullivan et al., 1995). This 13-item scale is developed for both non-clinical and clinical populations. Subjects reflect on past painful experiences and indicate the degree to which they experienced thoughts or feelings during pain on a 5-point scale (e.g., "I can't seem to keep it out of my mind", "I feel I can't stand it any more"). For the assessment of the extent to which the patient believes that s/he can gain control over pain (internal locus), that medical doctors or medication can change the pain situation (external locus), or that what will happen with the pain is a matter of chance, the Multidimensional Pain Locus of Control Scale (MPLC; Ter Kuile et al., 1993) might be of interest.

## Coping with pain

Pain coping is what people do to try to control or tolerate pain, regardless of the achieved success of these efforts. It refers to conscious, goal-directed and self-initiated actions, which can be cognitive (e.g., trying to relax through imagery) or behavioral (e.g., starting with a physical exercising program). Because of the wide diversity of cognitive coping strategies, mostly dealt with in the literature on pain coping, Fernandez (1986) introduced a classification system with three main categories: (1) imagery, (2) self-talk and (3) attention diversion. In imagery, the patient evokes images that can decrease the pain intensity through transformation of the pain into another sensation that can better be supported (loosening a tight ribbon around the painful area), or by images that are incompatible with the pain (often relaxing images such as the waves of the ocean, sunny beach). In self-talk, the focus is on the personal resourcefulness of dealing with pain, rather than the pain itself. In self-talk, a virtual dialogue with the pain is being held, in which pain can be personalized as an enemy or as a teacher (Hanson & Gerber, 1990). Finally, attention diversion is the process of directing the attention to competing stimuli, such as a mental task. Attention diversion seems to work best when the competing task has a positive valence (McCaul et al., 1992).

One of the difficulties in assessing pain coping is that most of the strategies used by patients are extremely idiosyncratic. In addition, it remains unclear how to differentiate between the "good" and the "bad" coping strategies (Tunks & Bellissimo, 1988). Nevertheless, Rosenstiel and Keefe (1983) designed the 50-item Coping Strategies Questionnaire (CSQ) aimed at assessing the use of six cognitive and two behavioral coping strategies including diverting attention, reinterpreting pain sensation, coping self-statements, ignoring pain sensations, praying or hoping, catastrophizing, increasing activity level and increasing pain behaviors. There are also two additional items tapping the perceived control over pain and the ability to decrease pain respectively. In spite of the theoretical shortcomings of the construct of coping, the CSQ has been repeatedly used in clinical studies to compare the use of certain coping strategies and functional adaptation in chronic pain patients. Generally, patients who catastrophize and who perceive low pain control appear to be more disabled and depressed (Turner, 1991). There is increasing evidence that the self-perceived efficacy of the individual's coping attempts, rather than coping itself, is clinically more relevant. With Stone and Neale's (1989) Daily Coping Inventory (DCI) adapted for chronic pain coping, Keefe et al. (1997) demonstrated that rheumatoid arthritis patients who reported high levels of coping efficacy in one day had lower levels of pain the next day.

## Pain-related fear

In an attempt to explain how and why some individuals develop a chronic pain syndrome, Lethem et al. (1983) introduced a "fear-avoidance" model. The central concept of their model is fear of pain. "Confrontation" and "avoidance" are postulated as the two extreme responses to this fear, of which the former leads to the reduction of fear over time. The latter, however, leads to the maintenance or exacerbation of fear, possibly leading to a phobic state. The avoidance results in the reduction of both social and physical activities, which in turn leads to a number of physical and psychological consequences augmenting the disability. A basic question that may be asked is what is the patient afraid of, or in other words, what is the nature of the perceived threat? The literature reflects this lack of clarity by discussing fear of pain, fear of work and physical activity, and fear of (re)injury as a result of movement.

The Pain Anxiety Symptoms Scale (PASS; McCracken et al., 1992) was developed to measure the cognitive, physiologic, and motoric aspects of fear of pain. It consists of 40 items with a 5-point Likert scale. The authors found significant correlations with measures of anxiety, cognitive errors, depression, and disability. In a second study (McCracken et al., 1993), it was shown that, in a group of chronic low-back pain patients, greater pain-related anxiety was associated with higher predictions of pain and less range of motion during a procedure involving a passive but painful straight leg raising test. The authors also showed that different types of pain-anxiety symptoms have different relations with pain coping responses as measured with the Coping Strategies Questionnaire. Cognitive anxiety responses (e.g., "I find it hard to concentrate when I hurt") negatively interfered with coping strategy use, whereas physiological anxiety responses appeared to enhance coping (McCracken & Gross, 1993). The authors also found a substantial overlap between the CSQ-factor "Catastrophizing" and fear of pain. This is of interest as previous studies found strong associations between catastrophizing attributions and depression.

Chronic pain patients may not only fear pain, but also activities that are expected to cause pain. In this case, fear is hypothesized to generalize to other situations that are closely linked to the feared stimulus. Vlaeyen (1991) found that a group of 50 chronic low back pain patients had elevated scores that were clinically significant on the "social phobia" and "agoraphobia" scales of the Fear Survey Schedule (FSS-III; Wolpe & Lang, 1964). More specifically, Waddell et al. (1993) developed the Fear-Avoidance Beliefs Questionnaire (FABQ), focusing on the patient's beliefs about how work and physical activity affect his/her low back pain. The FABQ consists of two scales, fear-avoidance beliefs of physical activity and fear-avoidance beliefs of work, of which the latter was consistently stronger in predicting work disability. The authors found that fear-avoidance beliefs about work are strongly related to disability of daily living and work lost in the past year, and more so than biomedical variables such as anatomical pattern of pain, time pattern, and severity of pain.

A more specific kind of fear-avoidance concerns fear of movement and physical activity that is (wrongfully) assumed to cause (re)injury. Kori et al. (1990) introduced the term "kinesiophobia" (kinesis = movement) for the condition in which a patient has "an excessive, irrational, and debilitating fear of physical movement and activity resulting from a feeling of vulnerability to painful injury or reinjury". These authors also developed the Tampa Scale for Kinesiophobia (TSK) as a measure for fear of movement/(re)injury. The TSK consists of 17 items, each of which is provided with a 4-point Likert scale. In a previous study using the Dutch version of the TSK, Vlaeyen et al. (1995a) found that fear of movement/(re)injury appears to be related to gender and compensation status, when variance due to current pain intensity was corrected for. However, even stronger associations were found with catastrophizing and depression, rather than with pain intensity and pain coping. Furthermore, subjects who report a high degree of fear of movement/(re)injury showed more fear and escape/avoidance when exposed to a simple movement consisting of lifting a 5.5 kg bag. They also quit lifting the bag significantly sooner than the less fearful patients. A subsequent study also showed that fear of movement/(re)injury is associated with changes in muscular reactivity (Vlaeyen et al., 1999).

In a recent validation study, Crombez et al. (1999) concluded that the TSK and both subscales of the FABQ (Physical and Work) were significantly related to self-reported disability. These instruments were also superior in predicting disability as compared to pain intensity, pain duration, and negative affect. The TSK was also a better predictor of disability than pain catastrophizing. The PASS was not significantly related to self-reported disability. The TSK, PASS and one subscale of the FABQ, i.e., the FABQ-Physical, were reliably associated with poor behavioral performance and their predictive value was higher than that of current pain intensity, pain duration, experienced pain increase, negative affect and catastrophizing (tested for TSK only).

## Assessment in the clinical setting

Most people, including the majority of health care professionals, will search for an underlying somatic pathology if a patient complains of pain. Often the assumption is that the underlying cause must first be corrected before the symptom can diminish. This is also often the view of the patient when first consulting a pain clinic or behavioral rehabilitation facility. The assessment of pain can be facilitated enormously when the therapist introduces an alternative biopsychosocial model from the beginning, making clear that individual and environmental responses following pain may in fact influence subsequent pain and disability. This means that the behavioral assessor holds an interactionist point of view that environmental, behavioral and organismic variables mutually interact. In clinical assessment, the functional analysis (Haynes & O'Brien, 1990) is the classic strategy that links the different constructs described above into one framework, represented by the behavioral equation SORC (Figure 13.1). R is the problematic behavior that is identified for modification, and in the case of pain inferred by pain behaviors ($R_b$), pain cognitions ($R_c$), and psychophysiological reactivity ($R_p$). The other components represent the controlling variables of which this response is a function. The immediate environmental variables are represented as S (the internal and external stimuli that precede R) and C (the internal and external consequences that follow R). Internal events are those that occur inside the body and which are detected by proprioception. External events occur outside the organism and are detected through perception. The organismic variable is represented by O and includes biological status and stable personality characteristics. The equation represents not a static but a dynamic, spiral system, in which consequences instigate new stimuli for subsequent SORC chains. As an example, a person with rheumatoid arthritis

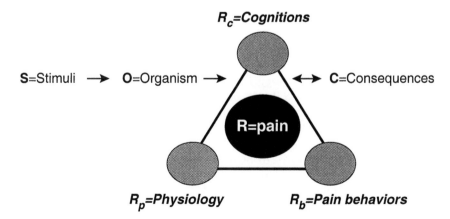

Figure 13.1. The SORC equation applied to pain (based on Vlaeyen, 1991)

(O) may encounter a daily stressor (S) which triggers muscular reactivity $(R_p)$, catastrophizing beliefs and feelings of helplessness $(R_c)$. The associated fears cause increased awareness of painful areas and result in an increase in protective pain behaviors. These elicit solicitous responses from family members (C), who unwittingly reinforce the patient's sick-role and disability.

In clinical situations, the interview can best be considered as the initial assessment tool which generates hypotheses on the elements of the SORC equation. The hypotheses can subsequently be tested by means of reliable and valid instruments which we described above. For more detailed information about interviewing pain patients, we refer to Fordyce (1976) and Turk et al. (1983).

# References

Ahles, T.A., Coombs, D.W., Jensen, L., Stukel, T., Maurer, L.H., & Keefe, F.J. (1990). Development of a behavioral observation technique for the assessment of pain behaviors in cancer patients. *Behavior Therapy, 21*, 449–460.

Arntz, A., & Schmidt, A. (1989). Perceived control and the experience of pain. In: A. Steptoe & A. Appels (Eds.), *Stress, personal control and health* (pp. 131–162). Chichester: Wiley.

Bandura, A. (1977). Self-efficacy: Towards a unifying theory of behavior change. *Psychological Review, 84*, 191–215.

Beecher, H.K. (1959). *Measurement of subjective responses*. New York: Oxford University Press.

Bergner, M., Bobbitt, R.A., Carter, W.B., & Gibson, B.S. (1981). The Sickness Impact Profile: Development and final revision of a health status measure. *Medical Care, 19*, 787–805.

Bouten, C.V.C., Verboeket-van de Venne, W.P.H.G., Westerterp, K.R., Verduin, M., & Janssen, J.D. (1996). Daily physical activity assessment: Comparison between movement registration and doubly labelled water. *Journal of Applied Physiology, 81*, 1019–1026.

Burckhardt, C.S., Clark, S.R., & Bennet, R.M. (1991). The Fibromyalgia Impact Questionnaire: Development and validation. *Journal of Rheumatology, 18*, 728–733.

Bussman, J.B.J., van de Laar, Y.M., Neleman, M.P., & Stam, H.J. (1998). Ambulatory accelerometry to quantify motor behaviour in patients after failed back surgery: A validation study. *Pain, 74*, 153–161.

Chapman, C.R., Oka, S., & Jacobson, R.C. (1997). Phasic pupil dilation response to noxious stimulation in humans. In: *Proceedings of the 8th World Congress on Pain, 8*, 449–458.

Craig, K.D., Hyde, S., & Patrick, C.J. (1991). Genuine, suppressed, and faked facial behavior during exacerbation of chronic low back pain. *Pain, 46,* 161–172.

Crombez, G., Baeyens, F., & Eelen, P. (1997a). Changes in facial EMG activity related to painful heat stimuli on the hand. *Journal of Psychophysiology, 11,* 256–262.

Crombez, G., Baeyens, F., Vansteenwegen, D., & Eelen, P. (1997b). Startle intensification by painful heat stimuli. *European Journal of Pain, 1,* 87–94.

Crombez, G., Eccleston, C., Baeyens, F., & Eelen, P. (1998). When somatic information threatens, pain catastrophizing enhances attentional interference. *Pain, 75,* 187–198.

Crombez, G., Vlaeyen, J.W.S., Heuts, P.H.T.G., & Lysens, R. (1999). Pain-related fear is more disabling than pain itself: Evidence on the role of pain-related fear in chronic back pain disability. *Pain, 80,* 329–339.

DeGood, D.E., & Shutty, M.S. (1992). Assessment of pain beliefs, coping and self-efficacy. In: D.C. Turk & R. Melzack (Eds.), *Handbook of pain assessment* (pp. 214–234). New York: Guilford.

Fairbank, J.C.T., Couper Mboat J., Davies, J.B.D., & O'Brien, J.P. (1980). The Oswestry Low Back Pain Disability Questionnaire. *Physiotherapy, 66,* 271–273.

Fernandez, E. (1986). A classification system of cognitive coping strategies for pain. *Pain, 26,* 141–152.

Feuerstein, M., Greenwald, M., Gamache, M.P., Papciak, A.S., & Cook, E.W. (1985). The Pain Behavior Scale: Modification and validation for outpatient use. *Journal of Psychopathology and Behavioral Assessment, 7,* 301–315.

Flor, H., Birbaumer, N., Schugens, M.M., & Lutzenberger, W. (1992a). Symptom-specific psychophysiological responses in chronic pain patients. *Psychophysiology, 29,* 452–460.

Flor, H., Miltner, W., & Birbaumer, N. (1992b). Psychophysiological recording methods. In: D.C. Turk & R. Melzack (Eds.), *Handbook of pain assessment* (pp. 169–190). New York: Guilford.

Follick, M.J., Ahern, D.K., & Aberger, E.W. (1985). Development of an audiovisual taxonomy of pain behavior: Reliability and discriminant validity. *Health Psychology, 4,* 555–568.

Fordyce, W.E. (1976). *Behavioral methods for chronic pain and illness.* St. Louis: Mosby.

Graham, F.K. (1979). Distinguishing among orienting, defense, and startle reflexes. In: H.D. Kimmel, E.H. Van Olst, & J.F. Orlebeke (Eds.), *The orienting reflex in humans* (pp. 137–167). Hillsdale, NJ: Lawrence Erlbaum Associates.

Hanson, R.W., & Gerber, K.E. (1990). *Coping with chronic pain: A guide to patient self-management.* New York: The Guilford Press.

Hardy, J.D., Wolff, H.G., & Goodell, H. (1967). *Pain sensations and reactions.* Baltimore: Williams and Wilkins.

Haynes, S.N., & O'Brien, W.H. (1990). Functional analysis in behavior therapy. *Clinical Psychology Review, 10,* 649–668.

Jensen, M.P., & Karoly, P. (1991). Control beliefs, coping efforts, and adjustment to chronic pain. *Journal of Consulting and Clinical Psychology, 59,* 431–438.

Jensen, M.P., & Karoly, P. (1992). Self-report scales and procedures for assessing pain in adults. In: D.C. Turk & R. Melzack (Eds.), *Handbook of pain assessment* (pp. 135–151). New York: Guilford.

Jensen, M.P., Karoly, P., & Huger, P. (1987). The development and preliminary validation of an instrument to assess patients' attitudes toward pain. *Journal of Psychosomatic Research, 35,* 149–154.

Jensen, M.P., Karoly, P., O'Riordan, E.F., Bland, F., Jr., & Burns, R.S. (1989). The subjective experience of acute pain: An assessment of the utility of 10 indices. *Clinical Journal of Pain, 5,* 153–159.

Jensen, M.P., Turner, J.A., Romano, J.M., & Karoly, P. (1991). Coping with chronic pain: A critical review of the literature. *Pain, 47,* 249–283.

Keefe, F.J., & Block, A.R. (1982). Development of an observation method for assessing pain behavior in chronic low back pain patients. *Behavior Therapy, 13,* 363–375.

Keefe, F.J., Affleck, G., Lefebvre, J.C., Starr, K., Caldwell, D.S., & Tennen, H. (1997). Pain coping strategies and coping efficacy in rheumatoid arthritis: A daily process analysis. *Pain, 69,* 35–42.

Kerns, R.D., Turk, D.C., & Rudy, T.E. (1985). The West Haven-Yale Multidimensional Pain Inventory (WHYMPI). *Pain, 23,* 345–356.

Kole-Snijders, A.M.J., Vlaeyen, J.W.S., Goossens, M.E.J.B., Rutten-Van Mölken, M.P.M.H., Heuts, P.H.T.G., van Breukelen, G., & van Eek, H. (1999). Chronic low back pain: What does cognitive coping skills training add to operant-behavioral treatment? Results of a randomized clinical trial. *Journal of Consulting and Clinical Psychology, 67,* 931–944.

Kori, S.H., Miller, R.P., & Todd, D.D. (1990). Kinesiophobia: A new view of chronic pain behavior. *Pain Management, Jan./Febr.,* 35–43.

Lang, P.J. (1995). The emotion probe: Studies of motivation and attention. *American Psychologist, 50,* 372–385.

Lazarus, R.S., Averill, J.R., & Opton, E.M. (1970). Towards a cognitive theory of emotion. In: M.B. Arnold (Ed.), *Feelings and emotions.* New York: Academic Press.

Lefebvre, M.F. (1981). Cognitive distortion in depressed psychiatric and low back pain patients. *Journal of Consulting and Clinical Psychology, 49,* 517–525.

LeReche, L., & Dworkin, S.F. (1988). Facial expressions of pain and emotions in chronic TMD patients. *Pain, 35,* 71–78.

Lethem, J., Slade, P.D., Troup, J.D., & Bentley, G. (1983). Outline of a fear-avoidance model of exaggerated pain perception: I. *Behaviour Research and Therapy, 21,* 401–408.

Lorenz, J., & Bromm, B. (1997). Event-related potential correlates of interference between cognitive performance and tonic experimental pain. *Psychophysiology, 34,* 436–445.

Lousberg, R., Schmidt, A.J.M., & Groenman, N.H. (1992). The relationship between spouse solicitousness and pain behaviour: Searching for more experimental evidence. *Pain, 51,* 75–80.

Margolis, R.B., Tait, R.C., & Krause, S.J. (1986). A rating system for use with patient pain drawings. *Pain, 24,* 57–65.

McCaul, K.D., Monson, N., & Maki, R.H. (1992). Does distraction reduce pain-produced distress among college students? *Health Psychology, 11,* 210–217.

McCracken, L.M., & Gross, R.T. (1993). Does anxiety affect coping with pain? *Clinical Journal of Pain, 9,* 253–259.

McCracken, L.M., Gross, R.T., Sorg, P.J., & Edmands, T.A. (1993). Prediction of pain in patients with chronic low back pain: Effects of inaccurate prediction and pain-related anxiety. *Behaviour Research and Therapy, 31,* 647–652.

McCracken, L.M., Zayfert, C., & Gross, R.T. (1992). The Pain Anxiety Symptoms Scale: Development and validation of a scale to measure fear of pain. *Pain, 50,* 67–63.

McDaniel, L.K., Anderson, K.O., Bradley, L.A., Young, L.D., Turner, R.A., Agudelo, C.A., & Keefe, F.J. (1986). Development of an observation method for assessing pain behavior in rheumatoid arthritis patients. *Pain, 24,* 165–184.

McGrath, P.J., Johnson, G., Goodman, J.T., Schillinger, J., Dunn, J., & Chapman, J.A. (1985). CHEOPS: A behavioral scale for rating postoperative pain in children. In: H.L. Fields, R. Dubner, & F. Cervero (Eds.), *Advances in pain research and therapy* (Vol. 9, pp. 395–402). New York: Raven Press.

Meenan, R.F., Gertman, P.M., & Mason, J.H. (1980). Measuring health status in arthritis: The Arthritis Impact Measurement Scales. *Arthritis and Rheumatism, 23,* 146–152.

Melzack, R. (1975). The McGill Pain Questionnaire: Major properties and scoring methods. *Pain, 1,* 277–299.

Melzack, R. (1987). The short form McGill Pain Questionnaire. *Pain, 30,* 191–197.

Melzack, R., & Wall, P.D. (1965). Pain mechanisms: A new theory. *Science, 150,* 978.

Öhman, A. (1979). The orienting response, attention and learning: An information-processing perspective. In: H.D. Kimmel, E.H. Van Olst, & J.F. Orlebeke (Eds.), *The orienting reflex in humans* (pp. 443–471). Hillsdale, NJ: Lawrence Erlbaum Associates.

Parker, H. Wood, P.L., & Main, C.J. (1995). The use of the pain drawing as a screening measure to predict psychological distress in chronic low back pain. *Spine, 20,* 236–243.

Parker, J., Smarr, K., Buescher, K., Phillips, L., Frank, R., Beck, N., Anderson, S., & Walker, S. (1989). Pain control and rational thinking: Implications for rheumatoid arthritis. *Arthritis and Rheumatism, 32*, 984–990.

Patrick, D.L., Deyo, R.A., Atlas, S.J., Singer, D.E., Chapin, A., & Keller, R.B. (1995). Assessing health-related quality of life in patients with sciatica. *Spine, 20*, 1899–1909.

Price, D.D., & Harkins, S.W. (1992). Psychophysical approaches to pain measurement and assessment (pp. 111–134). In: D.C. Turk & R. Melzack (Eds.), *Handbook of pain assesment*. New York: Guilford.

Reitsma, B., & Meijler, W.J. (1997). Pain and patienthood. *Clinical Journal of Pain, 13*, 9–21.

Richards, J.S., Nepomuceno, C., Riles, M., & Suer, Z. (1982). Assessing pain behavior: The UAB pain behavior scale. *Pain, 12*, 393–398.

Rojahn, J., & Gerhards, F. (1986). Subjective stress sensitivity and physiological responses to an aversive auditory stimulus in migraine and control subjects. *Journal of Behavioral Medicine, 9*, 203–212.

Roland, M., & Morris R. (1983). A study of the natural history of back pain. Part I: Development of a reliable and sensitive measure of disability in low-back pain. *Spine, 8*, 141–144.

Rosenstiel, A.K., & Keefe, F.J. (1983). The use of coping strategies in chronic low back pain patients: Relationship to patient characteristics and current adjustment. *Pain, 17*, 33–44.

Rudy, T.E., Turk, D.C., Brena, S.F., Stieg, R.L., & Brody, M.C. (1990). Quantification of biomedical findings of chronic pain patients: Development of an index of pathology. *Pain, 42*, 167–182.

Salén, B.A., Spangfort, E.V., Nygren, A.L., & Nordermar, R. (1994). The disability rating index: An instrument for the assessment of disability in clinical settings. *Journal of Clinical Epidemiology, 47*, 1423–1434.

Shutty, M.S., & DeGood, D.E. (1990). Patient knowledge and beliefs about pain and its treatment. *Rehabilitation Psychology, 35*, 43–54.

Skinner, B.F. (1953). *Science and human behavior*. New York: Macmillan.

Sokolov, Y.N. (1963). *Perception and the conditioned reflex*. Oxford: Pergamon Press.

Spanos, N.P., Rivers, S.M., & Gottlieb, J. (1978). Hypnotic responsivity, meditation, and laterality of eye movements. *Journal of Abnormal Psychology, 87*, 566–569.

Spanos, N.P., Radke-Bodorik, H.L., Ferguson, J.D., & Jones, B. (1979). The effects of hypnotic susceptibility, suggestions for analgesia, and utilization of cognitive strategies on the reduction of pain. *Journal of Abnormal Psychology, 88*, 282–292.

Spinhoven, P., ter Kuile, M.M., Linssen, A.C.G., & Ganzendam, B. (1989). Pain coping strategies in a Dutch population of chronic low back pain patients. *Pain, 37*, 77–83.

Stone, A., & Neale, J. (1984). New measure of daily coping: Development and preliminary results. *Journal of Personality and Social Psychology, 46,* 892–906.

Sullivan, M.J.L., Bishop, S.R., & Pivik, J. (1995). The pain catastrophizing scale: Development and validation. *Psychological Assessment, 7,* 281–292.

Ter Kuile, M.M., Linssen, A.C.G., & Spinhoven, Ph. (1993). The development of the Multidimensional Locus of Pain Control Questionnaire (MLPC): Factor structure, reliability, and validity. *Journal of Psychopathology and Behavioral Assessment, 15,* 387–404.

Tunks, E., & Bellissimo, A. (1988). Coping with the coping concept: A brief comment. *Pain, 34,* 171–174.

Turk, D.C., & Okifuji, A. (1996). Perception of traumatic onset, compensation status, and physical findings: Impact on pain severity, emotional distress, and disability in chronic pain patients. *Journal of Behavioral Medicine, 19,* 435–453.

Turk, D.C., & Rudy, T.E. (1989). A cognitive-behavioral perspective on chronic pain: Beyond the scalpel and syringe. In: C.D. Tollison (Ed.), *Handbook of chronic pain management* (pp. 222–236). Baltimore: Williams & Wilkins.

Turk D.C., Meichenbaum D., & Genest, M. (1983). *Pain and behavioral medicine. A cognitive-behavioral perspective.* New York: Guilford Press.

Turk, D.C., Wack, J.T., & Kerns, R.D. (1985). An empirical examination of the "pain-behavior" construct. *Journal of Behavioral Medicine, 8,* 119–130.

Turk, D.C., Okifuji, A., Sinclai, J.D., & Starz, T.W. (1996). Pain, disability and physical functioning in subgroups of fibromyalgia patients. *Journal of Rheumatology, 23,* 1255–1262.

Turk, D.C., Sist, T.C., Okifuji, A., Miner, M.F., Florio, G., Harrison, P., Massey, J., Lema, M.L., & Zevon, M.A. (1998). Adaptation to metastatic cancer pain, regional/local cancer pain and non-cancer pain: Role of psychological and behavioral factors. *Pain, 74,* 247–256.

Turner, J.A. (1991). Coping and chronic pain. In: M.R. Bond, J.E. Charlton, & C.J. Woolf (Eds.). *Proceedings of the VIth World Congress on Pain* (pp. 219–227). Amsterdam: Elsevier.

Vlaeyen, J.W.S. (1991). *Chronic low back pain: Assessment and treatment from a behavioral rehabilitation perspective.* Amsterdam: Swets and Zeitlinger.

Vlaeyen, J.W.S., Schuerman, J.A., Groenman, N.H., & Van Eek, H. (1987). Dimension and components of observed chronic pain behavior. *Pain, 31,* 65–75.

Vlaeyen, J.W.S., Snijders, A.M.J., Schuerman, J.A., Van Eek, H., Groenman, N.H. & Bremer, J.J.C.B. (1989). Chronic pain and the three systems model of emotions. A critical examination. *Critical Reviews in Physical and Rehabilitation Medicine, 2,* 67–76.

Vlaeyen, J.W., Pernot, D.F., Kole-Snijders, A.M., Schuerman, J.A., et al. (1990). Assessment of the components of observed chronic pain behavior: The Checklist for Interpersonal Pain Behavior (CHIP). *Pain, 43*, 337–347.

Vlaeyen, J.W.S., Geurts, S.M., Kole-Snijders, A.M.J., Schuerman, J.A., Groenman, N.H., & Van Eek, H. (1990a). What do chronic pain patients think of their pain? Towards a pain cognition questionnaire. *British Journal of Clinical Psychology, 29*, 383–394.

Vlaeyen, J.W.S., Pernot, H.F.M., Snijders, A.M.J., Schuerman, J.A., Groenman, N.H., & Van Eek, H. (1990b). Assessing the components of chronic pain behavior: The Checklist for Interpersonal Pain Behavior (CHIP). *Pain, 43*, 337–347.

Vlaeyen, J.W.S., Kole-Snijders, A.M.J., Boeren, R.G.B., Van Eek, H. (1995a). Fear of movement/(re)injury in chronic low back pain and its relation to behavioral performance. *Pain, 62*, 363–372.

Vlaeyen, J.W.S., Kole-Snijders, A.M.J., Rotteveel, A., Ruesink, R., & Heuts, P.H.T.G. (1995b). The role of fear of movement/(re)injury in pain disability. *Journal of Occupational Rehabilitation, 5*, 235–252.

Vlaeyen, J.W.S., Seelen, H.A.M., Peters, M., De Jong, P., Arnetz, E., Beisiegel, E., & Weber, W. (1999). Fear of movement/(re)injury and muscular reactivity in chronic low back pain patients: An experimental investigation. *Pain, 82*, 297–304.

Waddell, G., Newton, M., Henderson, I., Somerville, D., & Main, C. (1993). A Fear-Avoidance Beliefs Questionnaire (FABQ) and the role of fear-avoidance beliefs in chronic low back pain and disability. *Pain, 52*, 157–168.

Wolpe, J., & Lang, P.J. (1964). A fear schedule for use in behavior therapy. *Behaviour Research and Therapy, 2*, 27–30.

Zaslansky, R., Sprecher, E., Katz, Y., Rozenberg, B., Hemli, J.A., & Yarnitsky, D. (1996). Pain-evoked potentials: What do they really measure? *Electroencephalography and Clinical Neurophysiology: Evoked-Potentials, 100*, 384–392.

# 14 ASSESSMENT OF FATIGUE—THE PRACTICAL UTILITY OF THE SUBJECTIVE FEELING OF FATIGUE IN RESEARCH AND CLINICAL PRACTICE

Maurice Alberts, Jan H.M.M. Vercoulen and Gijs Bleijenberg

The feeling of fatigue is a universal phenomenon. For most of us it is a regular experience, a normal response of the body to physical or mental strains that may even be evaluated as pleasant. However, fatigue can also become a major complaint in a variety of physical and psychiatric illnesses such as multiple sclerosis (MS), rheumatoid arthritis, AIDS, cancer, cardial disorder, Parkinson, systemic lupus erythematosus (SLE), depression, and muscular diseases. Furthermore, fatigue can result from medical treatment as a side-effect. Complaints of fatigue directly relate to the quality of life and functional impairment in patients, but it also is a financial and economic problem for society, since fatigued employees have a decreased productivity and an increased usage of medical services (Chen, 1986; David et al., 1990). As figures on the prevalence of fatigue in the general population and in primary care vary between 10% and 25%, depending on the setting and the way it is measured, it obviously is a prominent problem that should not be underestimated (David et al., 1990; Fukuda et al., 1994).

Despite the high prevalence of fatigue and its increasingly acknowledged negative effect on the patient's well-being and daily functioning, the phenomenon remains poorly understood. Perhaps the incapacity to operationalize fatigue in unambiguous terms led Muscio to state in 1921 "that the term be absolutely banished from scientific discussion, and consequently that attempts to obtain a fatigue test be abandoned." Since that time, diverse research disciplines have studied the biological, behavioral, and sociological aspects of fatigue, but still no widely accepted definition and assessment method exists. A renewed interest in fatigue as a complaint was recently established with the description of the chronic fatigue syndrome (CFS). The American Centers for Disease Control proposed a conceptual framework and research guidelines in order to encourage more systematic and comprehensive assessment of fatigue in studies on CFS and related illnesses (Fukuda et al., 1994). Definitions of different types of fatigue are given by these authors.

Prolonged fatigue is defined as self-reported, persistent fatigue lasting one month or longer, and chronic fatigue as a self-reported, persistent or relapsing fatigue lasting six consecutive months or more. Clinically evaluated cases of unexplained severely disabling chronic fatigue meeting additional criteria of co-occurring symptoms is defined as CFS. In the concept of CFS, fatigue refers to a severe mental and physical exhaustion, which differs from somnolence or lack of motivation and which is not attributable to exertion or diagnosable disease. These guidelines are useful in the differentiation between long lasting fatigue and acute fatigue occurring in normal circumstances (for example in occupational or traffic situations). Acute fatigue often is relieved by adequate coping behavior, such as resting, and is not the focus of this chapter.

# The assessment of fatigue

The aim of this non-exhaustive review is to illustrate several applications of the measurement of fatigue in different types of research and to provide some insight into the possibilities and limitations of fatigue instruments. Being a subjective phenomenon, fatigue can only be measured indirectly through the use of self-report techniques. Fatigue may be assessed as a general concept (unidimensional) or as a multidimensional concept. Table 14.1 provides an overview of the characteristics and psychometric qualities of the unidimensional fatigue instruments and Table 14.2 summarizes those of the multidimensional instruments. The most frequently used questionnaires and other techniques, such as self-observation and interviews, are discussed here. In subsequent paragraphs fatigue instruments are presented in certain types of research. Each instrument, however, may be useful in other applications of fatigue as well.

## EPIDEMIOLOGICAL STUDIES

Epidemiological studies have been performed to establish the prevalence of excessive fatigue in the general population or in primary care patients. For example, the 11-item Fatigue Questionnaire (FQ) was developed for such purposes (Chalder et al., 1993). The time frame is the preceding week and the FQ contains two subscales: seven items address *physical fatigue and its consequences* (e.g. "are you lacking in energy?", "do you have problems with tiredness?"), and four items address *mental fatigue* (e.g., "do you have difficulty concentrating?"). A cut-off score between 3 and 4 (in case of bimodal scoring) was

Table 14.1. Unidimensional fatigue instruments

| Instrument | Fatigue-scale (no. items) | Reponse-format | Time frame | Reliability | Validity | Comment |
|---|---|---|---|---|---|---|
| POMS | fatigue-inertia (7) | 5-point scale | past week | 0.89 | Several norm scores and studies support the predictive and construct validity | widely used, subjective fatigue, incorporated into measures of mood states. |
| FSS | fatigue severity (9) | 7-point scale | right now (?) | 0.81–0.89 | construct:? discriminant: + sensitivity: ± cut-off score ≥ 4 | frequently used, impact of fatigue – momentary – rather than severity of subjective fatigue (the FSS is the main factor of the FAI). |
| MIVE | Vital Exhaustion (23) | 3-point scale | variable | 0.90/0.86 | construct: + discriminant: + sensitivity: ? cut-off score: ≥8 | VE incorporates fatigue and some aspects of depression, but is presented as a distinct concept. |
| FACT-F | fatigue (13) | 5-point scale | past 7 days | 0.93–0.95 | construct: – discriminant: + sensitivity: ? norm scores: ± | fatigue independently or in the broader context of quality of life. |
| MFQ | mental fatigue (9) | 5-point scale | last month | 0.85/0.93 | construct: – discriminant: + sensitivity: – norm scores of small groups are available | only instrument assessing severity of mental fatigue exclusively, close resemblance with the PFRS-cognition difficulty subscale. |

Table 14.2. Multidimensional fatigue instruments

| Instrument | Dimensions (no. items) | Reponse-format | Time frame | Reliability | Validity | Comment |
|---|---|---|---|---|---|---|
| FQ | physical fatigue (11)<br>mental fatigue (4) | 4-point scale | last week | 0.85<br>0.82<br>(0.89 for the<br>total scale) | construct: +<br>discriminant: ±<br>sensitivity: +<br>cut-off score 3–4,<br>norm scores: − | two-dimensional instrument,<br>used in several studies. |
| FAI | global fatigue severity (11)<br>situation specific fatigue (6)<br>consequences (3)<br>response to rest/sleep (2) | 7-point scale | past<br>2 weeks | 0.92<br>0.77<br>0.70<br>0.85 | construct: +<br>discriminant: +<br>sensitivity: ?<br>norm scores: + | expanded version of the FSS<br>adding a MS-specific fatigue<br>subscale and two other<br>subscales, fatigue is defined<br>in the instruction |
| CIS | subjective fatigue (8)<br>concentration (5)<br>motivation (4)<br>activity (3) | 7-point scale | past<br>2 weeks | 0.88<br>0.92<br>0.83<br>0.87 | construct: +<br>discriminant: +<br>sensitivity: +<br>cut-off score ≥ 35<br>norm scores: + | subjective fatigue and<br>related behavioral aspects. |
| MFI | general fatigue (4)<br>physical fatigue (4)<br>concentration (4)<br>motivation (4)<br>activity (4) | 5-point scale | lately/<br>previous<br>days | average 0.84 | construct: +<br>discriminant: +<br>sensitivity: ±<br>norm scores: +<br>cross-cultural: + | subjective fatigue and<br>related behavioral aspects<br>of the past days. |
| PFRS | fatigue(12)<br>cognitive difficulty (11)<br>emotional distress (15)<br>somatic symptoms (16) | 7-point scale | past week | 0.96<br>0.95<br>0.95<br>0.88 | construct: +<br>discriminant: ±<br>sensitivity: +<br>norm scores: ± | physical fatigue, cognitive<br>difficulties and symptoms<br>regarding emotional distress<br>and somatic distress. |

determined to distinguish fatigued cases from non fatigued cases. Results of a community survey in southern England indicate that 18% of respondents experienced substantial fatigue lasting six months or longer, confirming the magnitude of the complaint in the general population (Pawlikowska et al., 1994). Other applications of the FQ will be discussed in subsequent sections.

Another epidemiological study assessing the prevalence of fatigue as a common health problem in a primary care setting and its relationship with psychiatric morbidity, illness behavior, and outcome is discussed in more detail in Box 14.1.

---

**Box 14.1    The prevalence of fatigue in primary care and its relationship with psychiatric comorbidity and illness behavior**

Cathébras et al. (1992) studied 686 patients in two primary care clinics. Ninety-three patients (13.6%) were considered fatigued according to the patients' presentation of complaints or the physicians' recording of complaints. Fifty-eight percent of these patients were recently fatigued (i.e. less than 6 months) and 42% were chronically fatigued (i.e. more than 6 months). Forty-five percent of the fatigued patients had depressive comorbidity. The 593 non-fatigued patients served as a comparison group.

Fatigued patients had greater emotion worry (the belief that one has or is vulnerable to a serious emotional problem) and more willingly acknowledged a psychosocial contribution to their complaints than non-fatigued patients. Chronic fatigued patients compared to recently fatigued patients reported more illness worry (hypochondrical beliefs) and tended to make fewer psychosocial attributions for their complaints at initial assessment. At follow up chronic fatigued patients (still) had higher illness worry and exhibited stronger somatic attributions. The apparent difference in attributional style was explained by a greater somatic focus in patients with chronic fatigue and was not due to a higher prevalence of psychiatric disorder in chronic fatigued patients.

Fatigued patients with depressive comorbidity experienced higher illness worries and higher emotional worries than non-depressed patients, who were indistinguishable from other groups on most measures. The authors conclude that in (less than) half of the fatigued patients psychiatric distress and somatic amplification may contribute to the experience of fatigue.

## PREVALENCE AND COMPARISON OF FATIGUE IN DIFFERENT DISEASES

Many studies have investigated the extent to which fatigue is present as a disabling symptom in a variety of primarily chronic diseases. Fatigue instruments in these studies should be able to distinguish the severity of fatigue in distinct groups. For example, a cross-sectional study provided a characterization of fatigue in MS patients compared to CFS patients and healthy controls (Vercoulen et al., 1996a). A central questionnaire in this study was the multidimensional Checklist Individual Strength (CIS-20) (Vercoulen et al., 1994), a 20-item self-report instrument referring to the previous two weeks and addressing the *subjective experience of fatigue* (8 items, e.g. "I feel tired"), *concentration* (5 items, e.g. "I have trouble to concentrate"), *motivation* (4 items, e.g. "I feel no desire to do anything"), and *physical activity level* (3 items, e.g. "I don't do much during the day"). The study showed that fatigue and associated aspects are serious problems affecting daily functioning in MS patients as compared to healthy controls. However, CFS patients had higher scores than MS patients on subjective fatigue and concentration problems.

The Multidimensional Fatigue Inventory (MFI-20) (Smets et al., 1995) is developed in the research area of cancer treatment to evaluate fatigue in patients undergoing radiotherapy. The MFI closely resembles the CIS with 17 identical items and comparable subscales; the MFI distinguishes the subscales *"general fatigue"* (4 items) and *"physical fatigue"* (4 items), whereas the CIS combines these into one subscale "subjective experience of fatigue". The main difference between both instruments is the time frame covered. Compared to the CIS, the MFI assesses momentary fatigue as the items refer to the experiences of the previous days. Extensive research on the validity of the internal structure and a cross-cultural comparison between Dutch and Scottish cancer patients receiving radiotherapy support the multidimensional character and the universality of the concept of fatigue (Smets et al., 1996).

Other questionnaires also have been used in comparative studies. For example, Packer et al. (1994) applied the Fatigue Severity Scale (discussed in the section on fatigue as an outcome variable in treatment studies) to measure the severity of fatigue in patients with MS, CFS, and postpolio-syndrome compared to a healthy group. All patient groups were more fatigued than the control group. The FQ was not able to differentiate the intensity of physical fatigue of CFS patients and patients with neuromuscular disorders, but both groups were significantly more fatigued than patients with affective disorders (Wessely & Powell, 1989).

## NATURAL COURSE OF FATIGUE

Regardless of the origin, fatigue complaints may vary in time. Fatigue may dissolve suddenly, re-occur unexpectedly, or the intensity may change. Instruments assessing the natural course of fatigue or the effects of treatment should be sensitive to changes over time.

Recently, two longitudinal studies used multidimensional question-naires to assess changes in fatigue to determine the prognosis of CFS patients (Ray et al., 1997; Vercoulen et al., 1996b). In both studies fatigue at follow up was applied as a dependent (criterion) variable for which predictors at initial assessment were sought. Box 14.2 describes the study of Vercoulen et al. (1996b) which illustrates the ability to measure changes over time of the CIS-20. In the study of Ray et al.

---

**Box 14.2    Predictors of the natural course of fatigue in Chronic Fatigue Syndrome**

Vercoulen et al. (1996b) performed a longitudinal study on 246 self referred CFS-patients to determine spontaneous improvement and factors predicting fatigue severity and improvement. At initial assessment a multidimensional assessment of behavioral, cognitive, emotional and social functioning was performed. Fatigue was mea-sured with the Checklist Individual Strength (CIS). All measures were repeated after a follow up interval of 18 months and self-reported change was determined.

At initial assessment fatigue severity of the CFS patients was sig-nificantly higher than that of healthy subjects. At follow-up 3% of the patients reported complete recovery, and 17% improvement. The ability of the CIS-20 to measure changes over time was con-firmed as fatigue intensity of recovered patients had significantly lowered to the level of healthy subjects and improved patients had lower scores than at initial assessment, but still higher than healthy subjects, whereas the fatigue intensity of non-improved patients remained unchanged. In a stepwise multiple regression analysis fatigue at follow up — the dependent variable — was predicted by fatigue severity, self-efficacy, and functional impairment at initial assessment. As self-efficacy also appeared the strongest predictor for self-reported improvement, tadditional analyses (cross-lagged panel) were performed to evaluate the causal direction between self-effi-cacy and fatigue. It was concluded that negative self-efficacy causes fatigue instead of fatigue causing negative self-efficacy.

(1992) the Profile of Fatigue Related Symptoms (PFRS) was employed, a 54-item questionnaire developed to capture the heterogeneous range of symptoms associated with CFS. In line with the CIS and the FQ, two separate factors address *physical fatigue* (12 items) and *cognitive difficulty* (11 items). Unfortunately, two clearly "mental fatigue" items belong to the physical fatigue subscale. The remaining two subscales evaluate *general psychological distress* (15 items referring to anxiety, depression, and anger), and additional *somatic symptomatology* (16 items referring to a diversity of somatic complaints, such as back pain and a sore throat). The ability to measure changes in time was supported as fatigue scores of 137 CFS patients changed in concordance with a direct rating of overall change.

## FATIGUE AS AN OUTCOME VARIABLE IN TREATMENT STUDIES

In studies evaluating the effectiveness of therapy for specific diseases, the severity of fatigue can be assessed as an outcome (effect) variable. Fatigue instruments used in such studies should be responsive to clinically significant change due to treatment effects.

A frequently used instrument is the 9-item Fatigue Severity Scale (FSS; Krupp et al., 1989) which was developed to facilitate research concerning fatigue in neurologic and related disorders. The FSS was administered to SLE patients, MS patients, and healthy adults. A score of 4 or higher is regarded as the cut-off indicating severe fatigue as only 5% of healthy controls rate their fatigue at this level, compared to 60–90% of patients with medical disorders. SLE patients and MS patients had similar degrees of fatigue severity exceeding that of healthy controls. Ambiguous evidence exists concerning the sensitivity to detect clinical expected changes due to treatment effects. Austin et al. (1996) found significant improvement on FSS-scores in SLE patients receiving telephone counseling interventions aiming to improve the health outcomes (see Box 14.3). Another study evaluating the effects of two commonly used medications for MS found no significant changes in FSS-scores in either condition (Krupp et al., 1995). Other applications of the FSS have been reported in patient groups with sleep disorders (Lichstein et al., 1997), polio (Schanke, 1997), Lyme disease (Ravdin et al., 1996) and CFS (Packer et al., 1994). The FSS is a useful research and clinical instrument because of its briefness and easy scoring. However, at least six of the nine items address behavioral consequences of fatigue (for example "fatigue interferes with carrying out certain duties and responsibilities"). Therefore, the FSS should be considered a unidimensional measure of

---

**Box 14.3   Fatigue as a measure of health outcome in SLE patients receiving telephone counselling interventions.**

Austin et al. (1996) performed a controlled study to evaluate the relative effectiveness of two psycho-educational telephone counseling strategies for improving the functional status of SLE patients. No comparison was made with a "usual care" control group, but with previous patients receiving no formal telephone counseling or a client centered approach. Patients were randomly assigned to the condition "treatment counselling" (TC) or "symptom monitoring" (SM). Health outcome measures were fatigue (Fatigue Severity Scale) and functional status (physical, affect, and pain subscales of the Arthritis Impact Measurement Scales 2). Mediating factors were "patient-physician communication", self-efficacy, and social support. Fifty-five patients completed the baseline assessment, intervention program, and the 6-month follow up assessment.

Patients in both conditions did not differ on sociodemographic or disease characteristics (duration, type of medication). The main findings were that physical function and social support significantly improved in the TC condition compared to the SM condition. Fatigue, self-efficacy, and affect were significantly improved for the combined TC and SM groups, but no difference was found between conditions. The only mediating factor strongly associated with better health outcome was self-efficacy, suggesting that telephone counseling may be effective because it improves the patient's confidence in the ability to control fatigue rather than because of improvements in communication or social support. The study provided some support to including routine telephone contact in guidelines for the management of SLE.

---

the *impact of fatigue* on daily functioning rather than a measure of the intensity of fatigue itself.

The successor of the FSS, the Fatigue Assessment Instrument (FAI; Schwartz et al., 1993) differs from most other fatigue instruments as fatigue is explicitly defined in the instruction as "a sense of tiredness, lack of energy or total body give-out". The FAI was administered to several small groups of patients (with Lyme disease, MS, dysthymia, CFS, post-Lyme chronic fatigue, and SLE) and healthy controls. The main factor of the questionnaire strongly resembles the FSS and is named "*global fatigue severity*" (11 items). All patient groups had higher fatigue scores than healthy subjects. The second factor, "*situation specific fatigue*", contains six items describing whether one's fatigue is sensitive to particular circumstances like temperature, stress, depression, long periods of inactivity, or positive experiences. This subscale showed stronger ability to detect significant changes due to medication treatment in MS patients than the FSS (Krupp et al., 1995). The remaining two factors, "*psychological consequences of fatigue*" and "*whether one's fatigue responds to sleep or rest*", of respectively three and two items only, appear to provide little extra information on the dimensionality of fatigue.

Examples of another instrument applying fatigue as an outcome measure are found in two studies evaluating the effect of cognitive behavior therapy in CFS patients. The FQ appeared sensitive to detect clinically significant changes in fatigue (Butler et al., 1991; Deale et al., 1997).

## FATIGUE AS AN ELEMENT OF QUALITY OF LIFE

A complex but important issue in patient-oriented research is quality of life (QOL). A detailed elaboration on this matter can be found elsewhere in this book (see chapters 16 and 17). The experience of fatigue and its consequences constitutes an important element of quality of life.

An instrument incorporating fatigue in the broader context of psychological well-being (mood states) is the Profile of Mood States (POMS; McNair et al., 1981). The subscale fatigue/inertia provides a solid uni-dimensional measure of the *intensity of subjective fatigue* during the past week and consists of 7 synonym items: exhausted, weary, worn out, listless, sluggish, bushed, and fatigued. Applications of the POMS-fatigue inertia subscale are widespread. For example, it was used as one of the process variables evaluating the effect of a psychiatric group intervention on the reduction of psychological distress in patients with malignant melanoma (Fawzy et al., 1990). At six-months' follow-up the fatigue scores in the intervention group were significantly less than those of the control group. Although the fatigue/inertia subscale is rather short, the entire POMS (65 items) may take some time to complete. Therefore, when the interest is solely in a measure of fatigue — not mood states — one might consider using the 37-item shortened POMS (Shacham, 1983) which contains a 5-item fatigue/inertia subscale with equally good qualities as the original subscale.

## CONCEPTUAL ANALYSIS

While reviewing the literature, a striking observation is that several fatigue instruments are developed in specific research areas. Considerable differences exist regarding the instruction, time-frame, (number of) items, response format, total length, dimensionality, psychometric qualities, and availability of normscores (Tables 14.1 and 14.2). This jeopardizes the comparability of studies. Nevertheless, similarity exists in the concepts being measured. At least three dimensions can be distinguished: (1) The *subjective feeling of fatigue* is the core of most instruments. Synonyms like "weak", "tired", "fatigued", or "(lack of) energy" are used in virtually all questionnaires. The subscales of the CIS/MFI and the POMS appear the most unambiguous; (2) The *impact of fatigue*, either in general ("do you have problems with tiredness") or more specifically related to daily activities ("fatigue interferes with my work, family or social life"). The FSS provides an appropriate measure of limited length; and (3) *Cognitive consequences* (difficulty concentrating and difficulty in thinking clearly) are often reported in relationship to excessive fatigue. The FQ, CIS/MFI, and the PFRS contain separate subscales addressing the severity of these complaints, but items differ considerably.

Unfortunately, none of the existing fatigue instruments contains separate subscales for these three dimensions of fatigue. In order to overcome the dissimilarities between fatigue instruments and to improve comparability between studies, a standard questionnaire should be developed addressing aforementioned dimensions by means of separate subscales.

## ALTERNATIVE FATIGUE INSTRUMENTS: DIARY AND INTERVIEW

Evidently, investigations of fatigue rely primarily on retrospective self-report questionnaires. However, problems arise with this type of measurement and other instruments should be considered in certain circumstances.

The longer the time frame covered by the instrument, the less valid the information obtained due to deficiencies in human recollection. Some instruments avoid this bias by evaluating the instantaneous presence of fatigue (e.g. "how fatigued do you feel at this moment?"). These measures, however, are vulnerable to fluctuations in fatigue due to particular circumstances. For example, a CFS patient may feel modestly fatigued (average score) at the start of a research examination but can become completely exhausted within a few hours (high score). To overcome these problems a concurrent self-observation instrument was developed (Figure 14.1) (Vercoulen et al., 1996a). Over two weeks patients rate their fatigue four times daily on a scale of 0 (no fatigue) to 4 (very severe fatigue) on a prescheduled diary. The Daily Observed Fatigue (DOF) score varies between 0 and 16. The advantages of this mode of scoring is that a general retrospective estimation over a long period is avoided and that it allows to reliably assess fluctuations in fatigue. Other advantages include the possibility to evaluate fatigue scores day by day, or to count the number of days that patients are free of complaints. Furthermore, the influence of special days (weekend-days, holidays or birthdays) is easily revealed and can be taken into account.

A disadvantage inherent to questionnaires is that they rely on the ability of the patients to appraise all items and to evaluate ambiguous terms that may mean different things to different individuals. In some circumstances a structured interview may provide a more accurate

| Date : ............... <br> Time : | breakfast <br> .... hrs | lunch <br> .... hrs | diner <br> .... hrs | bedtime <br> .... hrs | |
|---|---|---|---|---|---|
| **1a. Did you feel fatigued the past few hours?** | 0 1 2 3 4 | 0 1 2 3 4 | 0 1 2 3 4 | 0 1 2 3 4 | **Fatigue / pain** <br> 0 = no <br> 1 = a little bit <br> 2 = considerable <br> 3 = severe <br> 4 = very severe |
| **b. Did you have pain the past few hours?** | 0 1 2 3 4 | 0 1 2 3 4 | 0 1 2 3 4 | 0 1 2 3 4 | |
| **c. By marking a box behind one of the complaints below, you can indicate that you suffered from it. If you were not bothered by the complaint you should leave the box unmarked.** | | | | | |
| - headache | 0 | 0 | 0 | 0 | |
| - musclepain | 0 | 0 | 0 | 0 | |
| - depressed mood | 0 | 0 | 0 | 0 | |
| - difficulty paying attention | 0 | 0 | 0 | 0 | |
| - irritable/nervous | 0 | 0 | 0 | 0 | |
| - abdominal complaints | 0 | 0 | 0 | 0 | |
| - forgetfulness | 0 | 0 | 0 | 0 | |
| - other complaints | 0 | 0 | 0 | 0 | |
| **d. How active have you been the past few hours?** | 0 1 2 3 4 | 0 1 2 3 4 | 0 1 2 3 4 | 0 1 2 3 4 | **Activity** <br> 0 = not at all <br> 1 = a little <br> 2 = considerable <br> 3 = active <br> 4 = very active |

Figure 14.1. Example of a self-observation symptom checklist.

assessment method. This was demonstrated, for example, by Meesters and Appels (1996) with the assessment of Vital Exhaustion (VE), a mental state characterized by unusual fatigue, increased irritability, and feelings of demoralization. Overlap with depression occurs for common somatic and vegetative symptoms, but depressed affect (sadness) and cognitions (feelings of guilt and lower self-esteem) are mainly absent in VE. VE reflects a relatively recent breakdown in adaptation to stress and was found to act as a short-term risk factor of manifest heart disease. VE can be assessed by the Maastricht Questionnaire (MQ) (Appels et al., 1987) or the Maastricht Interview for Vital Exhaustion (MIVE), in which 23 items are evaluated as positive, negative or unknown (Meesters & Appels, 1996). This comparison study in patients hospitalized because of myocardial infarction and healthy controls indicated that the discriminating power of the interview was much higher than that of the questionnaire. As the questionnaire is prone to a considerable amount of false positive results, the interview is preferably used for case selection in clinical or experimental research. However, in case of screening for the existence of VE in large populations, the questionnaire is a far less time-consuming device.

## Subconcepts of fatigue

Fatigue is not an isolated phenomenon occurring on its own. Behavioral and cognitive aspects influence the process of the experience and perpetuation of fatigue. For this reason a comprehensive assessment of fatigue implies measurement of several subconcepts simultaneously. The importance of some subconcepts (activity level, self-efficacy, and causal attributions), the measurement of these subconcepts and relationship with fatigue are discussed below.

ACTIVITY

*Importance*: Physical activity is related to psychological and physiological well-being. Excessive inactivity has been known to cause mood disturbances and maladaptive physiological changes (Winningham et al., 1994) and exercise is useful for the prevention and treatment of illness (Clearing-Sky, 1988; Dubbert, 1992). Additional information concerning the assessment of activity can be found in chapter 12.

*Relationship with fatigue*: A negative relationship between physical activity and fatigue is reported in a diversity of patient groups, including patients with end stage renal disease on chronic haemodialysis

(Brunier & Graydon, 1993), older adults with rheumatoid arthritis (Belza et al., 1993), cancer patients (Dimeo et al., 1997), and CFS patients (Vercoulen et al., 1997).

*Instruments*: In the aforementioned studies different instruments were used to assess activity level; a composite score estimating the energy expenditure of "daily" physical activities related to housework, work outside the home, and leisure (Belza et al., 1993; Brunier & Graydon, 1993), a maximal physical performance on a treadmill stress test (Dimeo et al., 1997), a general question classifying subjects themselves as very active, moderately active or quite inactive (Chen, 1986), and a matchbox sized motion-sensing devise (actometer) (Vercoulen et al., 1997).

Virtually all fatigue questionnaires contain items referring to activity, for example "exercise brings on my fatigue" (FAI). Furthermore, the CIS and the MFI employ specific subscales that inquire after reduced activity.

*Validity of self-reported activity level*: Vercoulen et al. (1997) investigated to what extent subjective rating on self-report instruments adequately reflects the actual amount of physical activity performed as measured by a motion-sensing devise (actometer). Self-report questionnaires requiring general subjective interpretations over a prolonged period (e.g. "have you been very active, moderately active or not at all active the past month?") appeared to be an expression of the patient's view about activity and may be biased by cognitions concerning illness and disability rather than actual activity. Questionnaires requiring simple ratings of specified activities, such as the subscales "walking" and "mobility" of the Sickness Impact Profile (Bergner et al., 1981) are more acceptable substitutes for the costly and time-consuming method of direct activity assessment using an actometer.

## CAUSAL ATTRIBUTIONS

*Importance*: Most patients have ideas about the origin of their complaints (causal attributions, see also chapter 9). These ideas are influenced by past experiences and may direct future expectations and may guide the patient's behavior towards resolving their complaints. Moreover, attributional style influences the illness presentation and the prognosis.

*Instruments*: Attributions are not evaluated in the fatigue questionnaires themselves. In addition to the FQ, questions were asked concerning the reason respondents think they are fatigued. These causes were classified as physical (for example, flu, recent operation, anaemia); psychosocial (related to work, family, or lifestyle); psychological (anxiety, stress, or depression); environmental (weather, pollution); and CFS (Pawlikowska et al., 1994). Similar categories of attributions are found in other questionnaires such as the Causal Attribution List (Vercoulen et al., 1996a), the subscale disease conviction of the Illness Behavior Questionnaire (Pilowsky & Spence, 1983), and the Symptom Interpretation Questionnaire (Robbins & Kirmayer, 1991).

*Relationship with fatigue*: In the general population and in primary care, the majority of patients with a relatively short duration of fatigue tend to attribute their complaints to psychosocial or environmental causes (Cathébras et al., 1995; Pawlikowska et al., 1994). Patients with a short duration of fatigue and seeking a somatic explanation for their complaints reported more neurological and psychiatric symptoms, but did not have a worse prognosis. For these patients acute fatigue probably has an obvious cause (such as a viral infection) and is relieved by adequate coping behavior (for example resting). However, when fatigue becomes long lasting (chronic), neither the cause nor the resolution of the complaint is evident. Over time, chronic fatigued patients may experience increasing pressure to find a socially acceptable explanation for their inabilities, i.e., physiological rather than psychological, regardless of the lack of evidence for an organic disease process. Persistent somatic attributions might be indicative for broader underlying illness-schemata expressing the fear that the illness is unpredictable, chronic, and incurable (Wessely et al., 1998). Patients also may have the idea that certain activities produce fatigue or even are damaging and should be avoided (Vercoulen et al., 1997). Prospective studies of patients with chronic fatigue indicate that holding strong somatic attributions is associated with worse prognosis (Cope et al., 1994; Sharpe et al., 1992; Vercoulen et al., 1996b; Wilson et al., 1994) and worse treatment effect (Butler et al., 1991).

## SELF-EFFICACY

*Importance*: Chronic fatigued patients may experience a feeling of not being in control of their complaints (negative self-efficacy) or they may think they can influence their complaints (positive self-efficacy). The significance of self-efficacy as a predictor of health behavior and health outcome is increasingly acknowledged.

*Instruments*: Two instruments addressing fatigue related self-efficacy were used in previously mentioned studies (Austin et al., 1996; Vercoulen et al., 1996a). Both self-efficacy scales are modifications from pain cognition lists and contain five items (Table 14.3). A more

**Table 14.3.** Fatigue related self-efficacy instruments

---

FSES (Austin et al., 1996):
1. I am certain that I can decrease my fatigue quite a bit when I want.
2. I am certain that I can continue most of my daily activities in spite of fatigue.
3. I am certain that I can keep fatigue from bothering my sleep.
4. I am certain that I can lower my fatigue at least a little even without taking pills.
5. I am certain that I can greatly lower my fatigue even without taking pills.

Self-efficacy Scale (Vercoulen et al., 1996a):
1. Do you think you can control your complaints?
2. No matter what I do, I can't change my complaints.
3. I think I will be able to influence my fatigue positively.
4. I feel helpless against my fatigue.
5. Because of my positive attitude I feel able to deal with my fatigue.

---

general measure of self-efficacy is the internal attributions subscale of the Multidimensional Health Locus of Control questionnaire (Wallston et al., 1978) which evaluates to what extent patients feel that their health is determined by their own behavior or capacities.

*Relationship with fatigue*: Longitudinal studies consistently report that positive self-efficacy expectations mediate a better outcome in patients with chronic fatigue complaints. Self-efficacy was strongly associated with improved health outcome in a study evaluating telephone counseling methods in patients with SLE (Austin et al., 1996). Self-efficacy also was an important predictor of fatigue severity and the strongest predictor of chronicity in a study on the natural course of CFS (Vercoulen et al., 1996b). Outcome (impairment) was predicted by a low internal locus of control in a follow up study on CFS patients (Ray et al., 1997). In two cross-sectional studies investigating psychosocial factors in MS patients a close relationship was found between self-efficacy and fatigue (Schwartz et al., 1996; Vercoulen et al., 1996a) .

DEPRESSION AND FUNCTIONAL IMPAIRMENT

Depression and functional impairment are two subconcepts that also are strongly associated with fatigue. Both subconcepts will be discussed briefly here.

## DEPRESSION

Considerable overlap exists between the subjective experiences of chronic fatigue and depressive mood. As fatigue is one of the somatic symptoms characteristic for a clinical depression, it is addressed in the Beck Depression Inventory, the Hamilton Depression Rating scale and the Zung. The central element in a depressive mood state, however, is the general lack of interest or pleasure in daily activities that normally are enjoyed. This motivational component usually is unaffected in patients with excessive fatigue. Nevertheless, long lasting fatigue may become the cause of a depressive disorder (Wessely et al., 1998).

In CFS, depression is not an essential factor involved in the perpetuation of complaints. Several longitudinal studies on the natural course of CFS did not find depression as a predictor variable for the outcome of the illness (Clark et al., 1995; Vercoulen et al., 1996b; Wilson et al., 1994). Furthermore, in a controlled study of the effects of antidepressive therapy no changes in severity of fatigue or depression were observed in depressed and non-depressed CFS patients. Apparently, the processes underlying the presentation of depressive symptoms in CFS patients with depressive comorbidity differ from those of patients with major depressive disorder (see Box 14.4).

## FUNCTIONAL IMPAIRMENT

Chronic fatigue is strongly associated with functional impairment experienced by patients (Kroenke et al., 1988; Vercoulen et al., 1996b). A reduction in exercise tolerance negatively influences the self-care ability, household activities, social activities, and the pursuit and enjoyment of leisure activities. Most fatigue instruments contain items that refer to functional limitations, but a more comprehensive assessment is provided by, for example, the Sickness Impact Profile (Bergner et al., 1981) or the Rand-36 (Ware & Sherbourne, 1992). The SIP measures the influence of complaints in different areas of daily functioning such as eating, sleeping, walking, home-making, work, recreation, ambulation, and social interactions. While the complete SIP is a voluminous instrument, one might consider selecting the subscales referring to physical functioning or psychosocial functioning only. The Rand-36 is a shorter health status questionnaire addressing dimensions such as physical functioning, social functioning, mental health, pain, and general well-being.

> **Box 14.4    Fatigue as an outcome variable in a study assessing the effects of antidepressant therapy in chronic fatigue syndrome.**
>
> Antidepressant therapy is commonly proposed as a treatment in CFS since a proportion of patients have depression or overlapping symptoms. In a randomized, double-blind, placebo-controlled study the effect of fluoxetine on the severity of fatigue, depression and other characterisitics of CFS patients was assessed (Vercoulen et al., 1996c). Forty-four depressed patients were randomly assigned to receive fluoxetine or a placeo therapy. For 52 non-depressed patients the same procedure was followed. The design allowed to distinguish any direct effect of fluoxetine on fatigue from indirect effects mediated by an improvement in depression. Pre-treatment, post-treatment and follow-up measures were performed.
>
> Fluoxetine therapy did not have a beneficial effect on the severity of fatigue, the severity of depression and other outcome measures in both depressed and non-depressed patients. Methodological aspects as differences in pre-treatment depression severity, non-compliance or a too low effective dosage could not account for the unexpected results. Apparently, the processes underlying the presentation of depressive symptoms in CFS patients with depressive comorbidity differ from those of patients with major depressive disorder.

## A MODEL OF FATIGUE IN CHRONIC FATIGUE SYNDROME

A model was empirically designed to gain insight into and understanding of the dynamics of behavioral and cognitive processes involved in the experience of fatigue in CFS patients (see Figure 14.2) (Vercoulen et al., 1998). "Self-efficacy" and "focusing on bodily symptoms" had a direct causal effect on fatigue. Furthermore, the tendency to attribute complaints to a somatic cause mediates a lower physical activity level, which in turn directly effects the experience of more severe fatigue. Depression was excluded from the model, confirming earlier findings that depression in CFS is not a fundamental subconcept in CFS. Furthermore, the model did not fit the data for MS patients, suggesting that the underlying processes of the persistence of fatigue may be different in distinct groups.

Like any model, this model is a simplification of reality. Factors such as social functioning and the relationship between the patient and his environment were not tested but evidently play an important role in the perpetuation of the subjective feeling of fatigue.

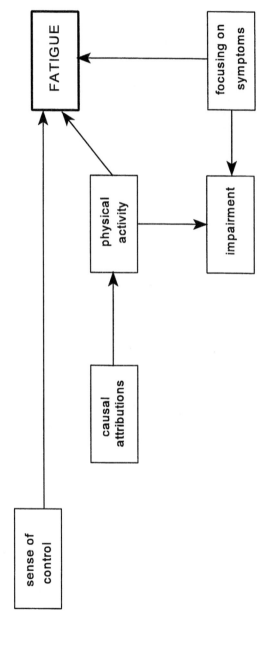

Figure 14.2. Model of factors involved in the continuation of fatigue in CFS patients.

# How to optimize the choice of appropriate measures for specific research questions?

In the diversity of measurement methods and tools it is difficult to find the instrument that provides the most appropriate measure of fatigue. Besides the psychometric qualities of the instruments (Tables 14.1 and 14.2) other issues must be considered.

Firstly, one has to choose between a unidimensional or a multidimensional assessment of fatigue. Multidimensional instruments provide a more comprehensive description of the different components of fatigue, but they take more time to complete compared to unidimensional instruments.

Secondly, one has to decide on the most appropriate time frame. The shorter the time frame the more the instrument becomes a measure of current fatigue. This might be particularly suitable for studies concerned with acute fatigue, for example after intensive physical or mental exercise. With longer time frame coverage the instrument becomes more appropriate for measurement of chronic conditions of fatigue occurring in several physical and mental disorders. However, it remains questionable whether adequate recall is possible for such long periods as the past month. Researchers might make changes to the time frame in the instructions of existing fatigue instruments to suit their own purposes, although this will hamper comparisons across studies.

Thirdly, one has to choose which important subconcepts should be measured in addition to fatigue. Two individuals with the same overall fatigue score may differ on other dimensions. One fatigued person may have such strong functional impairment that s/he depends on professional or family support for daily routines, while another fatigued person might be able to perform the basic activities himself. Whenever the level of physical functioning is important, one should consider a measure addressing functional limitations (e.g., SIP), or activity level (e.g., CIS activity). If illness beliefs or cognitions are of primary interest one should consider using a self-efficacy scale or a measure of causal attributions.

## Assessment of fatigue in the clinical setting

In primary care fatigue is one of the three main reasons for visiting a general practitioner (Lamberts, 1991). Physicians have to deal with fatigued patients every day and normally have limited time to spare. To evaluate the intensity of fatigue, physicians have to rely on their experience in this field and on the competence of the patients in describing their complaints. Even for experienced physicians this is a hazardous task since varying terms are used in the description of fatigue amongst patients and doctors. Synonyms like "tired", "exhausted", "no energy", "run-down", "feeling weak" or "worn-out" may mean different things to different individuals.

---

**Shortened Fatigue Questionnaire (SFQ)**

Name           :
Gender         :
Date of birth  :
Date of today  :

---

On this page you will find four statements indicating how you have been feeling **the past two weeks**.

You can answer each question by placing a mark in one of the seven boxes. The position of the marking indicates to what extent you feel the statement applies to you.

For example: if you think the statement is completely true, you should place a mark in the left box, like this:

yes, that is true | X | | | | | | | no, that is not true

If you think the answer is not 'yes, that's true' but also not 'no, that is not true', you should mark the box that best corresponds with your feeling. For example like this:

yes, that is true | | | | | X | | | no, that is not true

Please answer all the statements and place only one mark at each statement.

1. I feel tired — yes, that is true | | | | | | | | no, that is not true

2. I am tired very quickly — yes. that is true | | | | | | | | no, that is not true

3. I feel fit — yes, that is true | | | | | | | | no, that is not true

4. Physically I feel exhausted — yes, that is true | | | | | | | | no, that is not true

---

Figure 14.3. The Shortened Fatigue Questionnaire: instruction and items.

Hence, a short, self-explanatory instrument with good psychometric qualities was developed to assess fatigue in a clinical setting: the "Shortened Fatigue Questionnaire" (SFQ; Alberts et al., 1997). CIS and MFI data were available from 1772 respondents of three patient groups (patients with CFS, functional bowel disorder and cancer) and three normal groups (students, service personel and healthy controls). Using factor analysis (principal component analysis), item analysis and theoretical considerations, a set of four items was selected that had good internal consistency in all groups (Cronbach's alpha varied from 0.83 to 0.90) and that was able to differentiate several patient groups (CFS, MS and functional bowel disorder) from each other and from healthy groups. Special attention was given to a practical format, both for patient and physician. The SFQ consists of two separate pages (Figures 14.3 and 14.4). Patients are asked to fill out the front page that contains an instruction about the time frame (past two weeks), an example of how to score the 7-point scale, and finally, the four items "I feel tired", "I am tired very quickly", "I feel fit", and "Physically I feel exhausted". The answers are automatically duplicated on the underlying page (scoring-form) from where the physician can read the item-scores (ranging from 1–7) and can easily calculate the total score (ranging from 7–28). In addition to the total fatigue score, the diagnosis or main complaint can be recorded. Furthermore, SFQ scores of comparison groups are displayed which makes a practical evaluation of the patient's score possible. One can think of many applications. Applying the questionnaire repeatedly allows the physician to observe the natural course of the fatigue or to examine the occurrence of fatigue as a side-effect from treatment. Furthermore, the SFQ might be used as an aid in diagnosing CFS.

The psychometric qualities of the SFQ were tested in a follow up study among CFS patients with a relatively short duration of complaints. Results indicate that the reliability is good (Cronbach's alpha is 0.92) and that SFQ scores of recovered, improved, and unchanged CFS patients can be distinguished. The SFQ is a practical instrument for usage in daily medical practice or in clinical scientific studies.

## Conclusion

Fatigue is a frequently encountered symptom causing problems in a variety of primarily chronic diseases. As a subjective experience fatigue

## Score form SFQ

**Name**          :

**Gender**        :

**Date of birth**  :

**Date of today**  :

Chief complaint  :...................................................................

Date of origin      :.............(month)................(year)

Diagnosis            :...................................................................

| Groups | average age | << low | < avg. | = avg. | > avg. | >> high |
|---|---|---|---|---|---|---|
| *Healthy groups* | | | | | | |
| healthy adults | 37 | 4 | 4 | 5- 8 | 9-14 | ≥15 |
| students normal circumst. | 22 | 4 | 5-7 | 8-14 | 15-21 | ≥22 |
| students demanding circum. | 21 | ≤5 | 6-9 | 10-17 | 18-23 | ≥24 |
| servicemen at rest (normal) | 21 | 4 | 5-6 | 7-14 | 15-22 | ≥23 |
| servicemen in field exercise | 21 | ≤5 | 6-11 | 12-18 | 19-24 | ≥25 |
| | | | | | | |
| *Patient groups* | | | | | | |
| cancer | 61 | 4 | 5-12 | 13-21 | 22-27 | 28 |
| functional bowel disease | 41 | ≤ 6 | 7-12 | 13-21 | 22-27 | 28 |
| multiple sclerosis | 36 | ≤12 | 13-19 | 20-26 | 27 | 28 |
| chronic fatigue syndrome | 38 | ≤22 | 23-25 | 26-27 | 28 | 28 |

| 1. I feel tired | yes,that is true | 7 | 6 | 5 | 4 | 3 | 2 | 1 | no, that is not true |
|---|---|---|---|---|---|---|---|---|---|

| 2. I am tired very quickly | yes, that is true | 7 | 6 | 5 | 4 | 3 | 2 | 1 | no, that is not true |
|---|---|---|---|---|---|---|---|---|---|

| 3. I feel fit | yes, that is true | 1 | 2 | 3 | 4 | 5 | 6 | 7 | no, that is not true |
|---|---|---|---|---|---|---|---|---|---|

| 4. Physically I feel exhausted | yes, that is true | 7 | 6 | 5 | 4 | 3 | 2 | 1 | no, that is not true |
|---|---|---|---|---|---|---|---|---|---|

**Total score SFQ:** .....................

Figure 14.4. The Shortened Fatigue Questionaire: scoring form.

can only be measured indirectly by methods relying on self-report by the patients. As cognitive and behavioral factors play an important role in the process of the experience of fatigue a multidimensional assessment of fatigue and important subconcepts is imperative.

# References

Alberts, M., Smets, E.M.A., Vercoulen, J.H.M.M., Garssen, B., & Bleijenberg, G. (1997). "Verkorte vermoeiheidsvragenlijst": Een praktisch hulpmiddel bij het scoren van vermoeidheid [Shortened Fatigue Questionnaire: A practical aid for the assessment of fatigue]. *Nederlands Tijdschrift voor Geneeskunde, 141*, 1526–1530.

Appels, A., Höppener, P., & Mulder, P. (1987). A questionnaire to assess premonitory symptoms of myocardial infarction. *International Journal of Cardiology, 17*, 15–24.

Austin, J.S., Maisiak, R.S., Macrina, D.M., & Heck, L.W. (1996). Health outcome improvements in patients with systemic lupus erythematosus using two telephone counseling interventions. *Arthritis Care and Research, 9*, 391–399.

Belza, B.L., Henke, C.J., Yelin, E.H., Epstein, W.V., & Gilliss, C.L. (1993). Correlates of fatigue in older adults with rheumatoid arthritis. *Nursing Research, 42*, 93–99.

Bergner, M., Bobbit, R.A., Carter, W.B., & Gilson, B.S. (1981). The Sickness Impact Profile: development and final version of a health status measure. *Medical Care, 19*, 787–805.

Brunier, G.M., & Graydon, J. (1993). The influence of physical activity on fatigue in patients with ESRD on haemodialysis. *ANNA Journal, 20*, 457–461.

Butler, S., Chalder, T., Ron, M., & Wessely, S. (1991). Cognitive behaviour therapy in chronic fatigue syndrome. *Journal of Neurology, Neurosurgery, and Psychiatry, 54*, 153–158.

Cathébras, P.J., Robbins, J.M., Kirmayer, L.J., & Hayton, B.C. (1992). Fatigue in primary care: Prevalence, comorbidity, illness behavior, and outcome. *Journal of General Internal Medicine, 7*, 276–286.

Cathébras, P., Jacquin, L., le-Gal, M., Fayol, C., Bouchou, K., & Rousset, H. (1995). Correlates of somatic causal attributions in primary care patients with fatigue. *Psychotherapy and Psychosomatics, 63*, 174–180.

Chalder, T., Berelowitz, G., Pawlikowska, T., Watts, L., Wessely, S., Wright, D., & Wallace, E.P. (1993). Development of a fatigue scale. *Journal of Psychosomatic Research, 37*, 147–153.

Chen, M.K. (1986). The epidemiology of self-perceived fatigue among adults. *Preventive Medicine, 15*, 74–81.

Clark, M.R., Katon, W., Russo, J., Kith, P., Sintay, M., & Buchwald, D. (1995). Chronic fatigue: Risk factors for symptoms persistence in a 2.5-year follow-up study. *American Journal of Medicine, 98*, 187–195.

Clearing-Sky, M. (1988). Exercise: Issues for prescribing psychologists. *Psychology & Health, 2*, 189–207.

Cope, H., David, A., Pelosi, A., & Mann, A. (1994). Predictors of chronic "postviral" fatigue. *Lancet, 344*, 864–848.

David, A., Pelosi, A., McDonald, E., Stephens, D., Ledger, D., Rathbone, R., & Mann, A. (1990). Tired, weak, or in need of rest: Fatigue among general practice attenders. *British Medical Journal, 301*, 1199–1202.

Deale, A., Chalder, T., Marks, I., Wessely, S. (1997). Cognitive behavior therapy for chronic fatigue syndrome: A randomized controlled trial. *American Journal of Psychiatry, 154*, 408–414.

Dimeo, F., Stieglitz, R.D., Novelli Fischer, U., Fetscher, S., Mertelsmann, R., & Keul, J. (1997). Correlation between physical performance and fatigue in cancer patients. *Annals of Oncology, 8*, 1251–1255.

Dubbert, P.M. (1992). Exercise in behavioral medicine. *Journal of Consulting Clinical Psychology, 60*, 613–618.

Fawzy, I.F., Cousins, N., Fawzy, N.W., Kemeney, M.E., Elashoff, R., & Morton, D. (1990). A structured psychiatric intervention for cancer patients. *Archives of General Psychiatry, 47*, 720–725.

Fukuda, K., Straus, S.E., Hickie, I., Sharpe, M.C., Dobbins, J.G., Komaroff, A.L., & the International Chronic Fatigue Syndrome Study Group (1994). The chronic fatigue syndrome: A comprehensive approach to its definition and study. *Annals of Internal Medicine, 121*, 953–959.

Kroenke, K., Wood, D.R., Mangelsdorff, A.D., Meier, N.J., & Powell, J.B. (1988). Chronic fatigue in primary care. Prevalence, patient characteristics, and outcome. *Journal of the American Medical Association, 260*, 929–934.

Krupp, L.B., LaRocca, N.G., Muir Nash, J., & Steinberg, A.D. (1989). The fatigue severity scale. Application to patients with multiple sclerosis and systemic lupus erythematosus. *Archives of Neurology, 46*, 1121–1123.

Krupp, L.B., Coyle, P.K., Dosscher, N.P., Miller, A., Cross, A.H., Jandorf, M.A., Halper, J., Johnson, B., Morgante, L., & Grimson, R. (1995). Fatigue therapy in multiple sclerosis: Results of a double-blind, randomized, parallel trial of amantadine, pemoline, and placebo. *Neurology, 45*, 1956–1961.

Lamberts H. (1991). *In het huis van de huisarts [Within the home of the general practitioner]*. Verslag van het Transitieproject. Lelystad: Meditekst.

Lichstein, K.L., Means, M.K., Noe, S.L., & Aguillard, R.N. (1997). Fatigue and sleep disorders. *Behaviour Research and Therapy, 35*, 733–740.

McNair, D.M., Lorr, M., & Droppleman, L.F. (1981). *Profile of mood states*. San Diego, CA: Educational and Industrial Testing Service.

Meesters, C., & Appels, A. (1996). An interview to measure vital exhaustion. I. Development and comparison with the Maastricht Questionnaire. *Psychology & Health, 11*, 557–571.

Packer, T.L., Sauriol, A., & Brouwer, B. (1994). Fatigue secondary to chronic illness: Postpolio syndrome, chronic fatigue syndrome, and multiple sclerosis. *Archives of Physical Medicine and Rehabilitation, 75*, 1122–1126.

Pawlikowska, T., Chalder, T., Hirsch, S.R., Wallace, P., Wright, D.J., & Wessely, S.C. (1994). Population based study of fatigue and psychological distress. *British Medical Journal, 308*, 763–766.

Pilowsky, I., & Spence, N.D. (1983). *Manual for the illness behaviour questionnaire (IBQ). (2nd Ed.).* Adelaide: University of Adelaide.

Ravdin, L.D., Hilton, E., Primeau, M., Clements, C., & Barr, W.B. (1996). Memory functioning in Lyme borreliosis. *Journal of Clinical Psychiatry, 57,* 282–286.

Ray, C., Jefferies, S., William, R., & Weir, C. (1997). Coping and other predictors of outcome in chronic fatigue syndrome: A 1-year follow-up. *Journal of Psychosomatic Research, 4,* 405–415.

Ray, C., Weir, W.R.C., Phillips, S., & Cullen, S. (1992). Development of a measure of symptoms in chronic fatigue syndrome: The profile of fatigue related symptoms (PFRS). *Psychology & Health, 7,* 27–43.

Robbins, J.M., & Kirmayer, L.J. (1991). Attributions of common somatic symptoms. *Psychological Medicine, 21,* 1029–1045.

Schanke, A.K. (1997). Psychological distress, social support and coping behaviour among polio survivors: A 5-year perspective on 63 polio patients. *Disability and Rehabilitation, 19,* 108–116.

Schwartz, J.E., Jandorf, L., & Krupp, L.B. (1993). The measurement of fatigue: A new instrument. *Journal of Psychosomatic Research, 37,* 753–762.

Schwartz, C.E., Coulthard-Morris, L., & Zeng, Q. (1996). Psychosocial correlates of fatigue in multiple sclerosis. *Archives of Physical Medicine and Rehabilitation, 77,* 165–170.

Shacham, S. (1983). A shortened version of the Profile of Mood States. *Journal of Personality Assessment, 47,* 305–306.

Sharpe, M., Hawton, K., Seagroatt, V., & Pasvol, G. (1992). Follow up of patients presenting with fatigue to an infectious diseases clinic. *British Medical Journal, 305,* 147–152.

Smets, E.M., Garssen, B., Bonke, B., & De-Haes, J.C. (1995). The Multidimensional Fatigue Inventory (MFI): Psychometric qualities of an instrument to assess fatigue. *Journal of Psychosomatic Research, 39,* 315–325.

Smets, E.M., Garssen, B., Cull, A., & de-Haes, J.C. (1996). Application of the multidimensional fatigue inventory (MFI-20) in cancer patients receiving radiotherapy. *British Journal of Cancer, 73,* 241–245.

Vercoulen, J.H.M.M., Swanink, C.M.A., Fennis, J.F.M., Galama, J.M.D., Van der Meer, J.W.M., & Bleijenberg, G. (1994). Dimensional assessment of chronic fatigue syndrome. *Journal of Psychosomatic Research, 38,* 383–392.

Vercoulen, J.H.M.M, Hommes, O.R., Swanink, C.M.A., Jongen, P.J.H., Fennis, J.F.M., Galama, J.M.D., Van der Meer, J.W.M., & Bleijenberg, G. (1996a). The measurement of fatigue in patients with multiple sclerosis: A multidimensional comparison with patients with chronic fatigue syndrome and healthy subjects. *Archives of Neurology, 53,* 642–649.

Vercoulen, J.H.M.M., Swanink, C.M.A., Fennis, J.F.M., Galama, J.M.D., Van der Meer, J.W.M., & Bleijenberg, G. (1996b). Prognosis in chronic fatigue syndrome: A prospective study on the natural course. *Journal of Neurology, Neurosurgery and Psychiatry, 60,* 489–494.

Vercoulen, J.H.M.M., Swanink, C.M.A., Zitman, F.G., Vreden, S.G.S., Hoofs, M.P.E., Fennis, J.FM., Galama, J.M.D., Van der Meer, J.W.M., & Bleijenberg, G. (1996c). Randomised, double-blind, placebo-controlled study of fluoxetine in chronic fatigue syndrome. *Lancet, 347,* 858–861.

Vercoulen, J.H.M.M., Bazelmans, E., Swanink, C.M.A., Fennis, J.F.M., Galama, J.M.D., Jongen, P.J.H., Hommes, O., Van der Meer, J.W.M., & Bleijenberg, G. (1997) Physical activity in chronic fatigue syndrome: Assessment and its role in fatigue. *Journal of Psychiatric Research, 31,* 661–673.

Vercoulen, J.H.M.M., Swanink, C.M.A., Galama, J.M.D., Fennis, J.F.M., Jongen, P.J.H., Hommes, O., Van der Meer, J.W.M., & Bleijenberg, G. (1998). The persistence of fatigue in chronic fatigue syndrome and multiple sclerosis: The development of a model. *Journal of Psychosomatic Research, 45,* 507–517.

Wallston, K.A., Wallston, B.S., & DeVellis, R. (1978). Development of the Multidimensional Health Locus of Control (MHLC) Scales. *Health Education Monographs, 6,* 160–170.

Ware, J.E., Sherbourne, C.D. (1992). The RAND-36 Short-form Health Status Survey: 1. Conceptual framework and item selection. *Medical Care, 30,* 473–481.

Wessely, S., Hotopf, M., & Sharpe, M. (1998). *Chronic fatigue and its syndromes.* Oxford: Oxford University Press.

Wessely, S., & Powell, R. (1989). Fatigue syndromes: A comparison of chronic "postviral" fatigue with neuromuscular and affective disorders. *Journal of Neurology, Neurosurgery and Psychiatry, 52,* 940–948.

Wilson, A., Hickie, I., Lloyd, A., Hadzi Pavlovic, D., Boughton, C., Dwyer, J., & Wakefield, D. (1994). Longitudinal study of outcome of chronic fatigue syndrome. *British Medical Journal, 308,* 756–759.

Winningham, M.L., Nail, L.M., Burke, M.B., Brophy, L., Cimprich, B., Jones, L.S., Pickard Holley, S., Rhodes, V., St-Pierre, B., & Beck, S. (1994). Fatigue and the cancer experience: The state of the knowledge. *Oncology Nursing Forum, 21,* 23–36.

# 5 HEALTH STATUS MEASUREMENT

Joop W. Furer, Christane König-Zahn and Bert Tax

Health is a comprehensive and complex concept for which no generally accepted definition is available. Extensive discussions are held about what should be excluded from the concept (either as a cause or a result of (poor) health), what elements or dimensions should be distinguished within the concept and how elements or dimensions would be interrelated. Its complexity leaves room for various approaches. For example, several approaches may be recognized in five outcome measures of treatment or health care interventions. This set of five has a long history and is known as "the five Ds": death—disease—disability—discomfort—dissatisfaction (Elinson, 1972). These five Ds reflect a development in time: initially, methods were completely determined by a biomedical approach, gradually socio-medical and psychological approaches were added as well.

When founding the World Health Organisation (WHO) in 1946, the United Nations member states adopted the most widely accepted health definition to date: "Health is a state of complete physical, mental and social well-being and not merely the absence of disease or infirmity".

The WHO definition covers two important issues in the debate about health concepts. The first refers to positive and negative health concepts. The positive health concept can be seen as a stage in a development which was described by McDowell and Newell (1987) as follows: first health status was considered in terms of survival, which was followed by a stage emphasizing the absence of disease, then came a period that characterized health as the ability of the individual to fulfil his daily activities, followed by the present focus on positive themes such as happiness, social and emotional well-being and quality of life. One of the advantages of a positive health concept is that it describes health in terms of what it really is. In the negative health concept, health is defined as a negation of disease: absence of disease implies health. The latter is the implicit assumption of curative medicine and many questionnaires include to a greater or lesser extent questions about (symptoms of) disease. Still, the positive concept has several disadvantages: it is difficult to delimit its content, it is practically unattainable and its relations with pathology are obscure. The second issue relates to the dimensionality of health. As was mentioned earlier, the WHO distinguished a *physical*, a *mental* and a *social* dimension. It was broadly welcomed that a narrow concept including only a physical dimension was left behind (Wilkin et al., 1992). However, the controversy remained as to whether social health is conceptually equal to the other two dimensions or whether it should be seen as a derivative of physical and mental health (Stewart & Ware, 1992; Ware, 1986).

Another general issue of confusion is caused by the fact that morbidity concepts have been developed from three distinct frames of reference, i.e., the biomedical, behavioral and social. The biomedical frame of reference deals with measurable disorders of organ structures or functions, considering ill-health as *"disease"*. The behavioral deals with the subjective experience of disorder, considering ill-health as *"illness"*. Finally, the social frame of reference deals with the consequences of illness and health on social functioning and on society as a whole. In this frame of reference, ill-health is considered as *"sickness"*. Surely, the three frames of reference do not completely coincide. Thus, although suffering from a serious, medically diagnosed disease, one may feel healthy and full of vitality and may be able to completely fulfil one's social obligations.

Although consensus may still have a long way to go, research cannot wait for an all-explaining definition; thus, although not being perfect, the WHO definition is as yet the guideline for many studies. For example, the World Organization of General Practitioners/Family Physicians (WONCA, 1995) defines "health status" as: "the defined well-being of a person in terms of physical, mental, and social condition or function."

## Precursors of health status measurement

The following applications of health status measurement can be distinguished (Bergner, 1987): (1) examination of the health status of general populations; (2) examination of the effects of clinical interventions; (3) examination of the effects of changes in the health care delivery system; and (4) examination of the effects of health promotion activities.

Many developments have stimulated the use of health status measurement and have contributed to its present state. One precursor of current questionnaires was developed to collect anamnestic patient data in clinical practice as efficiently as possible, i.e., without taking too much of the physician's time. The questionnaire was completed by the patient in the waiting room and the physician saw the answers before seeing the patient. This questionnaire—the Cornell Medical Index (CMI; Brodman et al., 1949)— was developed as a list of symptoms for medical purposes only. Later it was used all over the world in scientific research, for example to detect mental disorders in general populations.

Another contribution was the development of selection instruments during World War II for relatively healthy—i.e., not ill—recruits. The task was to determine the mental and physical health status of recruits on a large scale and extensive use was made of the recruits' subjective assessment. One of the scales that was developed was the Neuropsychiatric Screening Adjunct (NSA; Star, 1950), parts of which may be found in a number of more recent instruments.

After the Second World War the WHO health definition gave a powerful impetus to politicization of the health concept by setting the highest possible health standards for all world citizens following the atrocities of the war. The consequence was an increased need of national health departments to make progress towards this goal.

Subsequently, the expansion of the health care system called for an overall picture of people's need for care. Combined with the belief that society could be molded, an analysis of people's needs would make clear where care provisions had to be adjusted. Similar to the health survey for recruit selection, national health surveys were held for the benefit of health care policy-making. Although one or two Health Examination Surveys (HES) were carried out, i.e., from a disease frame of reference, lower costs were an important reason for carrying out national Health Interview Surveys (HIS) (from an illness frame of reference). Large-scale Health Interview Surveys about mental health were held by Gurin et al. (1960), while Bradburn and Caplovitz (1965) examined psychological well-being.

Side-effects of medical innovations stimulated also the application of broad health status measurement. In the second half of the 20th century, several biomedical technological innovations have been fairly successful from a medical-technical point of view, although they did not pay much attention to the patient's well-being. Other medical achievements reduced mortality caused by diseases, but the result was a big increase of chronically ill patients. Since these patients could not expect further benefit within a disease frame of reference, the focus of attention shifted to their well-being, functional status and ability to continue their social activities. Consequently, the need was felt to determine the "outcome" in these areas by using appropriate indicators. Another development away from the narrow biomedical model was stimulated by a growing awareness that drugs had side-effects, and that undergoing therapies or utilizing the health care system had unintended side-effects as well. These are some important reasons why outcome studies preferred, and still prefer, to use broad evaluation indicators. Finally, it should be mentioned that the political arena has been constantly pressing doctors in health systems to achieve an adequate balance between costs and benefits of new (and old) interventions, therapies and regulations, with the aim to achieve effectiveness with regard to a broad spectrum of health aspects.

## Subconcepts of health status

Many researchers developed questionnaires reflecting only a small selection from the reservoir of health concepts. Others made an effort to design a comprehensive health status measure.

One very comprehensive effort was made in the seventies by the RAND Corporation (Stewart & Ware, 1992) preliminary to the Health Insurance Experiment (HIE). Measures had to be developed in order to examine the effect of various types of health insurance on the use of health services. For the purposes of that study, all the questionnaires available in the United States at that time (1975) in the field of physical, mental and social health were thoroughly examined and tested for their usefulness. Finally, four health dimensions were operationalized, striving to achieve conceptually unambiguous dimensions and a minimum of mutual overlap. Given the research question, the questionnaires that were compiled and revised for the HIE had to be sufficiently sensitive to changes in the health status of the general population, i.e., a relatively healthy population.

In addition to indicators covering the three dimensions of the WHO health definition, a general health perception was also added. The subconcepts distinguished within the dimensions are represented in Table 15.1.

Each dimension used both positive and negative subconcepts. Thus, psychological health included both "psychological distress" and "presence of psychological well-being" (Stewart & Ware, 1992). Conceptually as well as empirically, psychological health was inter-

Table 15.1.  Content of instruments used by the Health Insurance Experiment

| Physical health | Psychological health | Social health | General health perception |
| --- | --- | --- | --- |
| *Functional limitations* morbidity physical activity role function self care general | *Psychological distress* anxiety depression loss of behavioral and emotional control | *Social activities* social contacts group participation | *Health past/ present* prior health current health |
| *Physical abilities* | *Psychological well-being* positive affects emotional ties | | *Future health* health outlook health worry/ concern resistance/ susceptibility sickness orientation |

preted as an hierarchical model in which "psychological distress" and "psychological well-being" were the extremes of a single dimension (with a strong negative correlation). "Psychological distress" consisted of three distinct subconcepts (with strong positive intercorrelations) whilst "well-being" consisted of two distinct subconcepts (with a strong positive correlation).

Over the years, several short questionnaires including several dimensions and several subconcepts per dimension have been derived from more extensive questionnaires. A recent example and also the leading questionnaire at the moment is the RAND SF-36 (Ware & Sherbourne, 1992).

An effort to construct a comprehensive instrument to measure clinical symptoms of psychological distress in the general population (i.e., *not* in clinical patients) was made by Dohrenwend et al. (1980). Their motivation grew out of their experiences with available questionnaires and their evaluations of these instruments. The criticism was that current questionnaires measured non-specific psychological distress without establishing relations with psychopathological concepts; that they were based on serious symptoms of in-patients; that they came from highly divergent concepts and yet showed very high intercorrela-

Table 15.2.  The PERI Symptom Scales (Dohrenwend et al., 1980)

| Non-specific (demoralization) | Specific (psychopathology) | |
|---|---|---|
| Dread | Somatic problems | Rigidity |
| Anxiety | Guilt | Sexual problems |
| Sadness | Enervation | Reasons for drinking |
| Helplessness/hopelessness | False beliefs & | Problems due to drinking |
| Psychophysiological | perceptions | Active expression of hostility |
| symptoms | Manic | Passive aggressive behavior |
| Perceived physical health | characteristics | Perceived hostity from others |
| Poor self-esteem | Suicidal ideation | Antisocial history |
| Confused thinking | & behavior | Approval of rule breaking |
| | Insomnia | |
| | Distrust | |

tions; and that they did not distinguish between a state of general malaise versus psychopathological symptoms. Based on theoretical considerations and empirical findings the authors selected eight non-specific psychological distress scales and 17 psychopathology scales (see Table 15.2). The 25 scales are part of the Psychiatric Epidemiology Research Interview (PERI).

Although the non-specific scales met the criteria of both clinical content validity (as judged by experts) and internal reliability, their intercorrelations proved to be too high. Combined, these non-specific psychological distress scales constitute the construct called "demoralization". Next, a short "demoralization" scale was designed for the construct based on a theoretical and empirical foundation. Many questionnaires criticized by Dohrenwend et al. (1980) used items derived from the eight "non-specific distress" scales. These latter instruments, as well as their "demoralization" scale and colleagues were referred to by Dohrenwend as "thermometers" to indicate psychological health status. Similar to "running a temperature", they only indicate that something is wrong, without explaining *what* exactly.

The psychopathological symptom scales have not been fully developed, which should be deplored since few researchers have ventured to provide a critical overview of concepts such as carried out by Dohrenwend and his colleagues.

Researchers have also started looking for relevant subconcepts for the three dimensions. Table 15.3 presents an overview of the subconcepts that were found in our selection of frequently used questionnaires. Three examples are disease-specific: the Arthritis Impact Measurement Scales (AIMS; Meenan, 1982), the Asthma Quality of Life Questionnaire (AQLQ; Juniper et al., 1992) and the European Organization for Research and Treatment of Cancer QLQ-C30 (EORTC; Study Group, 1993). Many questionnaires have been designed to study a single dimension or subconcept and are meant to be used with various groups (generic). The examples presented here are the Katz Index or ADL (Katz et al., 1963), the McGill Pain Questionnaire (MPQ; Melzack, 1975), the Center for Epidemiologic Studies—Depression Scale (CES-D; Radloff, 1977) and the General Health Questionnaire (GHQ; Goldberg, 1972). The multidimensional generic measures cover a greater number of health dimensions usually with a greater number of subconcepts for the separate dimensions. The questionnaires vary considerably in size: the Dartmouth COOP Functional Health Assessment Charts (COOP; Nelson et al., 1987) consist of six one-item scales, the RAND 36-item Health Survey (SF-36; Ware & Sherbourne, 1992) has 36 questions to cover eight subconcepts, the Nottingham Health Profile (NHP; Hunt et al., 1986) consists of 38 questions to cover six subconcepts and the Sickness Impact Profile (SIP; Bergner et al., 1976) contains 136 questions referring to nine subconcepts. Thus, the number of questions varies considerably for the dimensions and subconcepts involved. The nature and number of subconcepts as well as the number of questions differ substantially between instruments, as Table 15.3 shows.

## The assessment of health status

An overwhelming majority of the huge number of instruments designed to measure health status are self-completed or interview administered. A minority of the instruments are based on the assumption that the respondent/client/patient's opinion is inadequate because of either lack of understanding or inability. These instruments are completed by an observer who has been studying the patient for some time or who has talked with the patient. One example is the Montgomery-Åsberg Depression Rating Scale (MÅDRS; Montgomery & Åsberg, 1979) designed to measure the intensity of depression in psychiatric patients. An observation scale designed to detect changes in psychiatric patients' health status by having them observed by nurses is the Nurses' Observation Scale for Inpatient Evaluation (NOSIE; Honigveld & Klett, 1965). Its subscales include: self-care; motor retardation; depression; irritability; manifest psychosis; social interests; and social skills.

Tabel 15.3. Schematic summary of the contents of the health status measuring devices

| | Generic instruments (multidimensional) | | | | Generic instruments (unidimensional) | | | | Disease/condition-specific instruments (multidimensional) | | |
|---|---|---|---|---|---|---|---|---|---|---|---|
| | COOP | NHP | SIP | SF 36 | KATZ | MPQ | CES-D | GHQ | AIMS | AQLQ | EORTC |
| **Physical** | | | | | | | | | | | |
| General health perception | 1 | – | – | 5 | – | – | – | – | – | – | 2 |
| Physical health/function | 1 | 8 | – | 10 | – | – | – | – | 5 | 11 | 5 |
| Mobility | – | – | 22 | – | – | – | – | – | 4 | – | – |
| Dexterity | – | – | – | – | – | – | – | – | 5 | – | – |
| ADL/IADL | – | – | 23 | – | 6 | – | – | – | 12 | – | – |
| Energy/vitality | – | 3 | – | 4 | – | – | – | – | – | – | – |
| Eating | – | – | 9 | – | – | – | – | – | – | – | – |
| Sleep | – | 5 | 7 | – | – | – | – | – | – | – | 2 |
| Pain | – | 8 | – | 2 | – | 20 | – | – | 4 | – | – |
| Symptoms | – | – | – | – | – | – | – | – | – | 12 | 5 |
| **Mental** | | | | | | | | | | | |
| Mental health/well-being | 1 | 9 | 9 | 5 | – | – | – | – | – | 5 | 4 |
| Cognitive function | – | – | 10 | – | – | – | – | – | – | – | – |
| Communication | – | – | 9 | – | – | – | – | – | – | – | – |

(continued)

Tabel 15.3. Schematic summary of the contents of the health status measuring devices (*continued*)

| | Generic instruments (multidimensional) | | | | Generic instruments (unidimensional) | | | | Disease/condition-specific instruments (multidimensional) | | |
|---|---|---|---|---|---|---|---|---|---|---|---|
| | COOP | NHP | SIP | SF 36 | KATZ | MPQ | CES-D | GHQ | AIMS | ALQ | EORTC |
| Anxiety | – | – | – | – | – | – | – | – | 6 | – | – |
| Depression | – | – | – | – | – | – | 20 | – | 6 | – | – |
| Symptoms | – | – | – | – | – | – | – | 30 | – | – | – |
| **Social** | | | | | | | | | | | |
| Social health/function | 1 | 5 | 20 | 2 | – | – | – | – | 4 | – | 2 |
| Role function | 1 | – | 27 | 7 | – | – | – | – | – | – | 2 |
| **Health change** | 1 | – | – | 1 | – | 9 | – | – | – | – | – |

Other instruments were developed to express the respondents' psychiatric condition in terms of diagnoses, containing standardized questions for the respondent and ratings from the interviewer. Examples include the Present State Examination (PSE; Wing et al., 1974), which was later incorporated into the Schedules for Clinical Assessment in Neuropsychiatry (SCAN; Wing et al., 1990), and the Structured Clinical Interview for DSM-III-R (SCID; Spitzer et al., 1987).

In order to give an impression of the great diversity of available self-report questionnaires seven instruments will be briefly described below. They are questionnaires that have been used extensively in health (care) studies. Several of them focus on a broad range of health disorders and diseases; they are called generic questionnaires. As a rule, they can be applied to any category of patients or even non-patients. Disease-specific or condition-specific questionnaires deal with a single disease or condition. One of the first generic questionnaires was the Index of Daily Living, which was developed by Katz as early as the 1950s. It is an observation scale designed to measure aspects of individual physical performance. Two other examples cover the psychological dimension; the GHQ developed in the 1960s as a screening instrument, and the Center for Epidemiological Studies-Depression Scale (CES-D) developed in the 1970s for epidemiological research. Examples of generic questionnaires measuring a greater number of dimensions include the SIP, also developed in the 1970s and for several years one of the most popular instruments, and the SF-36, which is gradually replacing the SIP. Finally, two disease-specific questionnaires are presented: the AIMS, which was made suitable for a specific group of patients by adjusting a generic instrument (i.e., the Index of Well-Being), and the AQLQ. A special feature of the latter is that respondents are asked to answer only questions about limitations of activities that are relevant to themselves. Publications referred to in descriptions of the measures have been limited to key articles published by the authors who developed the measures.

## GENERIC QUESTIONNAIRES

- *The Index of Independence in Activities of Daily Living (Index of ADL)*

The ADL was one of the earliest measures of functional independence (Katz et al., 1963). It is a generic measure focusing on one, i.e., the physical, dimension. It was developed to provide predictive information on the course of an illness as well as to determine any effects of treatment in chronically ill and aging populations. Designed as a measure of basic functions, it measures performance rather than ability. Functions are hierarchically related and are rated on a Guttman-type scale. The scale summarizes an individual's performance in six functions: bathing; dressing; toileting; transfer; continence; and feeding. ADL performance is rated on a three-point scale by an observer. Ratings are dichotomized into "independence" and "dependence" and then converted into a graded index of activities. ADL performance is summarized as grades A to G, A being the most independent grade and G being the most dependent.

- *The General Health Questionnaire (GHQ)*

Initially, the GHQ was designed to identify respondents with non-psychotic psychiatric illnesses by assessing the severity of their psychiatric disturbance. It was developed as a screening test aimed at detecting psychiatric disorders among respondents in community settings and non-psychiatric clinical settings. It is also used to estimate the prevalence of psychiatric disorders and as a generic measure of psychological health status.

The GHQ is based on the assumption of psychiatric disturbance "being evenly distributed throughout the population in varying degrees of severity ... ranging from severe disorder to a hypothetical normality ..." (Goldberg, 1972). Individual scores on the GHQ are thought to be the quantitative estimate of an individual's current psychiatric disturbance. The emphasis is always on how the respondent's present state differs from his usual state. All items have four response categories, ranging from "less than usual" to "much more than usual".

The versions most frequently used are the GHQ-30, its short form, the GHQ-12, and the GHQ-28. The GHQ-28 comprises four subscales: somatic symptoms; anxiety and insomnia; social dysfunction; and severe depression. Overall scores, indicating the severity of psychological disturbance, can be calculated for all versions. Lower scores reflect better health. For the GHQ-28, four additional subscale scores can be calculated.

- *The Center For Epidemiological Studies-Depression Scale (CES-D)*

The CES-D was designed to assess current levels of depressive symptoms in the general population whereas other depression scales have been developed for use in clinical populations. Its emphasis is on the affective component, depressive mood (Radloff, 1977). The scale was intended for use in epidemiological studies in the general population.

The measure consists of 20 items selected from a number of previously validated depression scales. The CES-D includes questions on depressed mood, feelings of guilt and worthlessness, feelings of hopelessness and helplessness, psychomotor retardation, loss of appetite, and sleep disturbance. Respondents are asked to rate frequencies of symptoms over the past week on a 4-point Likert scale ranging from "rarely or none of the time (less than 1 day)" to "most or all of the time (5–7 days)". A sum score on the CES-D can be calculated, higher scores indicating the presence of depressive symptoms.

- *The Sickness Impact Profile (SIP)*

The SIP is a multidimensional generic health status instrument measuring subjectively perceived changes in behavior as a consequence of being sick. It was designed for use in populations with different cultural backgrounds as well as for patient groups differing in nature and severity of diseases. As behavior changes can be reliably reported and verified by observation while they are less prone to cultural bias, the focus of the SIP is on behavior rather than feelings. The behavioral aspects included in the instrument should represent a universal pattern of limitations that may be affected by any sickness, regardless of specific conditions, treatment, patient characteristics or prognosis (Bergner et al., 1976).

The questionnaire contains 136 statements covering the following subconcepts ("categories"): mobility; ambulation; body care and movement; eating; sleep and rest; emotional behavior; alertness/intellectual behavior; communication; social interaction; home management; work; and recreation. Respondents are asked to endorse those statements which apply to their situation and relate to their health status. In each category items are weighted, representing the differences in severity of behavioral limitations. Weights were obtained using equal-appearing interval scaling procedures. Sum scores are calculated for each category based on the weights of each statement and presented as a percentage of total possible dysfunction in that category. Three of the categories (ambulation, mobility, body care and movement) can be aggregated into a physical dimension and four others can be combined into a psycho-social dimension (social interaction, emotional behavior, alertness behavior, communication). Finally, an overall SIP score can be calculated. Higher scores reflect worse performance.

- *The RAND 36-Item Short Form Health Survey (SF-36)[1]*

The RAND SF-36 is a multidimensional generic questionnaire measuring health status in large populations and different (patient) groups for use in cross-sectional and longitudinal studies. It was developed by a team of RAND investigators as an alternative to longer measures included in the Medical Outcome Study (MOS) analyzing patient outcomes in different systems of medical care. The conceptual framework is based on the multidimensional WHO definition of health. Following the WHO definition of health, the SF-36 extends its range of measurement to include not only negative but also positive health states (Ware & Sherbourne, 1992).

The SF-36 includes eight subscales, ranging from two to ten items plus one item about changes in health. The subscales are: general health; physical functioning; bodily pain; vitality; mental health; social functioning; role limitation (physical); and role limitation (emotional). Response alternatives vary between 2-point to 6-point Likert scales. Subscale scores are calculated and transformed into a 0–100 scale, higher scores representing better health.

## SPECIFIC QUESTIONNAIRES

- *The Arthritis Impact Measurement Scales (AIMS)*

The AIMS is a multidimensional condition-specific index to measure the health status of arthritis patients according to the broad WHO notion of health. The approach chosen was derived from the Index of Well-Being and its adapted version used in the RAND Health Insurance Experiment. The existing measures were modified by shortening some scales while at the same time adding others in order to achieve a better assessment of health status areas that appeared to be particularly relevant to patients with rheumatic diseases (Meenan, 1982).

It consists of 45 items grouped into nine scales: mobility; physical activity; dexterity; activities of daily living; pain; anxiety; depression; social activity; and household activities. Its response alternatives range from yes/no answers to 6-point ratings of frequency or severity. They are Guttman-type; scale scores are calculated by adding the scores on all items within a section. Raw scores are converted into a standard range of 0–10, with 0 representing "good health" and 10 representing "poor health". A total health score can be derived by adding the resulting values for the six scales of mobility, physical activity, household activities, dexterity, pain and depression.

- The Asthma Quality of Life Questionnaire (AQLQ)

The AQLQ is a multidimensional condition-specific measure designed to determine the effects of treatment on quality of life in clinical trials in asthma. It assesses subjective aspects of health status, including both physical and emotional aspects, that might be impaired by asthma. It is based on the philosophy that a measure should reflect aspects of functioning that are important to individual patients with asthma (Juniper et al., 1992).

The test includes 32 items covering the subconcepts of activity limitation, symptoms, emotional function, and exposure to environmental stimuli. Assessment of activity limitations is patient-specific, i.e., the questions refer to a number of activities that are important to the patient involved. Items are rated on 7-point Likert scales for frequency or severity. Subscale scores are computed as mean scores on the scale, lower scores indicating greater impairment.

# How to optimize the choice of appropriate measures?

Important issues to be addressed in selecting appropriate health measures include: What is the objective of the assessment of health status? Which conceptual, psychometric and practical aspects are important? How do available measures match the requirements of the assessment?

## MEASUREMENT OBJECTIVES

The objectives of health measurement can be manifold. For example, its purpose may be to assess the health needs of different patient groups, to assess health outcomes following therapeutic interventions in patients, with specified chronic diseases, to facilitate doctor-patient communication in a specific clinical setting, or to monitor individual patients' health status. Some measures were initially developed as diagnostic tools although they are now being used to establish the prevalence of disease in epidemiological studies or as screening instruments. The target population may vary from more or less healthy individuals in a general population sample to severely sick in-patients. Obviously, measures designed for specific purposes or populations may not necessarily work in a different context.

## CONCEPTUAL, PSYCHOMETRIC AND PRACTICAL ASPECTS

Having identified the objective, it should be decided which *health concept* is relevant and which *subconcepts* should be emphasized. Table 15.3 illustrates the great variety of domains addressed by different health measures. The relative emphasis placed upon each subconcept should take account of the target population and, more specifically, the nature and impact of the health problem of interest. For example, most patients suffering from arthritis will have limitations of functional abilities and pain; for this patient group, any measure should include those elements (as is the case, for example, in the AIMS).

Consideration should also be given to whether the main emphasis should be on ill health or good health. If the target population is relatively healthy, measures mainly addressing negative aspects will generate highly skewed scores, whereas the same measures may yield varied and well-distributed scores in a sick target group.

Several health status measures have been developed from a purely professional perspective, while other researchers have used patients or the general public to generate the content of their measures. The content of the Katz Index of ADL was derived from observations by professionals regarding activities performed by a group of patients with hip fractures; the initial item pool for the NHP was collected from a survey of patients with various diseases who described the effects of ill-health; the items for the SIP were derived from interviews with healthy and ill lay-persons and with health professionals. It would seem plausible that measures developed from a patient perspective will appear more relevant to lay respondents and will be better accepted. On the other hand, measures developed mainly from a professional point of view might have a higher clinical utility.

Having defined the conceptual basis and the objectives of health status assessment, attention must be paid to the *psychometric properties* of the measure. The main properties to consider are validity, reliability and responsiveness to change. Again, the relative importance of each of these properties will depend on one's objectives when measuring health status. We will confine our brief overview to psychometric issues and terminology used by health researchers.

Validity means that measures must indeed measure what they purport to measure. Three major types of validity can be distinguished. The basic issue in studies of *construct validity* is whether the health measure relates to other measures in ways consistent with presented hypotheses. One of the criteria usually applied here is a high correlation between the questionnaire and similar indicators of the health concept—which is called convergent validity—and low correlations between the questionnaire and indicators of other (health) concepts, which is called discriminant validity. A thorough way of demonstrating concept validity is by using Campbell and Fiske's (1959) multitrait-multimethod techniques. The discriminatory power of an instrument, i.e., its ability to discriminate between mutually different groups of respondents (e.g., between patients and healthy individuals), is called "known-group validity".

An important issue is whether the questionnaire adequately represents the health concept. This representation is called *content validity*. This aspect of validity cannot be assessed using statistical or other quantitative methods. Rather, it is an estimate of whether a theoretical and usually highly abstract concept has been adequately defined and whether it is adequately represented in the items of the instrument.

*Criterion validity* is the degree to which a given measure produces results which correspond well to those obtained through the simultaneous use of a "gold standard" (concurrent validity) or which predict a future outcome or event (predictive validity). The main problem in assessing criterion validity is that a generally accepted "gold standard" is not usually available.

*Reliability* refers to the reproducibility of measurement. When measurements are repeated, questionnaires should produce similar results if the respondents' conditions have remained the same. The level of agreement between answers at different points in time is called *test-retest reliability*. Another aspect of reliability relates to the questionnaire as such and refers to the homogeneity of (a series of) questions, the *internal consistency* of a scale.

Although standardized terminology, methods and statistics are available to define validity and reliability, there is as yet no such thing for *responsiveness to change*. Responsiveness to change refers to "a questionnaire's ability to detect clinically important changes in a patient's status" (Deyo & Patrick, 1989), an important feature if the measuring instrument is to be used as an outcome measure. Responsiveness to change implies a mixture of validity and reliability: the instrument should measure clinically relevant changes in subjective health status (validity) and must be able to distinguish even minor changes, i.e., produce little noise (reliability).

PRACTICAL REQUIREMENTS

Relations between the scientific demands and the feasibility of measuring health status in practice may sometimes be strained. In terms of *practical implementation* it is important that the questionnaire is user-friendly, both for respondents and researchers. Several factors may contribute to this, including the length of the questionnaire, the complexity of the questions, answering formats, scoring procedures and the steps needed to calculate any scale scores. Naturally, the importance of these features will depend partly on the function of the questionnaire as well as on concrete study conditions. Questionnaires used in patient or client contacts will have to meet different requirements than those used in scientific research. A questionnaire used in daily practice must fit in with daily routines, taking up as little time as possible. Furthermore, if health care professionals wish to use information derived from a questionnaire immediately when meeting clients or patients, scale scores must be obtained and interpreted both easily and directly.

Thus, in order to make carefully considered decisions, the following questions should be clarified:

- What elements of health status are relevant to the research question? Which should be definitely included and what else might be of interest?
- Which target group is approached for measuring health status (e.g., specific age groups or patient categories)?
- Considering the aim of the study, what will be the right type of questionnaire to be used: generic, disease-specific, or a combination of the two?

The next step is to find a questionnaire that has been thoroughly tested on its psychometric qualities, is appropriate to the research questions and suitable for the intended study population. A more detailed discussion of these issues may be found in textbooks (Furer et al., 1995; Hutchinson et al., 1997; König-Zahn et al., 1993, 1994; McDowell & Newell, 1987; Wilkin et al., 1992).

# The assessment of health status in the clinical setting

In addition to scientific population studies, questionnaires are also used in clinical settings, serving more clinical, individual applications. Thus, hospitals frequently use observation lists. If questionnaires are used, they should be brief and easy to interpret, particularly in ambulatory care. An example of a very short instrument specifically designed to be used by general practitioners is the COOP/WONCA Charts. This measure has been developed for a quick assessment of patients' functional status and had to satisfy several requirements: it should provide reliable and valid data on several dimensions that were considered essential for individual performance (i.e., physical, mental, social); it should be possible to apply it as a matter of routine; it should be easy to interpret; and it should produce useful information. Following its development by Nelson and his colleagues (1987), the World Organization of General Practitioners/Family Physicians (WONCA) made it more widely known, thus promoting its implementation. It consists of a series of six charts measuring: physical fitness; daily activities; feelings; social activities; overall health; and changes in health. Each chart briefly states a question about the respondent's functional status during the last few weeks. All questions have five response categories, illustrating all functional levels by means of drawings. By standardizing both questions and drawings as part of a manual an effort has been made to achieve uniform usage worldwide (Van Weel et al., 1995). Applied either in one-time screening or repeated monitoring, the instrument is filled in by the patient (in the waiting-room) and is then assessed by the physician. The charts provide a quick and broad overview of a patient's health status, including information that might be lacking in a predominantly medical approach. Because of the brevity of the COOP/WONCA Charts—cf. their six one-item questions—it is recommended to keep more detailed and precise instruments in store (both generic and disease-specific or condition-specific) to be used when marked health changes have been detected.

To improve the recognition of mental problems in general practice, several procedural recommendations have been made. Zung (1990) advised general practitioners to use a "depression thermometer", i.e., a depression questionnaire that could be completed in the waiting room. If the score is high, the general practitioner would have to assess in a clinical examination whether there were sufficient grounds to make a diagnosis of depression and to identify the type of depression. Apart from its *screening function*, Zung believed that the depression questionnaire might also play a role in therapeutic treatment. By applying repeated measurements it would be possible to follow the developments of depression episodes, both in terms of the severity of depression—based on total scores—and the nature of the depression—based on shifts in item scores (for example, a more biological symptom profile moving towards a more psychological symptom profile). If used this way, the questionnaire will also have a *monitoring function*.

In monitoring the course of depression during psychotherapy or drug-induced therapy, both psychologists and psychiatrists frequently use the Beck Depression Inventory (BDI; Beck et al., 1988). The BDI consists of 21 items each made up of four statements which represent differences in intensity for attitudes or symptoms. The BDI's responsiveness to change appeared to be quite high: changes in BDI scores were highly consistent with changes in clinical ratings for hospitalized patients (Beck et al., 1988; Wilkin et al., 1992). Thus, the BDI seems to be a suitable instrument for monitoring in clinical practice. Wetzler and van Praag (1989) stated in their review that various depression questionnaires produced similar results and therefore they do not express a strong preference for any particular questionnaire. To study the effects of antidepressants they advise the MÅDRS observation scale (Montgomery & Åsberg, 1979).

## Examples of the application of different methods

In this final section we wish to focus our attention on (1) disease-specific and generic questionnaires, and on (2) the usefulness of generic instruments as a comparative standard.

One of the advantages of disease-specific questionnaires is that they may include health subconcepts that are specifically relevant to just one or a limited number of diseases. More generic subconcepts may be adjusted to match one specific disease in such a way that it is possible to follow the impact of that particular disease with greater precision. As questionnaires grow more specific, they will provide fewer opportunities to compare their results with other diseases. Generic questionnaires may lack refinement to be applied to specific diseases or conditions and even to include questions that may be irrelevant to them. On the other hand, the results of generic questionnaires may be used to compare the impact of a specific disease/condition to other diseases or conditions.

However, generic instruments often have similar discriminating power to disease-specific questionnaires, when applied to patients suffering from a single, specific disease. This was illustrated in a study where the Parkinson's Disease Questionnaire (PDQ; Peto et al., 1995) and the SF-36 were compared. The PDQ consists of 39 questions, including for example the subscales "bodily discomfort", and "stigma". Seven of the eight PDQ-39 subscales were able to make significant distinctions between four groups of patients with different severity of Parkinson's disease. The SF-36, a generic instrument, came very close to achieving a similar result: out of eight subscales, six SF-36 scales produced significantly discriminating results.

A more practical problem with specific questionnaires is that for each specific disease or condition a great deal of thorough designing and validating has to be done. Consequently, it is always advisable to include one or more generic instrument in the study to supplement a more specific instrument. Generic instruments tend to have solid foundations and lots of reference materials.

Applying generic questionnaires to various diseases and conditions has made it clear that they may produce highly differentiated results. Generic measures make it possible to compare the burden of various diseases and conditions on several dimensions and subconcepts. These comparisons were not possible until generally accepted generic instruments became available. An overview of descriptive data pertaining to specific diseases and conditions will be important parameters in deciding how health care resources should be employed.

The SF-36 is one of the generally accepted generic questionnaires used to describe the health status of various patient categories. Thus, the SF-36 manual presents scale scores for patients with hypertension, congestive heart failure, diabetes type II, myocardial infarction and clinical depression—in addition to data for the general population according to age, sex, etc. (Ware et al., 1993). Other sources have described patients suffering from migraine, depressives before and after drug-induced therapy, and Parkinson's disease. Inspection of the SF-36 manual clearly shows that, compared to the general population, the group of patients with hypertension demonstrates poorer health on only two scales, i.e., "role limitations-physical" and "physical functioning". Depressives (diagnosed according to a standard psychiatric interview) have low scores on many scales representing both mental health status and physical health condition. The extremely low scores found in a study by Peto et al. (1995) demonstrate that patients with Parkinson's disease are in very poor health, both mentally and physically.

These and similar comparisons illustrate the specific nature of health loss associated with particular diseases or conditions, identifying those diseases and conditions that will cause high amounts of physical and mental health degeneration. As a result, psychiatric disorders among other conditions are given high priority on the agenda of health research and health care policy.

## Notes

1.  Also known as the MOS 36-Item Short Form Health Survey (SF-36) and the Health Status Questionnaire (HSQ).

## References

Beck, A.T., Steer, R.A., & Garbin M.G. (1988). Psychometric properties of the Beck Depression Inventory: Twenty-five years of evaluation. *Clinical Psychology Review, 8*, 77–100.

Bergner, M. (1987). Health status measures: An overview and guide for selection. *Annual Reviews of Public Health, 8*, 191–210.

Bergner, M., Bobbitt, R.A., Kressel, S., Pollard, W.E., Gilson, B.S., & Morris, J.R. (1976). The Sickness Impact Profile: Conceptual formulation and methodology for the development of a health status measure. *International Journal of Health Services, 6*, 393–415.

Bradburn, N.M., & Caplovitz, D. (1965). *Reports on happiness: A pilot study of behaviour related to mental health.* Chicago: Aldine.

Brodman, K., Erdman, A.J., Lorge, I., Wolff, H.G., & Broadbent, T.H. (1949). The Cornell Medical Index: An adjunct to medical interview. *Journal of the American Medical Association, 140*, 530–534.

Campbell, D.T., & Fiske, D.W. (1959). Convergent and discriminant validation by the multitrait-multimethod matrix. *Psychological Bulletin, 56*, 81–105.

Deyo, R.A., & Patrick, D.L. (1989). Barriers to the use of health status measures in clinical investigation, patient care, and policy research. *Medical Care, 27*, (Suppl. 3), S254–268.

Dohrenwend, B.P., Shrout, P.E., Egri, G., & Mendelsohn, F.S. (1980). Nonspecific psychological distress and other dimensions of psychopathology. *Archives of General Psychiatry, 37*, 1229–1236.

Elinson, J. (1972). Methods of sociomedical research. In: H.E. Freeman et al. (Eds.), *Handbook of medical sociology* (pp. 483–500). Englewood Cliffs, NJ: Prentice Hall.

EORTC Study Group on Quality of Life (1993). The European Organisation for Research and Treatment of Cancer QLQ-C30: A quality-of-life instrument for use in international clinical trials in oncology. *Journal of the National Cancer Institute, 85*, 365–376.

Furer, J.W., König-Zahn, C., & Tax, B. (1995). *Het meten van de gezondheidstoestand: beschrijving en evaluatie van vragenlijsten. III. Psychische gezondheid,* [Measuring health status: Description and evaluation of questionnnaires III. Mental health] Assen, The Netherlands: Van Gorcum.

Goldberg, D.P. (1972). *The detection of psychiatric illness by questionnaire.* London: Oxford University Press.

Gurin, G., Veroff, J., & Feld, S. (1960). *Americans view their mental health.* New York: Basic Books.

Honigfeld, G., & Klett, C. (1965). The Nurses' Observation Scale for Inpatient Evaluation. A new scale for measuring improvement in chronic schizophrenics. *Journal of Clinical Psychology, 21,* 65–71.

Hunt, S.M., McEwen, J., & McKenna, S.P. (1986). *Measuring health status.* London: Croom Helm.

Hutchinson, A., Bentzen, N., & König-Zahn C. (Eds.) (1997) *Cross-cultural health outcome assessment: A user's guide.* Groningen: European Research Group on Health Outcome.

Juniper, E.F., Guyatt, G.H., Epstein, R.H., Ferrie, P.F., Jaeschke, R., & Hiller, T.K. (1992). Evaluation of impairment of health-related quality of life in asthma: Development of a questionnaire for use in clinical trials. *Thorax, 47,* 76–83.

Katz, S., Ford, A.B., Moskowitz, R.W., Jackson, B.A., & Jaffe, M.W. (1963). Studies of illness in the aged. The Index of ADL: A standardized measure of biological and psychosocial function. *Journal of the American Medical Association, 185,* 914–919.

König-Zahn, C., Furer, J.W., & Tax, B. (1993). *Het meten van de gezondheidstoestand: Beschrijving en evaluatie van vragenlijsten: I. Algemene gezondheid,* [Measuring health status: Description and evaluation of questionnaires I. General health] Assen, The Netherlands: Van Gorcum.

König-Zahn, C., Furer, J.W., & Tax, B. (1994). *Het meten van de gezondheidstoestand: Beschrijving en evaluatie van vragenlijsten: II. Lichamelijke gezondheid, sociale gezondheid,* [Measuring health status: Description and evaluation of questionnaires II. Physical and social health] Assen, The Netherlands: Van Gorcum.

McDowell, I., & Newell, I. (1987). *Measuring health: A guide to rating scales and questionnaires.* New York: Oxford University Press.

Meenan, R.F. (1982). The AIMS approach to health status measurement: Conceptual background and measurement properties. *Journal of Rheumatology, 9,* 785–788.

Melzack, R. (1975). The McGill Pain Questionnaire: Major properties and scoring methods. *Pain, 1,* 277–299.

Montgomery, S.A., & Åsberg, M. (1979). A new depression scale designed to be sensitive to change. *British Journal of Psychiatry, 134,* 382–389.

Nelson, E., Wasson, J., Kirk, J., Keller, A., Clark, D., Dietrich, A., Stewart, A., & Zubkoff, M. (1987). Assessment of function in routine clinical practice:

Description of the COOP Chart method and preliminary findings. *Journal of Chronic Disease, 40* (Suppl. 1), 55S–63S.

Peto, V., Jenkinson, C., Fitzpatrick, R., & Greenhall R. (1995). The development and validation of a short measure of functioning and well-being for individuals with Parkinson's disease. *Quality of Life Research, 4,* 241–248.

Radloff, L.S. (1977). The CES-D scale: A self-report depression scale for research in the general population. *Applied Psychological Research, 1,* 385–401.

Spitzer, R.L., Williams, J.B.W., & Gibbon, M. (1987). *Instruction manual for the Structured Clinical Interview for DSM-III-R.* New York: New York State Psychiatric Institute, Biometrics Research Department.

Star, S.A. (1950). The screening of psychoneurotics in the army: Technical development of tests. In: S.A. Stouffer (Ed.), *Measurement and prediction* (pp. 486–547). New York: Wiley.

Stewart, A.L., & Ware, J.E. (Eds.) (1992). *Measuring functioning and well-being: the Medical Outcomes Study approach.* Durham, NC: Duke University Press.

Van Weel, C., König-Zahn, C., Touw-Otten, F.W.M.M., van Duijn, N.P., & Meyboom-de Jong, B. (1995). *Measuring functional health status with the COOP/WONCA charts. A manual.* Groningen: NCH series no. 7, Northern Centre of Health Care Research.

Ware, J.E. (1986). The assessment of health status. In: L.H. Aiken & D. Mechanic (Eds.), *Applications of social science to clinical medicine and health policy* (pp. 204–228). New Brunswick, NJ: Rutgers University Press.

Ware, J.E., & Sherbourne, C.D. (1992). The MOS 36 Item Short-Form Health Survey (SF-36). I. Conceptual framework and item selection. *Medical Care, 30,* 473–483.

Ware, J.E., Snow, K.K., Kosinski, M., & Gandek, B. (1993). *SF-36 Health Survey; Manual and interpretation guide.* Boston, MA: The Health Institute.

Wetzler, S., & Van Praag, H.M. (1989). Assessment of depression. In: S. Wetzler (Ed.), *Measuring mental illness: Psychometric assessment for clinicians* (pp. 69–88). Washington, DC: American Psychiatric Press.

Wilkin, D., Hallam, L., & Doggett, M.-A. (1992). *Measures of need and outcome for primary health care.* Oxford: Oxford University Press.

Wing, J.K., Cooper, J.E., & Sartorius, N. (1974). *The measurement and classification of psychiatric symptoms.* New York: Cambridge University Press.

Wing, J.K., Babor, T., Brugha, T., Burke, J., Cooper, J.E., Giel, R., Jablenski, A., Regier, D., & Sartorius, N. (1990). SCAN: Schedules for Clinical Assessment in Neuropsychiatry. *Archives of General Psychiatry, 47,* 589–593.

WONCA Classification Committee (1995). An international glossary for general/family practice. *Family Practice, 12,* 31–69.

Zung, W.W.K. (1990). The role of rating scales in the identification and management of the depressed patient in the primary care setting. *Journal of Clinical Psychiatry, 51,* S72–S76.

# 6 QUALITY OF LIFE ASSESSMENT

Jolanda de Vries

The focus of this chapter will be on the assessment of quality of life (QOL). According to the World Health Organisation Quality of Life group, QOL should be defined as "a person's perception of his/her position in life within the context of the culture and value systems in which s/he lives and in relation to his/her goals, expectations, standards, and concerns. It is a broad-ranging concept incorporating, in a complex way, the person's physical health, psychological state, level of independence, social relationships, personal beliefs, and relationship to salient features of the environment" (WHOQOL group, 1994, p. 28).

This definition reflects the view that QOL refers to a subjective evaluation which is embedded in a cultural, social, and environmental context. Although some researchers have already noted these aspects, it is the first time that they have been incorporated into a definition. Moreover, QOL is a very broad multidimensional concept, going beyond the WHO's definition of health which states that health is "a state of complete physical, mental, and social well-being and not merely the absence of disease of infirmity" (WHO, 1958). For this same reason, QOL cannot simply be equated with terms like functional status or health status, mental state, or well-being. As Ware (1991, p. 776) has put it: "It has become fashionable to talk about functional status and well-being as if they were synonymous with quality of life. Quality of life, however, is a much broader concept."

Many measures are claimed to assess QOL. However, strictly speaking, these often concern health status measures that focus on the influence of disease on a person's physical, psychological, and social functioning. Health status measures are only subjective in the sense that they are completed by patients themselves. In contrast, QOL measures, besides being completed by patients, are subjective in the sense that patients are also asked to evaluate the aspects of QOL (e.g., "How satisfied …?"/"How bothered …?").

Thus, a serious problem when studying QOL with health status measures is that lower levels of functioning are equated with lower QOL, resulting in a confounding between morbidity or physiological changes and QOL as subjective satisfaction. For example, the health status of a 31-year-old drug user with stage 2 HIV infection may be low. However, this person may have adapted to his situation to such an extent that he evaluates his QOL as quite satisfactory (O'Boyle, 1994). The use of objective indicators is therefore insufficient to adequately understand an individual's QOL.

## Review of the literature

After World War II there was an increasing awareness that people's QOL was not necessarily related only to material wealth. This idea instigated a number of studies into the detection of indicators that reflect the overall "health" and well-being of the general population (Andrews & Withey, 1976; Campbell et al., 1976; Gurin et al., 1960). Subsequently, the number of studies into QOL and related aspects increased rapidly.

Because many researchers had their own ideas about what QOL encompassed, in many cases *ad hoc* measures were used. One disadvantage of these *ad hoc* measures is their unknown reliability and validity. Another serious problem concerns comparability. When different measures are used in various studies, the results from these studies are difficult to compare. In the 1990s, a call for the use of measures with good psychometric properties resulted in an increase of reliable and valid measures. However, a standard QOL measure that is used universally seems a utopian idea.

### QUALITY OF LIFE

For a long time, quantity of life, that is, keeping people alive as long as possible, was the primary aim in the medical sciences. In that context, mortality and morbidity were the only outcome measures and the primary focus of research (Bergner, 1989). However, medical and biotechnological procedures often also affect the patient's comfort implying that "living longer" may not necessarily mean "living better". Trade-offs between length of life and QOL are especially pronounced in cancer treatments such as chemotherapy. Not surprisingly, the assessment of QOL was instigated in particular in oncology where patients started to indicate that their QOL was also very important (Morrow et al., 1992). As a consequence, QOL considerations were added to previous claims which emphasized increased longevity and from then onwards, QOL started to gain ground and the goals of health care became twofold: medical interventions should increase the duration of life *and* improve the QOL (Ware et al., 1981). In addition to the growing need to make effects of medical treatment more explicit, Van Knippenberg et al. (1991) mentioned three other factors that contributed to the increase in QOL studies. First, the fact that life expectancy is increasing. Second, impressive medical technological progress. And finally, the need for indicators of patients' well-being to include psychological as well as social aspects.

Because the focus in medical research is primarily on medication and treatment for influencing state of health, all nonmedical outcomes that are considered are thought of as QOL outcomes and labeled as such by clinicians (Bergner, 1989). Physicians further preferred measures for use in patient groups to be as objective as possible and thus QOL was operationalized as functional or health status (also referred to as health-related QOL). As a consequence, most so-called QOL measures actually assess performance or frequency of behavior and feelings instead of the patient's subjective evaluation of aspects of life (satisfaction). However, during the last few years the number of "real" QOL measures and studies has increased (see Boxes 16.1, 16.2 and 16.3 for examples).

## Subconcepts

In QOL assessment the emphasis is on mental and social aspects of life. For instance, according to Powers and Goode (in Goode, 1990), QOL "is primarily a product of relationships between people in each life setting" (p. 43). Schalock (1990) indicated that social indicators alone are insufficient to measure individuals' perceived QOL and that it should be measured together with psychological indicators that focus on a person's subjective reactions to life experiences. While QOL can be divided into a social and a psychological component, the concept can also be considered in alternative ways. For example, Liu (1974) defined QOL as the output of two aggregate input factors: physical and spiritual. Andrews and Withey (1976, p. 12) stated that QOL "is not just a matter of the conditions of one's physical, interpersonal and social setting, but also a matter of how these are judged and evaluated by oneself and others."

Most measures reflect the multidimensionality of QOL. This is important because, although a person may be confined to a wheelchair,

**Box 16.1    Quality of life of cancer patients: An example of a psychosocial evaluation study**

Pruijn and Van den Borne (1987) conducted an evaluation study examining the effectiveness of aftercare by fellow-sufferers. They used structured interviews with two types of cancer patients: Hodgkin's patients ($N$=216) and breast cancer patients with amputation of a breast ($N$=282). All respondents had undergone treatment during the past three years. Among the information gathered, extensive questions were asked about social comparisons and contact with fellow sufferers. For more than half of both patient groups the first personal contact with another patient with the same disease was during the stay in hospital or during first treatment. It appeared that 109 Hodgkin (51%) and 156 breast cancer patients (55%) indicated to have had contact with one or more fellow sufferers through the media, face-to-face, or by telephone at some point in time after the diagnosis. Concerning the significance that the patients themselves attached to their contact with fellow sufferers, the following picture emerged. The contact was considered meaningful by half of the persons in both patient groups. A majority of the patients were satisfied with the contacts they had with fellow sufferers. In the case where the patient was not satisfied with this contact, the dissatisfaction was due to negative experiences such as recurrence of the disease, deterioration in health status, or death of the contact person. Furthermore, 34% of the Hodgkin's and 17% of the breast cancer patients said that they had obtained more knowledge about their disease and treatment through their fellow sufferer. In addition, half of the patients indicated that through the contact with a fellow sufferer their self-confidence was at least somewhat confirmed. They also had the idea that they had acquired more control over their situation. Moreover, it had helped them to solve practical problems (38% of the breast cancer patients and 25% of the Hodgkin's patients). Contact with a fellow sufferer had also made them conscious of the fact that other people with the same disease had the same problems as well as the same feelings of uncertainty and fear. Aspects for which contacts with fellow sufferers had been particularly important were, for instance, getting a better perspective on one's own situation, feeling understood, and being able to talk about problems and concerns.

---

**Box 16.2    Quality of life of oesophageal cancer patients: An example of a medical intervention study**

Van Knippenberg et al. (1992) reported the results of a study on oesophageal cancer patients. A number of indicators of subjective QOL were filled out before and after a surgical operation in which parts of the oesophagus and the stomach were removed and the digestive tract was reconstructed. The results showed that post-operative, as compared to the pre-test, global evaluations (the total situation in the previous three months and three days; prevailing mood and physical well-being during the previous three days) remained the same. With respect to the respondents' activity level, psychological distress, and swallowing problems, the scores decreased. Finally, the physical symptoms of the patients had increased.

---

s/he nevertheless can have a good psychological well-being or sense of social support. This diversity of experience cannot be captured with a scale that only assesses one dimension (Fitzpatrick et al., 1992).

A whole range of aspects influences the choice of the dimensions that one should measure in a study. Fletcher et al. (1992) mention the following aspects: the severity and nature of a disease; the expected benefits and adverse effects of treatment; (considerations such as) the length of the study; the availability of suitable instruments; and the environment in which assessment will take place. Irrespective of these aspects, but in accordance with the WHO definition of health (1958), there are a few domains that are usually included in QOL studies: the physical, mental, and social domain. In addition, especially in clinical trials, often disease-related and treatment-related symptoms are included (e.g., Morrow et al., 1992).

Gerson (1976) identified two opposite approaches to QOL: individual versus transcendental. In the individual approach, the emphasis is on the person's control over his/her circumstances, freedom from constraint, etc. In the transcendental approach, the emphasis is on the degree to which individuals carry out their role in the larger social order, be it the country of residence or the world.

Over time the position has been taken that QOL must be studied from the perspective of the individual. For instance, Badura and Waltz (1984) defined QOL as the way the individual feels and Sartorius (1987) defined it in terms of the distance between a person's actual

**Box 16.3    Quality of life of sarcoidosis patients: An example of a descriptive study**

Drent and colleagues (1995) reported on research into the QOL of sarcoidosis patients. Sarcoidosis is a disseminated granulomatous disease of unknown origin. Depending on the organs involved and the severity of granulomatous inflammation, symptoms can vary considerably. Patients can be asymptomatic or present with symptoms such as cough, dyspnea, chest pain, skin lesions, joint and muscle pain. In addition, patients often suffer from systemic symptoms such as fever, weight loss, and fatigue (Drent et al., 1998). One of the aims of the project was to assess the impact of sarcoidosis on QOL.

Within this project a number of studies were performed. In one study, 64 sarcoidosis patients completed the WHOQOL-100 and a symptom checklist. Patients were divided into two groups: patients with actual symptoms and patients who were asymptomatic. The WHOQOL-100 revealed a number of areas in which sarcoidosis patients, especially those with current symptoms, experienced problems.

Surprisingly, both patient groups—including patients who had reported no actual symptoms—suffered from fatigue, sleeping problems and impaired general QOL compared to a matched healthy control group. So, sarcoidosis patients who had considered themselves asymptomatic demonstrated an impaired QOL as well.

A number of differences in QOL were found between the patient groups with and without current symptoms. Besides the physical problems mentioned above, patients with current symptoms suffered from impaired QOL mainly with respect to their level of independence. This area includes problems with patients' mobility, working capacity, and activities of daily living. Moreover, the patient group with symptoms had low levels of positive feelings and problems with recreation compared with the asymptomatic group. The areas in which QOL of these patients is impaired indicate that sarcoidosis has a considerable impact on daily life, even in patients with a relatively mild impairment of pulmonary function tests (Wirnsberger et al., 1998).

position and his or her goals. In addition, Andrews (1991, p. 2) defined QOL as "how individuals themselves evaluate their lives."

Another issue that is implicit in the WHO definition of health and definitions of QOL is the measurement of positive QOL factors. QOL is a concept with a positive connotation that encompasses positive and negative factors.

## TYPES OF QUALITY OF LIFE MEASURES
QOL instruments can be divided into generic, disease-specific, and domain-specific questionnaires.

Generic instruments are broad multidimensional measures, which are designed to measure QOL in diverse patient groups, age groups, and sometimes also in healthy persons (Fitzpatrick et al., 1992). In other words, generic instruments purport to be broadly applicable across types and severities of disease, across different medical treatments or health interventions, and across demographic and cultural subgroups (Patrick & Deyo, 1989). An example of a generic instrument is the World Health Organization Quality of Life assessment instrument (WHOQOL-100; WHOQOL group, 1995a).

Disease-specific QOL instruments are developed to measure QOL in specific diagnostic groups or patient populations such as rheumatoid arthritis, often with the goal of measuring responsiveness to treatment or clinically important changes (Patrick & Deyo, 1989). They focus on problems that are specific for these particular diseases or areas of function (Fitzpatrick et al., 1992). An example of a disease-specific instrument is the Diabetes Quality of Life Measure (DQOL; Diabetes Control and Complications Trial Research Group, 1988) for diabetes patients. The development of disease-specific measures has become a major topic in QOL literature. However, in many cases it has not been established that specific measures give significant incremental information beyond what is provided by a general approach (Kaplan, 1985). This has been demonstrated, for instance, by Kantz et al. (1992) in a study with osteoarthritis patients.

A third category of instruments is developed for use in specific categories of diseases like cancer and thus fall in between generic and disease-specific measures. They are generic in the sense that they are intended for use in all patients with diseases in a particular category (e.g., lung cancer patients, breast cancer patients, prostate cancer patients) but are disease-specific in that they can only be used for patients with a specific type of disease (e.g., cancer).

Most researchers propose to use both generic instruments and disease-specific measures (e.g., Bowling, 1995; Ware, 1991). Generic measures are necessary to compare outcomes across different populations and interventions, particularly for cost-effectiveness studies. Disease-specific measures assess the special states and concerns of specific diagnostic groups. Patrick and Deyo (1989) have mentioned three different strategies: the use of (i) separate generic and specific measures; (ii) modified generic measures (i.e., adapted for use in a particular study); and (iii) disease-specific supplements. The preferred strategy depends on project aims, methodological concerns, and practical constraints.

Domain-specific measures only assess one QOL domain such as psychological health. These instruments are used when the investigator is only interested in a particular aspect of QOL.

# How the Quality of Life is assessed

QOL is assessed by means of self-report questionnaires and (semi-structured) interviews. However, some self-report questionnaires can also be used in an interviewer-assisted or interviewer-administered approach. This is important if a respondent is not able to read or write due to cultural, educational, or health reasons, or because s/he is nervous about completing questionnaires (Fletcher et al., 1992).

SELF-REPORT QUESTIONNAIRES
In health-related QOL studies the major focus is on the development and use of measures with adequate psychometric qualities instead of *ad hoc* assessment. This emphasis has boosted the development of generic, and especially disease-specific, measures. A number of them will be reviewed.

*Generic measures*
Two examples of generic questionnaires will be discussed: The Congruity Life Satisfaction (CLS; Meadow et al., 1992) measure and the World Health Organization Quality of Life assessment instrument (WHOQOL-100; WHOQOL group, 1995a).

The CLS measures subjective well-being with 10 items. As far as is known, this measure is only used in general population studies. The respondents have to answer these items on a 6-point Likert type scale ranging from "Very dissatisfied" to "Very satisfied", yielding an overall life satisfaction score. The reliability and construct validity of the instrument seems to be fairly good (Sirgy et al., 1995).

At the beginning of the 1990s, the WHO started a project entitled "The assessment of QOL in health care" which aimed to develop cross-culturally an instrument that measures QOL in a very broad sense. The instrument, called the WHOQOL, is applicable to chronically ill persons, individuals living under stress and healthy persons. It has originally been developed in 15 collaborative centers all over the world, namely in Australia, Croatia, England, France, (North and South) India, Israel, Japan, the Netherlands, Panama, Russia, Spain, Thailand, USA, and Zimbabwe.

The construction process of the instrument consisted of the following steps. First, an expert panel on QOL consisting of representatives of the field centers developed a working definition of QOL and a list of facets (and definitions) of QOL. As already mentioned in the introduction, QOL was defined here as "a person's perception of his/her position in life within the context of the culture and value systems in which s/he lives and in relation to his/her goals, expectations, standards, and concerns. It is a broad-ranging concept incorporating, in a complex way, the person's physical health, psychological state, level of independence, social relationships, personal beliefs, and relationship to salient features of the environment" (WHOQOL group, 1994, p. 28).

Subsequently, discussion groups were held in each field center. The members of these groups were asked to discuss the meaning of the term QOL and which facets they thought belonged to it. After adapting the initial list of QOL facets incorporating the remarks of the members of the discussion groups, at least six focus groups were run in each field center consisting of lay persons, persons suffering from a chronic illness, and health professionals. The members of these focus groups were asked whether they felt particular facets had been omitted from the list or whether some facets present did not belong to the list. In addition, the definitions of the various facets were discussed. Finally, the participants were asked to suggest items for probing into the facets. On the basis of the transcripts of the focus groups and the criteria set for writing items, the pilot version of the instrument was developed and then tested (WHOQOL group 1994, 1995b).

In the next step, the WHOQOL pilot instrument was administered to at least 250 ill and 50 healthy persons in each center. The analysis plan aimed to examine the content validity of the WHOQOL domains and facets, to select the best questions for each facet, and to establish the WHOQOL's internal consistency and discriminant validity (WHOQOL group, 1995b). Based on these analyses, the so-called WHOQOL-100 or WHOQOL Field Trial Form (WHOQOL group 1995a) was developed.

The WHOQOL-100 consists of 100 items assessing 24 facets of QOL within six domains (physical health, psychological health, level of independence, social relationships, environment, and spirituality/religion/personal beliefs) and a general evaluative facet called overall quality of life and general health. Thus, each facet is represented by four items. The response scale is a 5-point Likert scale. This instrument can also be used as interviewer-assisted or interviewer-administered (de Vries, 1996) and has adequate psychomethric properties (de Vries & Van Heck, 1997).

*Disease-specific measures*
As examples of disease-specific measures, the following two questionnaires will be briefly discussed here: the CARDIAC (Faris & Stotts, 1990) and the Diabetes Quality of Life Measure (DQOL; Diabetes Control and Complications Trial Research Group, 1988).

Faris and Stotts (1990) have developed a QOL measure for patients suffering from percutaneous transluminal coronary angioplasty. It taps two domains: satisfaction and importance. Example items are "How satisfied are you with your physical independence (ability to do things for yourself, get around)?" for satisfaction and "How important is your physical independence (ability to do things for yourself, get around) to you?" for importance. Although the CARDIAC is reliable and well-known, it is not a widely used instrument (Bowling, 1995).

The DQOL is a measure for insulin-dependent diabetes mellitus patients. It consists of 46 core items covering three topics: satisfaction, impact, and worry. The latter is divided into worry about the disease and social/vocational worrying. "How satisfied are you with the time you spend exercising?" is an example of a "satisfaction" item. An illustrative "impact" item is "How often do you find that your diabetes interrupts your leisure time activities?" "How often do you worry about whether you will pass out?" is an example of a "worry" about diabetes item. When considered appropriate, 16 questions concerning school and family relationships can be added. The response scales are 5-point Likert type scales. The reliability and validity of the DQOL appears to be good, although some doubt has been cast on its additional value above a generic QOL measure (Bowling, 1995).

## INTERVIEWER-BASED QUESTIONNAIRES
### Generic measures

Two examples of instruments within this category are the Schedule for the Evaluation of Individual Quality of Life (SEIQOL; O'Boyle et al., 1993) and the Subjective Domains of Quality of Life scale (SDQLM; Bar-on & Amir, 1993).

The SEIQOL is an individual measure developed for healthy adults of all ages, although it can also be used in patient populations. The scale can only be administered in patients not suffering from impaired cognitive functions or motivational states, since respondents must have the insight to indicate which factors determine their lives. The procedure goes as follows. First, the respondent is asked in a structured interview to mention the five domains that s/he feels are the most salient to his/her QOL. In addition, the respondent has to give an exact description of what each domain implies. Subsequently, the respondent is requested to rate on a vertical scale ranging from 0 to 100 his/her current levels of functioning/satisfaction on each of the five selected domains. These extremes are anchored with the terms "Best possible" and "Worst possible". This procedure yields five independent continuous measurements. Finally, judgment analysis is applied to quantify the relative importance of each of the five domains for his/her QOL. The SEIQOL appears to have good validity and reliability (Browne et al., 1994; O'Boyle, 1994).

The SDQLM has been developed for a study with hypertensives. In this semi-structured interview respondents create their own QOL scale using the corrective evaluation. Patients have to mention their three most important QOL domains. Subsequently, they have to define the qualitative optimal, current, and dysfunctional levels. Finally, the patients are asked to evaluate their current functioning in the domains of their QOL on a scale from 1 to 6. The instrument appears to be sensitive to change and has a good internal consistency and construct validity (Amir & Bar-on, 1996).

### Disease-specific measures

The extended Dutch version of the Lancashire Quality of Life Profile (extended LQOLP; Van Nieuwenhuizen & Schene, 1996) is a revised version of the LQOLP as developed by Oliver and colleagues (e.g., 1997). Although the developers of the extended LQOLP perceive their instrument as domain-specific, it will be discussed in this paragraph because it covers a whole range of QOL domains and is specifically developed for severely mentally ill people. Using both the bottom-up (opinion of patients) and top-down (opinion of expert) as well as the concept-mapping procedure, the domain "life-regard" was added. Furthermore, items from the original LQOLP that in pilot testing appeared irrelevant or inapplicable to the majority of the respondents were removed (Van Nieuwenhuizen, 1998).

The final extended LQOLP taps 11 domains with 63 items: (i) fulfilment; (ii) positive self-esteem; (iii) negative self-esteem; (iv) framework; (v) living situation; (vi) safety; (vii) finances; (viii) leisure and social participation; (ix) health; (x) family relations; and (xi) negative affect. The extended LQOLP appears to be applicable to severely mentally ill persons. Patients seem to like the interview and when asked whether they were willing to be reinterviewed, 91% of the 423 patients responded positive, 6% were in doubt, and only 3% refused. In addition, the measure seems to be applicable for evaluation of mental health care (Van Nieuwenhuizen, 1998). The mean administration time is 62 minutes (sd=25). The instrument appears to have a good internal consistency and test-retest reliability. Moreover, preliminary results seem to indicate that the extended LQOLP is a sensitive instrument. The content, construct, and discriminant validity of the interview also seem good (Van Nieuwenhuizen, 1998).

## Choosing appropriate Quality Of Life measures

To optimize the choice of the appropriate QOL measure, the following considerations should be taken into account. Time is obviously an important precondition because it is nearly always a constraint. Depending on the time interviews or questionnaires might take from respondents, that is, patient burden, shorter or longer measures can be used. Generally, longer measures have a better reliability and assess more aspects of QOL, thus presenting a more detailed picture of the problems that respondents might experience. For instance, the WHOQOL-100 provides information about 24 different aspects of QOL that belong to six domains. The WHOQOL-Bref, containing only 26 items, only provides information at domain level and the number of domains is reduced to four physical health and level of independence (were two separate domains), psychological health and spirituality/religion/personal beliefs (were two separate domains), social relationships, and environment. So, the diversity and specificity of the information assessed with the short version is less but the time it takes respondents to complete the questionnaire, and thus the patient burden, is also reduced.

Another obvious precondition is the research setting. If the setting gives respondents privacy to talk, it is also possible to choose a measure based on interviews. If respondents have to complete a measure in a waiting room, interviews are less appropriate. In addition, the length of the instrument is restricted to the average time persons have to spend in the waiting room before they see their physician.

An important question is whether the results have to be comparable with other patient groups or healthy persons. If so, a generic instrument should be used. Moreover, the generic instrument should not have been developed only for use with sick persons if the comparison group consists of healthy individuals, because several of the core domains in QOL may be of little relevance to healthy persons. QOL measures that are exclusively based on domains such as physical health and self-care may not be broad enough to provide an adequate assessment in well persons (Patrick & Erickson, 1993).

The choice of assessment instrument is also related to the type of study and the availability of measures in the target language. In intervention studies, QOL of the patients should be the central point of focus. The measure chosen should be designed for use at the individual level. On the other hand, in clinical trials and related studies, a comparison between the experimental and control group is the purpose. In such instance, a measure that is sensitive to change is needed.

Researchers should preferably use a measure originally developed in their own culture or language. Nearly all existing measures are developed within the context of one particular language, only afterwards being translated into other languages. Although elaborate translation methodologies may be used, this can never erase the fact that such measures were originally designed to fit one particular culture. Therefore, such instruments remain culture-specific. In addition, it should be kept in mind that a measure can be psychometrically sound in a language other than its original, while missing important aspects that are specific for the particular cultural setting involved or containing aspects that are redundant in other cultures. One will never find out if this actually is the case unless researchers start to look at these possibilities with an open mind and let lay persons tell whether they are on the right trail (de Vries, 1996). One does not know which QOL facets are missing unless one looks for them (e.g., Fletcher et al., 1992). Furthermore, weights ascribed to aspects of QOL in one particular context might differ from weights stemming from other contexts

(Fletcher et al., 1992). In a cross-cultural study the culture-specific issue is even more important.

Finally, the psychometric properties of instruments are important selection criteria. Needless to say, measures that have a good reliability and validity should be preferred.

## Assessment in the clinical setting

The current popularity of measuring QOL is instigated by the recognition that it is an important outcome measure of medical treatment and a supplement to traditional biological end-points such as mortality (Hays & Shapiro, 1992). Information concerning QOL can add to medical knowledge (Moinpoir et al., 1989). This is one of the reasons for the increase in QOL studies and the development of new disease-specific instruments.

It is anticipated that QOL measures will be applied more frequently in clinical trials, in establishing baseline scores in a range of QOL areas, and when examining changes in QOL over the course of medical treatment. This holds particularly when disease prognosis predicts only partial recovery or remission and treatment may be more palliative than curative. For epidemiological research, instruments will allow detailed QOL data to be gathered on a particular population and used for predicting morbidity and mortality.

QOL assessment will also be useful in other types of intervention studies such as psychosocial interventions aiming at improving coping or social support. In addition, individual patient studies can be conducted to make the specific areas of QOL in which a patient experiences problems visible. In these two types of studies the distinction between health status and QOL as described in the introduction is especially important because both might provide different results and recommendations.

For clinical practice, adequate QOL instruments can assist the physician's understanding of how a disease affects a patient's QOL and it may help the clinician in making judgments about the areas in which a patient is most affected by disease. Information on a patient's QOL can assist the doctor in making treatment decisions and will also change and improve the interaction between patient and doctor. These changes will give more meaning and fulfilment to the work of the doctor and should lead to the patient being provided with more comprehensive health care. Because a complete form of assessment, covering different aspects of patients' functioning, is being carried out, patients may find their health care more meaningful which in turn might improve compliance. Routine use of QOL instruments will also improve and complete the recording of patient data, and enable communication of valuable information between professionals. In developing countries, where resources for health are limited, interventions aimed at improving QOL can be both effective and inexpensive (WHO, 1993).

At the international level, the availability of an international QOL assessment instrument such as the WHOOQL will make it possible to carry out multi-center studies and to compare the results obtained in different parts of the world. Such research has important benefits, permitting questions to be addressed that would not be possible in single-site studies. For example, a comparative study in two or more countries on the relationship between health care delivery and QOL requires an assessment yielding cross-culturally comparable scores. Particularly when studying rare disorders, the possibility of gathering data in several centers/countries may be important to reach an adequate number of patients. Multi-center collaborative studies can also provide simultaneous multiple replications of a finding, adding considerably to the confidence with which research results can be accepted. The availability of a cross-culturally comparable QOL measure will also facilitate comparative international epidemiological studies, thus furthering the understanding of diseases and the development of treatment methods (WHOQOL group, 1994).

# References

Amir, M., & Bar-on, D. (1996). Hypertension and quality of life: The disease, the treatment or a combination of both. *Psychology & Health, 11*, 685–695.

Andrews, F.M. (1991). Stability and change in levels and structure of subjective well-being: USA 1972 and 1988. *Social Indicators Research, 25*, 1–30.

Andrews, F.M., & Withey, S.B. (1976). *Social indicators of well-being: Americans' perceptions of life quality*. New York: Plenum Press.

Badura, B., & Waltz, M. (1984). Social support and the quality of life following myocardial infarction. *Social Indicators Research, 14*, 295–311.

Bar-on, D., & Amir, M. (1993). Re-examining quality of life of hypertensives: A new, self-structured measure. *American Journal of Hypertension, 6*, S62–S66.

Bergner, M. (1989). Quality of life, health status, and clinical research. *Medical Care, 27,* S148–S156.

Bowling, A. (1995). *Measuring disease: A review of disease-specific quality of life measurement scales.* Buckingham, UK: Open University Press.

Browne, J.P., O'Boyle, C.A., McGee, H.M., Joyce, C.R.B., McDonald, N.J., O'Malley, K., & Hiltbrunner, B. (1994). Individual quality of life in the healthy elderly. *Quality of Life Research, 3,* 235–244.

Campbell, A., Converse, P.E., & Rodgers, W.L. (1976). *The quality of American life.* New York: Sage.

de Vries, J. (1996). *Beyond health status: Construction and validation of the Dutch WHO Quality of Life instrument.* Thesis. Tilburg: Tilburg University.

de Vries, J., & Van Heck, G.L. (1997). The World Health Organization Quality of Life assessment instrument (WHOQOL-100): Validation study with the Dutch version. *European Journal of Psychological Assessment, 13,* 164–178.

Diabetes Control and Complications Trial Research Group (1988). Reliability and validity of a diabetes quality of life measure for the diabetes control and complications trial (DCCT). *Diabetes Care, 11,* 725–732.

Drent, M., Wirnsberger, R.M., Breteler, M.H.M., Kock, L.M.M., de Vries, J., & Wouters, E.F.M. (1998). Quality of life and depressive symptoms in patients suffering from sarcoidosis. *Sarcoidosis Vasculitis and Diffuse Lung Diseases, 15,* 59–66.

Faris, J.A., & Stotts, N.A. (1990). The effect of percutaneous transluminal coronary angioplasty on quality of life. *Progress in Cardiovascular Nursing, 5,* 132–140.

Fitzpatrick, R., Fletcher, A., Gore, S., Jones, D., Spiegelhalter, D., & Cox, D. (1992). Quality of life measures in health care. I: Applications and issues in assessment. *British Medical Journal, 305,* 1074–1077.

Fletcher, A., Gore, S., Jones, D., Fitzpatrick, R., Spiegelhalter, D., & Cox, D. (1992). Quality of life measurements in health care. II: Design, analysis, and interpretation. *British Medical Journal, 305,* 1145–1148.

Gerson, E.M. (1976). On "quality of life". *American Sociological Review, 41,* 793–806.

Goode, D.A. (1990). Thinking about and discussing quality of life. In: R.L. Schalock (Ed.), *Quality of life: Perspectives and issues* (pp. 41–57). Washington, DC: American Association on Mental Retardation.

Gurin, G., Veroff, J., & Feld, S. (1960). *Americans view their mental health: A nationwide interview survey.* New York: Basic Books.

Hays, R.D., & Shapiro, M.F. (1992). An overview of generic health-related quality of life measures for HIV research. *Quality of Life Research, 1,* 91–97.

Kantz, M.E., Harris, W.J., Levitsky, K., Ware, J.E., & Davies, A.R. (1992). Methods for assessing condition-specific and generic functional status outcomes after total knee replacement. *Medical Care, 30,* MS240–MS252.

Kaplan, R.M. (1985). Quality-of-life measurement. In: P. Karoly (Ed.), *Measurement strategies in health psychology* (pp. 115–146). New York: Wiley.

Liu, B.-C. (1974). Quality of life indicators: A preliminary investigation. *Social Indicators Research, 1,* 187–208.

Meadow, H.L., Mentzer, J.T., Rahtz, D.R., & Sirgy, M.J. (1992). A life satisfaction measure based on judgement theory. *Social Indicators Research, 26,* 23–59.

Moinpour, C.M., Feigl, P., Metch, B., Hayden, K.A., Meyskens, F.L., Jr., & Crowley, J. (1989). Quality of life end points in cancer clinical trials: Review and recommendations. *Journal of the National Cancer Institute, 81,* 485–495.

Morrow, G.R., Lindke, J., & Black, P. (1992). Measurement of quality of life in patients: Psychometric analyses of the Functional Living Index-Cancer (FLIC). *Quality of Life Research, 1,* 287–296.

O'Boyle, C.A. (1994). The Schedule for the Evaluation of Individual Quality of Life (SEIQOL). *International Journal of Mental Health, 23,* 3–23.

O'Boyle, C.A., McGee, H.M., Hickey, A., Joyce, C.R.B., Browne, J., & O'Malley, K. (1993). *The Schedule for the Evaluation of Individual Quality of Life (SEIQOL): Administration manual.* Dublin: Royal College of Surgeons in Ireland.

Oliver, J.P.J., Huxley, P.J., Priebe, S., & Kaiser, W. (1997). Measuring the quality of life of severely mentally ill people using the Lancashire Quality of Life Profile. *Social Psychiatry and Psychiatric Epidemiology, 32,* 76–83.

Patrick, D.L., & Deyo, R.A. (1989). Generic and disease-specific measures in assessing health status and quality of life. *Medical Care, 27,* S217–S232.

Patrick, D.L., & Erickson, P. (1993). Assessing health-related quality of life for clinical decision-making. In: S.R. Walker & R.M. Rosser (Eds.), *Quality of life assessment: Key issues in the 1990s* (pp. 11–63). Lancaster: Kluwer Academic Press.

Pruijn, J.F.A., & Van den Borne, H.W. (1987). Self-care of cancer patients. In: N.K. Aaronson & J. Beckman (Eds.), *The quality of life of cancer patients* (pp. 265–274). New York: Raven Press.

Sartorius, N. (1987). Cross-cultural comparisons of data about quality of life: A sample of issues. In: N.K. Aaronson & J. Beckman (Eds.), *The quality of life of cancer patients* (pp. 19–24). New York: Raven Press.

Schalock, R.L. (1990). Attempts to conceptualize and measure quality of life. In: R.L. Schalock (Ed.), *Quality of life: Perspectives and issues* (pp. 141–148). Washington, DC: American Association on Mental Retardation.

Sirgy, M.J., Cole, D., Kosenko, R., Meadow, H.L., Rahtz, D., Cicic, M., Jin, G.X., Yarsuvat, D., Blenkhorn, D.K., & Nagpal, N. (1995). A life satisfaction measure: Additional validational data for the Congruity Life Satisfaction measure. *Social Indicators Research, 34,* 237–259.

Van Nieuwenhuizen, C. (1998). *Quality of life of persons with severe mental illness: An instrument.*Thesis. Amsterdam: University of Amsterdam.

Van Nieuwenhuizen, C., & Schene, A.H. (1996). *Extended Dutch version of the Lancashire Quality of Life Profile.* Amsterdam: University of Amsterdam.

Van Knippenberg, F.C.E., De Haes, J.C.J.M., & Trijsburg, R.W. (1991). Kwaliteit van leven in de medische setting. [Quality of life in the medical setting.] *Nederlands Tijdschrift voor de Psychologie, 46,* 93–96.

Van Knippenberg, F.C.E., Out, J.J., Tilanus, H.W., Mud, H.J., Hop, W.C.J., & Verhage, F. (1992). Quality of life in patients with resected oesophageal cancer. *Social Science and Medicine, 35,* 139–145.

Ware, J.E. (1991). Conceptualizing and measuring generic health outcomes. *Cancer, 67,* 774–779.

Ware, J.E., Brook, R.H., Davies, A.R., & Lohr, K.N. (1981). *Choosing measures for health status for individuals in general populations.* Santa Monica: Rand Corporation.

WHO (1958). *The first ten years of the World Health Organization.* Geneva: WHO.

WHO (1993). *WHOQOL study protocol.* Geneva: WHO (MNH/PSF/93.9).

WHOQOL group (1994). Development of the WHOQOL: Rationale and current status. *International Journal of Mental Health* [Special issue: Quality of Life Assessment: Cross-cultural Issues-2], *23,* 24–56.

WHOQOL group (1995a). *Field Trial WHOQOL-100 February 1995: Facet definitions and questions.* Geneva: WHO (MNH/PSF/95.1.B).

WHOQOL group (1995b). The World Health Organization Quality of Life assessment (WHOQOL): Position paper from the World Health Organization. *Social Science and Medicine* [Special Issue on Health-related quality of life What is it? and How should we measure it?], *41,* 1403–1409.

Wirnsberger, R.M., de Vries, J., Breteler, M.H.M., Van Heck, G.L., Wouters, E.F.M., & Drent, M. (1998). Evaluation of quality of life in sarcoidosis patients. *Respiratory Medicine, 92,* 750–756.

# ASSESSING THE UTILITY OF BEHAVIORAL MEDICINE INTERVENTIONS: QUANTIFYING HEALTH-RELATED QUALITY OF LIFE

William J. Sieber and Robert M. Kaplan

Health-related quality of life (HRQOL) is viewed by patients, clinicians, and society as an important outcome of medical technology and disease control. HRQOL assessment has become necessary for the evaluation of pharmaceutical treatments, medical interventions, and in the tracking of population health. Behavioral medicine clinicians and researchers will benefit from recent advances in the assessment of treatment effectiveness. This chapter is not intended as a review of all HRQOL instruments; instead it provides a review of concepts less likely to be familiar to clinicians – ideas that are quickly determining how we measure health and the impact of behavioral medicine interventions. Further, we consider the role of outcomes assessment in the larger resource allocation process. We conclude by discussing what should be considered when choosing and applying a measurement strategy for assessing quality of life in a behavioral medicine setting.

The term "quality of life" is used inconsistently. Quality of life (QOL) is a broad term often encompassing aspects of life not always directly relevant to a behavioral medicine clinician (i.e., standard of living, job satisfaction). The term "health-related quality of life" (HRQOL) clarifies the health focus of interest and narrows quality of life to aspects relevant to health. Although the term "functional status" is often used interchangeably with the term "health-related quality of life", there is a clear distinction between the two. Functional status is the objective degree of disability caused by an illness, whereas HRQOL also includes subjective evaluation of that disability, referred to as "handicap" by the World Health Organization (WHO, 1980). It may often include symptoms that may not affect functioning (Kaplan & Anderson, 1996). Though the term "health status" is used by many authors, we prefer HRQOL, because it more accurately conveys gradations of life quality and "health status" does not adequately convey these gradations.

It should also be noted that the popularity of the term "quality of life" for both patients and regulatory agencies has led to numerous established measures being relabeled as QOL measures. We prefer to think of HRQOL measures as assessing multiple domains of health, not as an aggregation of separate measures developed independently to assess various aspects of health (e.g., combining a measure of depression and a symptom checklist and referring to it as assessment of QOL). Thus, the discussion below includes only those measures that have been specifically designed to assess health-related quality of life.

## Current importance of health-related quality of life

Until recently, common sense and clinical intuition were used to determine treatment effectiveness. Documenting which treatments are efficacious and which are not has been relatively unstandardized. Assessing side effects of medication and examining areas of health that are not the primary focus of treatment seemed unwarranted and burdensome. However, accountability is now a priority in health care. Measuring outcomes in a way that allows broader comparison of interventions has become the standard of care. The United States serves as an important example of how the focus in health outcomes has transformed the health care system. American doctors perform more procedures than their colleagues in any other country in the world, yet there is little evidence that Americans enjoy better health than their peers in other industrialized countries. Brook and Lohr (1987) have suggested that between 30–50% of all medical procedures have little or no documented benefit. To wisely invest health care dollars, it has become clear that we need to measure the product of health care.

The topic of HRQOL has become increasingly popular in the clinical research literature over the past ten years, not only because of extended survival from once terminal diseases, but because traditional measures of mortality and other biological outcomes do not adequately measure effectiveness of interventions designed to improve life quality. There is also a growing appreciation for the need to use such measures to assess which services produce the greatest amount of health for the money spent. The drive to use newer, more expensive, technology will result in soaring costs. Since resources are limited, it is necessary to determine which interventions produce the most benefit relative to their costs (Kaplan, 1993).

A goal in assessing outcomes is to have the ability to evaluate the value of care (a measure of cost and quality of care), and to assist patients, payers, and providers in selecting treatments based on value. This leads to the question of how value will be defined. Professional societies and medical disciplines, including behavioral medicine, will be increasingly asked to document the value of their services. This is especially important to behavioral medicine because interventions can have such a broad impact: smoking cessation, diet, exercise, and pain management are but a few of the areas to target that affect a broad range of conditions and areas of disability. What remains to be seen is what processes (health care) lead to better outcomes. Understanding how best to provide such documentation is the focus of the remainder of this chapter.

# Methods of assessing health-related quality of life

One way to understand the numerous instruments available to assess HRQOL is by crossing two dimensions: the intended use of the information and the breadth of health domains covered in the measure. More specifically, instruments range in regard to their usefulness in individual treatment decisions, and whether the content of the assessment is limited to disease specific expectations or a broader understanding of overall health status. The focus here will be broader applicability and thus disease specific measures will not be reviewed (see Spilker, 1996).

The diversity of problems encountered in most behavioral medicine settings make generic measures a more flexible component of a standardized assessment battery. While HRQOL measures cover a broad range of functioning, disability, and distress, they are often cited as being insensitive to small changes in clinical status (as compared to disease specific measures). Yet, despite the high face validity of disease specific measures, the literature does not uniformly support their greater sensitivity. It is generally regarded as good practice to include both a disease-specific as well as a generic measure in both research and clinical work.

## PSYCHOMETRIC-BASED ASSESSMENT
Psychometric approaches to measuring HRQOL are perhaps the most familiar to those trained in the health sciences. These measures often require the respondent to indicate the frequency and/or intensity of symptoms or behaviors. Responses to individual questions are aggregated to create separate homogeneous scales (e.g., physical function,

social, and/or emotional function). Such scales have been successfully used to assess the outcomes of medical treatments and to compare patient outcomes under different systems of care (Deyo & Patrick, 1989; Spilker, 1996).

Strengths of psychometric measures include the fact that assessment of multiple dimensions of health appeal to clinicians and are familiar to those trained in this common assessment strategy. Limitations include the inability to integrate the information in economic analyses of treatment outcome, the subjectivity of reporting perceived ability, and that mortality cannot be incorporated into the data analysis (longitudinal analyses will often exclude any deaths in a sample of cancer patients and thus may bias the results). Clinical interpretation can be difficult, as comparison of different treatments may favor one group on some of the scales, while the comparison group scores more favorably on other scales.

Perhaps the most common outcome assessment procedure in contemporary health services research is the SF-36 (Ware & Sherbourne, 1992). A product of the RAND-sponsored Medical Outcomes Study (MOS), the Short Form 36 (SF-36) is a 36-item general health status assessment questionnaire that has substantial data on its reliability and validity on a wide variety of populations (Ware et al., 1994). For a complete description of this instrument and its applications, see Chapter 15 in this volume.

Stiggelbout et al. (1996) have developed an instrument that directly asks patients to rate their general attitude toward quality of life over quantity of life. The instrument is conceptually similar to the time trade-off method (see below) but is a self-administered paper and pencil questionnaire, not an interview format used in traditional time trade-off tasks. The questionnaire was constructed on the basis of semi-structured interviews with cancer patients, resulting in ten statements concerning tradeoffs between quality of life and length of life, quality of life and chance of survival, and the attitudes of subjects toward discontinuation of treatment. Each statement is rated on a 7-point Likert scale ranging from completely agree to completely disagree. A high score on the "Q" scale implies a limit to the acceptability of reductions in quality of life; a high score on the "L" scale suggests high striving for lengthening life, even if that is associated with reduced quality of life. It appeared that older patients more often stressed quality of life and were less concerned with prolonged survival than younger patients. The authors address issues for future refinement of this scale, but specifically designed the questionnaire to evaluate attitudes toward trade-off of quality versus quantity of life. They argue that just as patients are less willing than healthy subjects to trade-off length of life for quality of life, patients might be less willing to trade-off length of life for quality of life in actual situations than in hypothetical situations.

## UTILITY-BASED MEASURES

Behavioral medicine professionals are faced with many of the same challenges as other health care providers. Documenting the effectiveness of their interventions relative to other interventions offered by other providers will become increasingly important in the health care marketplace. In fact, a panel convened in 1993 by the US Department of Health and Human Services suggested that standardized outcomes analyses be conducted to evaluate the cost/effectiveness of medical care (Gold et al., 1996). One way to directly compare relative treatment effectiveness is to examine the impact of interventions on the utility gained. This requires certain characteristics of an assessment instrument. Utility-based measures address this requirement.

There are many controversies and concepts relevant to utility-based measurement, and we cannot review them all here. The interested reader is referred elsewhere for a more extensive discussion of the issues (Gold et al., 1996). Utility theory and measurement were developed, in part, as a normative model for individual decision making. Utilities are numbers that represent the strength of an individual's preference for various health outcomes under conditions of uncertainty. Preferences are the values people assign to different health outcomes when uncertainty is not a condition of measurement. These numbers reflect a person's level of subjective satisfaction, or desirability with different health states. The utility approach uses one or more scaling methods to assign numerical values on a scale of 0 (anchored as death) to 1.0 (anchored as optimum health). The resultant score thus allows morbidity and mortality to be combined into a single weighted measure, often referred to as (quality adjusted life years), or QALYs.

# Quality Adjusted Life Years

The benefits of health care can be expressed in terms of the years of life they produce, adjusted for reduced quality of life. The most popular term for this concept is "quality adjusted life years" (QALYs) (Weinstein & Stason, 1977), although other terms such as "well years" have also been used. For example, if a cigarette smoker died of heart disease at age 50 and we would have expected him to live to age 75, it might be concluded that the disease cost him 25 life years. If 100 cigarette smokers died at age 50 (and also had life expectancies of 75 years), we might conclude that 2,500 (100 men × 25 years) life years had been lost. However, we should not assume that these 25 years lost were disease-free or disability-free. That is, death is not the only outcome of concern; many cigarette smokers would be expected to suffer myocardial infarction or develop pulmonary diseases that would leave them somewhat disabled to varying degrees. Although they are still alive, the quality of their lives has diminished.

The use of a concept such as QALYs permits all degrees of disability to be compared to one another. The QALY combines data on the total life years gained from an intervention with data on the utility (or value) of health states for those years, to give a single measure of achievement or output. By calculating the cost per QALY gained for different clinical procedures or even different social problems, available resources can be directed toward interventions that maximize health gain (Chisholm et al., 1997). That is, a disease that reduces the quality of life by one-half will take away .5 QALYs over the course of 1 year. If it affects two people, it will take away 1.0 QALY (equal to 2 × .5) over a 1-year period. A medical treatment that improves the quality of life by .2 for each of five individuals will result in a production of 1 QALY if the benefit is maintained over a 1-year period. Using this system, it is possible to express the benefits of various programs by showing how many QALYs they produce (Kaplan & Anderson, 1996). Using this common metric of QALYs also allows one to introduce cost into the direct comparison of programs. Several alternative terms have been developed which are fundamentally similar to QALYs yet focus on different elements of utility. Healthy year equivalent (HYE; Mehrez & Gafni, 1989) and disability adjusted life years, or DALYs, are just two examples. Using this approach allows for comparison of behavioral medicine programs to other medical procedures on very different populations. Thus, this approach provides a framework within which to make policy decisions that require selection between competing alternatives.

As mentioned above, a number of methods are used to calculate utilities and preferences (Revicki & Kaplan, 1992). Standard gamble or lottery procedures are used to calculate utilities, while preferences can be generated by using visual analog rating scales or other scaling methods. Either holistic or decomposed approaches can be used to elicit health utilities. Each approach has its benefits and limitations, and each researcher or clinician must decide which approach best fits their situation. Again, given the focus on application of HRQOL to behavioral medicine, interested readers are referred elsewhere for more coverage on this issue (e.g., Gafni, 1994; Kaplan et al., 1993; Testa & Nackley, 1994; Torrance, 1987). However, some understanding of these two approaches should inform decisions about the choice of instruments.

## HOLISTIC APPROACH

The holistic method of calculating utilities involves having an individual assign utilities to a number of hypothetical health state scenarios. These scenarios describe important aspects of a health condition in terms of physical, psychological, and social functioning. These scenarios are presented to individuals and the relative preferences are elicited for each health state.

Two common holistic methods explicitly have patients consider decisions under uncertainty: standard gamble and time trade-off. The standard gamble offers a choice between two alternatives: Choice A—living in a suboptimal state of health with certainty, or Choice B—taking a gamble on a new treatment for which the outcome is uncertain. The subject is told that the new treatment will lead to perfect health with a given probability (p) or immediate death with a given probability (p-1). The subject can choose between remaining in a state that is intermediate between wellness and death, or take the gamble and try the new treatment. The probability (p) is varied until the subject is indifferent between the choices A and B. For example, a person is told to imagine they are blind and that a treatment which would enable the patient to regain their sight results in a .001% chance of death. If the patient chooses the treatment then the odds of death are increased to .1%, for example, and the patient is again asked to choose their current state of blindness or the treatment with risk of death involved. The risk continues to be increased until the patient no longer is willing to take the risk. The less risk a patient is willing to take to alleviate a health state the higher the utility of that health state.

A variety of problems with the gamble method have become apparent. Some believe that the standard gamble has face validity because it approximates choices made by medical patients (Mulley, 1989), yet treatment of most chronic diseases does not result in complete cure or death. Also, the cognitive demands of the task are high, as well as the time required to ascertain one individual's utility/preference.

Another common holistic method is referred to as time trade-off. Here, the subject is offered the choice of living for a defined amount of time in perfect health or a variable amount of time in an alternative state that is less desirable (e.g., moderate disability). Presumably, all subjects would choose a year of wellness versus a year with some health problem. However, by reducing the time of wellness and leaving the time in the sub-optimal health state fixed, an indifference point can be determined. For example, a subject may rate being in a wheelchair for two years as equivalent to perfect wellness for a year. The time trade-off is theoretically appealing because it is conceptually equivalent to a QALY. However, there is a concern whether the tasks can be clearly understood by the average subject (Kaplan, 1995).

DECOMPOSED APPROACH

In the decomposed approach, patients are asked a series of questions about their functioning in specific health domains. Based on their responses, individuals are assigned a utility value. The weights and utilities are developed from previous ratings by samples from the general population, or some other reference group. For example, the Health Utility Index (HUI; Torrance & Feeny, 1989) and the Quality of Well-being Scale (QWB; Kaplan & Bush, 1982) use a decomposed approach to generate preferences. In fact, the HUI and QWB represent hybrids of psychometric and utility-based measures.

The utility/preference approach has several advantages compared to the psychometric approach. First, it incorporates time and risk preferences for different health state outcomes into the measurement process, and scores are easily incorporated into economic analyses. Preference assessment has been successfully incorporated into numerous clinical trials. However, there is controversy over the definition of utilities/preferences and the methods used to derive these values. Preferences for some health states vary widely between individuals as well as a result of how the health states are described.

However, there are unresolved issues with deriving preferences. Namely, the duration of the disease state may influence the preference itself. For example, many patients would value an illness condition as more desirable if the assumption was made that the "stay" in that health state was short ("I can tolerate anything for a day"), and thus relative (and absolute) preferences may change as a result. Another issue is whose preferences are most useful. It appears that the patient's perspective is most important, though often studies will rely on physician's rating/preference primarily out of convenience of design. In addition, measured preferences have been reported to vary with the method of elicitation and respondent populations surveyed. In eliciting preferences for hypothetical health states from the general population, the subjective rating of a respondent's own health state should be considered in determining representative population groups.

## The Quality of Well-Being Scale (QWB)

While the SF-36 serves as an example of a psychometric instrument, the Quality of Well-Being Scale (QWB) is a preference-based instrument used with several different populations (Kaplan & Anderson, 1996). While the Health Utilities Index (HUI) is also a psychometrically sound instrument, our experience has been with the QWB and thus is described in more detail here. Interested readers are referred to Feeney and Torrance (1989) for information on the HUI. The QWB assesses a patient's objective level of functioning in three domains: mobility, physical activity, and social activity. A distinction is made between "functional ability" and "functional performance" (Anderson et al., 1989), namely a patient is asked to report activity performed rather than the patient's perception of what could possibly have been performed. The QWB concentrates on functional performance (or what the individual actually did) on the past six completed days.

In addition to these three domains, the QWB assesses the presence of a wide array of symptoms. On any particular day, nearly 80% of the general population is optimally functional, yet over an interval of six days, only 12% experience no symptoms (Kaplan et al., 1976). Even if these symptoms do not affect a patient's functioning, they do lower quality of life. For example, the QWB score is heavily driven by the wide array of symptoms assessed, as compared to functional performance (Kaplan et al., 1976). Our experience has shown that the QWB instrument is, in its operation, sensitive to the health-related issues that are most important to people, and it is thus capable of capturing even small variations in health status. It is in fact the importance of symptoms on the QWB that may make it more useful to the behavioral medicine clinician than most other generic measures.

One of the criticisms of the QWB is that it is more expensive and difficult to administer than competing measures such as the SF-36. The QWB is relatively long and complex because it has some branching and probe questions and requires a trained interviewer. The original QWB used a complex interviewer-administered questionnaire because self-administered questionnaires produced biases resulting in overesti-mates of health status (Anderson et al., 1986, 1988). However, refinements in questionnaire design may allow us to get around these problems.

## The Quality of Well-Being Scale, Self-Administered (QWB-SA)

Given the above mentioned criticisms, a self-administered QWB—referred to as the Quality of Well-Being Scale, Self-Administered (QWB-SA)—was developed that addresses some of these issues (Kaplan et al., 1996, 1997).

The QWB has several strengths has we wished to maintain. First, the QWB includes assessment of symptoms in addition to various areas of functioning. To help make the instrument more useful in the clinical setting the list of symptoms was expanded. The revised list of symp-toms and problems includes several mental health items and all items are arranged in a manner consistent with a medical "review of systems". Second, the QWB assesses functional status (versus perceived ability) in three areas: mobility, physical activity, and social function-ing. This perspective was maintained. Third, the QWB asks a patient to report on symptoms and activity over a 6-day period. To reduce recall bias, the QWB-SA assesses only the three days prior to completion of the questionnaire. Finally, the scoring of the instrument utilizes popula-tion-derived preference weights. Given the addition of several items to the QWB-SA, new preference weights were derived from ratings by a new sample of subjects. A series of studies have begun to establish the psychometric properties of this new measure. It is our expectation that the information derived from the QWB-SA should prove useful to clin-icians as well as to health care managers and policy makers (Ganiats et al., 1997; Sieber et al., 1997; Sieber et al., 2000).

## Quality of Life Time Without Symptoms of Toxicity or Treatment (Q-TWiST)

A recent development has offered another way to calculate QALYs (Gelber et al., 1996). The Q-TWiST methodology was originally devel-oped for cancer research and to describe Quality of Life Time Without

Symptoms and Toxicity of treatment. Instead of survival analysis that scores patients 1.0 for being alive and 0.0 for death, TWiST codes time with symptoms or toxity as 0.0. The Q-TWiST methodology is an extension of the TWiST method but adds quality of life to the evaluation. Thus, the term Q-TWiST is used for quality-time without symptoms and toxicity. In many ways, the Q-TWiST methodology is identical to quality-adjusted survival analysis. There are three steps to the Q-TWiST analysis. First, health states are defined. These health states typically represent the expected outcomes and side effects of treatment. Each of these states is assigned a utility score. The exact method for assigning utilities may differ from study to study. Sometimes the utilities are simply assigned by the investigators while in other cases the utilities are provided by patients.

The second step involves partitioning of the overall survival time. For example, one component of survival might be TWiST or the time without any symptoms or adverse effects. The second stage might be the time with severe symptomatic adverse effects. A third component might be the amount of time with reductions in wellness due to the progression of the disease. All of these occur prior to death. Usually, survival analysis is used to estimate the duration of these states. For example, in a study of patients with breast cancer the median survival time might be seven years. The analysis would estimate the portion of time spent in each of the defined states.

The third stage involves comparison of treatments using the Q-TWiST methodology. For each treatment group, duration of stay in state is multiplied by the utility and the Q-TWiST is calculated as the sum of TWiST plus the products of remaining utilities and health states. For example, suppose that patients have a median survival of seven years. Three of the years are spent without symptoms (TWiST). Two years are spent with adverse reaction to medication. The utility for this state is .7, so the adjusted years in this state equal 1.4 (obtained by multiplying 2 years × .7 quality weight). Then, the remaining two years are spent in a state of disease progression with a utility of .5. This results in one adjusted year (.5×2=1). So, the total Q-TWiST is 5.4 (obtained as (3 years × 1.0) + (2 years × .7) + (2 years × .5)). Q-TWiST analysis typically compares treatments using these adjusted survival times.

The Q-TwiST was developed for studies in cancer and AIDS. Recently, Schwartz and colleagues have adapted the method for other chronic diseases (Schwartz et al., 1995a, 1995b, 1997). The Schwartz adaptation of Q-TwiST allows the dimensions to be continuous rather than binary. The preference weighting system uses patient ratings, but can also integrate social costs and the provider perspective. Several studies have shown the value of the modified Q-TWiST for evaluations of outcomes in neurologic diseases such as multiple sclerosis (Schwartz et al., 1997) and epilepsy (Schwartz et al., 1995b).

## Assessment in the clinical setting

### CHOOSING THE RIGHT INSTRUMENT

HRQOL measures have the potential to become the new standard in medical practice. Without these tests, patient functioning and well-being are unlikely to be discussed during a typical medical visit. A majority of patients feel it is appropriate and desirable to discuss psychological problems with their physicians, but few patients initiate these discussions even when they are experiencing problems (Good–Delvecchio et al., 1987). As a result, doctors are not well-informed about their patient's functional status, or HRQOL. Well-being, especially as it relates to psychological distress, often goes unrecognized and untreated. Collecting this information may be paramount to treatment success in behavioral medicine settings.

Medical personnel are sometimes concerned about the validity and importance of self-rated health collected through self-administered surveys, often preferring physiological and biomedical outcomes. There is a tradition of using highly technological apparatus to obtain extremely precise estimates of aspects of pathology and impairment. However, the majority of clinical measurements used for diagnosis and treatment-response monitoring are low technology and require use of questions (i.e., clinical history) very similar in style to those used in HRQOL scales. In addition, providers are often uncertain about the responsiveness of these questionnaires to detect small, clinically relevant changes (Deyo & Patrick, 1989; Revicki, 1992). On the other hand, those concerned with health care resource allocation and the assessment of the cost-effectiveness of interventions often criticize health status questionnaires for not incorporating mortality, duration of survival, or patient preferences into health outcomes (Feeny & Torrance, 1989; Kaplan et al., 1989). The task is to address these criticisms.

While clinical medicine attempts to do the best for an individual person, regardless of cost, the public concern is with reducing the burden of disease suffered by populations and its ethical standpoint is one of utilitarianism. However, since populations are made up of individuals and the burden of an illness in a population is the sum total of disease experienced by individuals, there should be some common ground on how to satisfy both clinical and public health medicine goals. Thus, the goal for providers of behavioral medicine should be to use a health status measure that is responsive to clinically meaningful differences in clinical symptoms and functional status, while providing information useful for determining where such changes are cost-effective for population-based health care.

One step toward this goal is the regular use of a HRQOL measure in everyday behavioral medicine practice. Such assessments would help ensure that important dimensions of health are consistently considered, would help track changes in health over time, and thus provide potentially useful information in treatment decisions. Such an assessment should provide a view of the patient's complete status, in order to detect unforeseen effects of treatment. Disease-specific measures do not have this breadth. As an instrument becomes more specific to a disease or particular function, it may no longer meet the goals of population-based assessment. Disease specific measures aid in identifying patient behaviors that exacerbate a chronic illness and may provide helpful information, but their specificity precludes their sole use as an HRQOL instrument.

To make this approach practical, assessment should vary in length according to the application. Comparability between treatments and populations would be enhanced if short forms (of more disease-specific symptoms) were imbedded within longer forms assessing more global function. This would allow a portability in both contributing to a normative database (e.g., generic questions), and tailoring the assessment to the particular disease being treated.

From both clinical and public health perspectives, outcome measures are needed that are responsive to changes in services or treatments. The lack of direct congruence between measures of disease activity and subjective feelings of distress is a reflection of the complexity of factors that determine well-being and HRQOL. As clinical practice is concerned with a holistic approach to patients, HRQOL may provide an appropriate way of tapping into patients' experiences. Standardized questionnaires may prove very helpful for those patients who find it hard to verbalize their feelings and for those health professionals who find it difficult to explore the patient's wider experiences.

Deverill et al. (1998) propose three criteria for an acceptable QALY-type measure. First, it must be practical in that it can be completed in a reasonably short time, facilitating a high response rate to the questions. Second, it must have adequate test-retest and inter-rater reliability. Third, it must have construct and empirical validity (gives results as expected with other measures of the construct). These authors state that QALY measures are rarely used correctly in economic analyses.

## Administration and issues determining frequency of assessment

If administration of some standardized HRQOL instrument is accepted into behavioral medicine practice, how frequently should these assessments occur? There are no clear guidelines on how frequently health outcome measures should be given. Some measures ask respondents about an extended time period (e.g., one month), though this increases the likelihood of recall bias and inaccurate reporting. The best evidence suggests that people do relatively well at recalling health events for an interval of approximately one week or less (Kaplan et al., 1978). Thus, shorter intervals will provide a better approximation of current health status, though some events (e.g., symptoms, function) may not be captured if the interval is too short (e.g., 24 hours).

Once a measure and assessment window is selected, the question of how frequently a measure should be used depends on the problem under study. For chronic health conditions, assessment yearly may be appropriate. On the other hand, acute or episodic illnesses might be expected to change considerably over a brief time interval, and thus weekly assessment may be more appropriate. Generally, a matching between the sensitivity of the measure, the burden in completing it (i.e., length of questionnaire, requirement of face-to-face interview in clinic), and the variability of the disease or patient's health status should occur.

### WHAT DOMAINS OF HEALTH TO ASSESS?

There is great value in using disease-specific measures of symptoms and problems unique to specific diseases in parallel with generic measures. One must be careful when selecting a disease-specific measure. A comparison of outcomes between two treatments using a disease-specific measure may be biased if the measurement includes a list of side effects likely to be experienced from one treatment but not the other; conversely, using only a generic measure without a broad assessment of symptoms may be insensitive to unanticipated side effects of either treatment. While it is important to assess function, most people report little or no dysfunction, yet report reduced HRQOL due to the presence of one or more symptoms. Thus, a generic measure that includes a broad spectrum of symptoms may be ideal.

Most health status measures (e.g., SF-36, QWB, HUI) begin with the World Health Organization definition of health as a complete state of physical, mental, and social well being, and not merely the absence of disease (WHO, 1948). This definition has led many investigators to assume that a general measure must include separate scales for physical, mental, and social health. In fact, some reviewers of the literature have gone as far as reviewing the quality of measures by recording whether there was a separate scale for each of these dimensions. However, this reliance on the labeling of subscales will likely misrepresent the actual content covered on many instruments.

For example, previously the QWB has been criticized because there is no subscale named "sensory function". However, the QWB includes symptoms for loss of vision, loss of hearing, impairment of vision (including wearing glasses or contact lenses), problems with taste and smell, and so on. Another example concerns mental health. Many authors note that the QWB excludes mental health content. Despite widespread interest in the model among practitioners in many different specialties, the QALY concept has received very little attention in the mental health fields until now. We believe that this reflects the widespread belief that mental and physical health outcomes are conceptually distinct. Ware and Sherbourne (1992) emphasized that mental and physical health are different constructs and that attempts to measure them using a common measurement strategy is like comparing apples to oranges. However, a measure without a mental health component does not necessarily neglect mental health. Mental health symptoms may be included and the impact of mental health, cognitive functioning, or mental retardation may be represented in questions about role functioning.

Consider the case of a person with depression. Depression may be a symptom reported by a patient just as a cough is reported by other patients. Depression without disruption of role function would cause a minor variation of wellness. If the depression caused the person to stay at home, his/her score would be lower, with severe depression leading to hospitalization resulting in a lower score still. Certainly, studies have shown the validity of the QWB assessing changes in mental health (see Patterson et al., 1994, 1997).

## CEILING AND FLOOR EFFECTS AND OTHER RELEVANT PSYCHOMETRIC ISSUES

Validity to the clinician is a straightforward concept: does the scale measure what it is intended to measure and compare well to a "gold standard" or criterion. However, criterion and construct validity pose certain dilemmas when assessing HRQOL; these important issues have been outlined earlier (Kaplan et al., 1976). Additional relevant performance statistics are the accuracy of the instrument: its sensitivity and specificity. While criticism is often directed toward health questionnaires as being based on a "soft" science, the primary method of data collection for physicians—medical history taking—is plagued by these same problems. The issue for behavioral medicine clinicians should be whether an instrument is sensitive enough to detect meaningful changes expected from an intervention. Using a measure which can detect these differences and be used to compare a population or intervention to other populations or interventions is ideal.

Other issues to consider in the selection of an assessment tool: Will the data collected be comparable to data collected on other populations? Is the data able to be used in decisions regarding resource allocation? Is there coverage of all domains of health that are relevant to this specific population? If the condition being assessed is expected to be stable, then is the measure reliable over time? Ebrahim (1995) suggests that the assessment of reliability and validity of health status measures is carried out inappropriately. Namely, that repeatability of a measure across a population does not adequately address the stability of the measure to assess changes over time for an individual. Has concurrent, construct and convergent validity been demonstrated with the particular disease/population being studied? Is the instrument responsive to observable increments in change? That is, is the instrument able to show an expected dose response curve? Is the instrument sensitive to changes within an individual over time? Are ceiling and floor effects a concern with this instrument or with this particular patient population?

Ceiling and floor effects have been studied in relation to several different measures. Some evidence suggests that perfect scores on the SF-36 and the SIP are common (Anderson et al., 1994). In contrast, perfect scores on the QWB are rare (Ganiats et al., 1997). Similarly, floor effects on a utility-based measure indicate mortality, not a psychometric problem as it would be on a traditional psychometric measure.

## INTERPRETATION AND USE OF DATA IN CLINICAL MANAGEMENT DECISIONS

As Remie and Garssen (1997) point out: should a cancer patient's high score on a depression questionnaire be considered abnormal or a healthy ability to acknowledge and disclose one's feelings and reactions to disease?

How does one interpret changes on an HRQOL scale? First, the clinician should not equate reported mean treatment/group differences with changes in an individual patient's score. Even after adjusting for possible mediating factors of age and gender, additional information is needed. Second, we believe the clinician must place a change in scores within the context of patient preferences (whether they be population-based or individually-derived). For example, does the patient more highly value the increased ability to ambulate or attach a greater value on symptom relief? A scale aimed to determine QALYs should have this ability.

Meyerowitz (1993) asks whether data drawn from large-scale studies play a meaningful role in clinical practice where the central concern is with a specific, unique individual. Unfortunately, studies have documented that physicians' perceptions of a patient's needs and concerns often differ from the patient's own report in terms of psychological distress and desire for information. In the absence of sound data, there is a high risk of making inaccurate judgments about what the patient wants. Therefore, an assessment tool that incorporates patients' preferences, either at a population or an individual level, seems most appropriate.

# Summary and conclusions

Numerous barriers must be overcome before HRQOL measures can be incorporated into clinical practice. The length and cognitive complexity of questionnaires are key issues. The ideal instrument should be quick to administer, sensitive to detect small changes in health, be interpretable by clinicians, and useful in the development of cost-effective population-based interventions.

The purpose of this chapter has been to summarize major methodological and practical issues associated with the construction and application of QALYs. In addition, we define the problems encountered by behavioral medicine practitioners who apply these measures. We concluded with some of the issues to be included in the application of QALYs in mental health care evaluation. These issues are particularly relevant to mental health care as interventions are explicitly aimed at improving life, rarely extending it. A critical issue in the future will be to increase utilization of existing HRQOL measures in clinical practice to help document the effectiveness of behavioral medicine interventions and position clinicians more prominently in the health care marketplace.

# References

Anderson, J.P., Bush, J.W., & Berry, C.C. (1986). Classifying function for health outcome and quality of life evaluation. *Medical Care, 24*, 454–469.

Anderson J.P., Bush J.W., & Berry, C.C. (1988). Internal consistency analysis: A method for studying the accuracy of function assessment for health outcome and quality of life evaluation. *Journal of Clinical Epidemiology, 41*, 127–37.

Anderson, J.P., Kaplan, R.M., & DeBon, M. (1989). Comparison of responses to similar questions in health surveys. In: F. Fowler (Ed.), *Health survey research methods* (pp. 13–21). Washington, DC: National Center For Health Statistics.

Anderson, J.P., Kaplan, R.M., & Schneiderman, J.L. (1994). Effects of offering advance directives on quality adjusted life expectancy and psychological well-being among ill adults. *Journal of Clinical Epidemiology, 47*, 761–772.

Brook, R.H., & Lohr, K.N. (1987). Monitoring quality of care in the Medicare program. Two proposed systems. *Journal of the American Medical Association, 258*, 3138–3141.

Chisholm, D., Healey, A., & Knapp, M. (1997). QALYs and mental health care. *Social Psychiatry and Psychiatric Epidemiology, 32*, 68–75.

Deverill, M., Brazier, J., Green, C., & Booth, A. (1998). The use of QALY and non-QALY measures of health-related quality of life: Assessing the state of the art. *Pharmacoeconomics, 13*, 411–420.

Deyo, R.A., & Patrick, D.L. (1989). Barriers to the use of health status measures in clinical investigation, patient care, and policy research. *Medical Care, 27(supp. 3)*, S254–S268.

Ebrahim, S. (1995). Clinical and public health perspectives and applications of health-related quality of life measurement. *Social Science and Medicine, 41*, 1383–1394.

Feeny, D.H., & Torrance, G.W. (1989). Incorporating utility-based quality of life assessment measures in clinical trials: Two examples. *Medical Care, 27*, S190–S204.

Gafni, A. (1994). The standard gamble method: What is being measured and how is it interpreted? *Health Services Research, 29*, 207–224.

Ganiats, T.G., Sieber, W.J., Barber, E., & Barrett-Connor, E. (1997). Initial comparison of four generic quality of life instruments. *Quality of Life Research, 6*, 648.

Gelber, R.D., Cole, B.F., Gelber, S., & Goldhirsch, A. (1996). The Q-TWiST method. In: B. Spilker (Ed.), *Quality of life in pharmocoeconomics in clinical trials* (2nd Ed., pp. 437–444). Philadelphia: Lippincott-Raven.

Gold, M.R., Siegel, J.E., Russel, L.B., & Weinstein, M.C. (1996). *Cost-effectiveness in health and medicine.* New York: Oxford University Press.

Good–Delvecchio, M.J., Good, B.J., & Cleary, P.D. (1987). Do patient attitudes influence physician recognition of psychosocial problems in primary care? *Journal of Family Practice, 25*, 53–59.

Kaplan, R.M. (1993). Application of a general health policy model in the American health care crisis. *Journal of the Royal Society of Medicine, 86*, 277–281.

Kaplan, R.M. (1995). Changed subject or wrong subject? *Psychology & Health, 10*, 277–280.

Kaplan, R.M., & Anderson, J.P. (1996). The general health policy model: An integrated approach. In: B. Spilker (Ed.), *Quality of life and pharmacoeconomics in clinical trials* (pp. 309–322). New York: Raven.

Kaplan, R.M., & Bush, J.W. (1982). Health-related quality of life measurement for evaluation research and policy analysis. *Health Psychology, 1*, 61–80.

Kaplan, R.M., & Litrownik, A.J. (1978). Further comments on multivariate methods in behavioral research. *Behavior Therapy, 9*, 474–476.

Kaplan, R.M., Bush, J.W., & Berry, C.C. (1976). Health status: Types of validity and the index of well-being. *Health Services Research, 11*, 478–488.

Kaplan, R.M., Feeny, D., & Revicki, D.A. (1993). Methods for assessing relative importance in reference based outcome measures. *Quality of Life Research, 2*, 467–475.

Kaplan, R.M., Ganiats, T.G., & Sieber, W.J. (1996). *The Quality of Well-being Scale Self-Administered.* Copyrighted material. San Diego, CA.

Kaplan, R.M., Sieber, W.J., & Ganiats, T.G. (1997). Comparison of the Quality of Well-being Scale with a self-administered questionnaire. *Psychology & Health, 12*, 783–791.

Kaplan, R.M., Anderson, J.P., Wu, A.W., Mathews, W.C., Kozin, F., & Orenstein, D. (1989). The Quality of Well-being Scale: Applications in AIDS, cystic fibrosis, and arthritis. *Medical Care, 27(Suppl 3)*, S27–S43.

Mehrez, A., & Gafni, A. (1989). Quality-adjusted life years, utility theory and healthy-years equivalents. *Medical Decision Making, 13*, 287–292.

Meyerowitz, B.E. (1993). Quality of life in breast cancer patients: The contribution of data to the care of patients. *European Journal of Cancer, 29A (Supp 1)*, 59–62.

Mulley, A.J. (1989). Assessing patients' utilities: Can the end justify the means? *Medical Care, 27*, S269-S281.

Patterson, T.L., Kaplan, R.M., Grant, I, Semple, S.J., Moscona, S., Koch, W.L., Harris, M.J., & Jeste, D.V. (1994). Quality of well-being in late-life psychosis. *Psychiatry Research, 63*, 169–181.

Patterson, T.L., Semple, S.J., Shaw, W.S., Halpain, M., Moscona, S, Grant, I., & Jeste, D.V. (1997). Self-reported social functioning among older patients with schizophrenia. *Schizophrenia Research, 27*, 199–210.

Remie, M., & Garssen, B. (1997). Non-expression of emotions in cancer patients. In: A.J.W. Boelhouwer (Eds.) *The (non) expression of emotions in health and disease* (pp. 237–245). Tilburg, The Netherlands: Tilburg University Press.

Revicki, D.A. (1992). Relationship between health utility and psychometric health status measures. *Medical Care, 30*, S274-S282.

Revicki, D.A, & Kaplan, R.M. (1992). Relationship between psychometric and utility-based approaches to the measurement of health-related quality of life. *Quality of Life Research, 2*, 477–487.

Schwartz, C.E., Cole, B.F., & Gelber, R.D. (1995a). Measuring patient-centered outcomes in neurologic disease. Extending the Q-TWiST method. *Archives of Neurology, 52*, 754–762.

Schwartz, C.E., Cole, B.F., Vickrey, B.G., & Gelber, R.D. (1995b). The Q-TWiST approach to assessing health-related quality of life in epilepsy. *Quality of Life Research, 4*, 135–141.

Schwartz, C.E., Coulthard-Morris, L., Cole, B., & Vollmer, T. (1997). The quality-of-life effects of interferon beta-1b in multiple sclerosis. An extended Q-TWiST analysis. *Archives of Neurology, 54*, 1475–1480.

Sieber, W.J., David, K., Adams, J., Kaplan, R.M., & Ganiats, T.G. (2000). Assessing the impact of migraine on health-related quality of life: An additional use of The Quality of Well-Being Scale – Self-Administered (QWB-SA). *Headache, 40*, 662–271.

Sieber, W.J., Ganiats, T.G., & Kaplan, R.M. (1997). Validation of a self-administered Quality of Well-being (QWB) scale. *Medical Outcomes Trust Bulletin, 5*, 2–3.

Spilker, B. (Ed) (1996). *Quality of life and pharmacoeconomics in clinical trials* (2nd ed.). Philadelphia: Lipincott-Raven Press.

Stiggelbout, A.M., DeHaes, C.J.M., Kiebert, G.M., Kievit, J., & Leer, J.H. (1996). Tradeoffs between quality and quantity of life: Development of the QQ questionnaire for cancer patient attitudes. *Medical Decision Making, 16*, 184–192.

Testa, M.A., & Nackley, J.F. (1994). Methods for quality of life studies. *Annual Review of Public Health, 15*, 535–559.

Torrance, G.W. (1987). Utility approach to measuring health-related quality of life. *Journal of Chronic Disease, 40*, 593–600.

Torrance, G.W., & Feeny, D. (1989). Utilities and quality-adjusted life years. *International Journal of Technology Assessment, 5,* 559–575.

Ware, J.E., & Sherbourne, C.D. (1992). The MOS 36-item short-form health survey (SF-36). I. Conceptual framework and item selection. *Medical Care, 30,* 473–483.

Ware, J.E., Kosinski, M., & Keller, S.D. (1994). *SF-36 physical and mental health summary scales: A user's manual.* Boston, MA: The Health Institute.

Weinstein, M.C., & Stason, W.B. (1977). Foundations of cost-effectiveness analysis for health and medical practice. *New England Journal of Medicine, 296,* 716–721.

World Health Organization (1948). *Constitution of the World Health Organization.* Geneva: WHO Basic Documents.

World Health Organization (1980). *World Health Organization manual.* Geneva: WHO Basic Documents.

# 8 MEASURES OF BLOOD PRESSURE AND HEART RATE VARIABILITY IN BEHAVIORAL RESEARCH ON CARDIOVASCULAR DISEASE

Willem J. Kop, David S. Krantz, Gayle Baker

Stress-induced changes in blood pressure (BP) and heart rate (HR) provide useful indices of autonomic nervous system activity (Krantz & Manuck, 1984). The autonomic nervous system (ANS) is intimately involved in the body's responses to environmental challenges such as physical activity and mental arousal. An extensive body of literature also exists demonstrating adverse short-term and long-term pathophysiological consequences of increases in ANS activity (Kop, 1999; Krantz et al., 1996; Williams et al., 1991). The ANS, which regulates activity of the cardiac muscle, glands, and smooth muscles, is divided into two efferent components: the sympathetic nervous system (SNS) and the parasympathetic nervous system (PNS). These two components of the ANS are involved in hemodynamic responses to physical and emotional stressors by direct nervous control of the blood vessels and heart muscle as well as indirect neurohormonal regulation of the cardiovascular system. The current scientific and lay literature emphasizes the effects of chronic and acute stress on the development of cardiovascular disorders such as hypertension and coronary artery disease. Increased activation of the SNS may result in adverse health outcome by directly affecting the pathophysiological processes responsible for disease progression (e.g., accelerated atherosclerosis) and in addition by elevating the workload of the cardiovascular system (e.g., increased BP). Measures of BP and HR responses to mental arousal may reveal important information about the pathophysiological mechanisms of stress-induced cardiovascular events and may improve the risk-stratification for adverse cardiovascular health outcome (Krantz et al., 1996). Therefore, cardiovascular measures are important and widely-used measurement tools employed in behavioral medicine research.

In this chapter we will limit our discussion to mental stress-induced responsiveness of blood pressure (BP) and heart rate variability (HRV). Excellent comprehensive reviews of cardiovascular assessment in behavioral medicine and the theoretical background thereof can be found elsewhere (for example: Guyton, 1991; Schneiderman et al., 1989). The first part of this chapter briefly reviews measures of HR, cardiac pump function, and BP, and how these measures are related to catecholamines and other neurohormones. In the last section, procedures for BP and HRV measurements will be discussed that may be used to assess ANS responses in laboratory and ambulatory settings. We will conclude with some suggestions for future research on ANS reactivity in the investigation of biobehavioral factors affecting cardiovascular disease progression.

## Hemodynamic effects of autonomic nervous system activity

Emotions such as fear and anger are accompanied by a pronounced "fight-or-flight" response of the sympathetic nervous system as indicated by increases in catecholamines—a finding initially documented by Cannon (1914). Below we will briefly review the hemodynamic system including BP and HR responses to mental stress, as well as the involvement of both direct ANS and indirect neurohormonal activation of the hemodynamic system.

HEART RATE
The rhythm of the heart is driven by changes in the membrane potentials of the sinus node which is located in the right atrium of the heart. The sinus node is innervated by the SNS and the nervus vagus of the PNS. Sympathetic innervation of the sinus node is mediated via adrenergic $\beta_1$ receptors and results in an increased HR, whereas vagal stimulation decreases HR via muscarinic cholinergic receptors. Factors that determine the rate of the heart beat are to be differentiated from factors involved in the force, or energy of contraction of the heart, and are referred to as chronotropic and inotropic factors, respectively. In addition to the adrenergic and cholinergic pathways, other neurotransmitters such as neuropeptide Y play a role in the chronotropic state of the heart. Autonomic efferent influences on the heart are modulated by afferent pathways of which the parasympathetic baroreceptor projections are most prominent. Both inotropic and chronotropic factors determine the force and speed of the pump function of the heart.

## CARDIAC PUMP FUNCTION

The heart's function as a pumping device for blood circulation was postulated by William Harvey in the late 18th century (similar theories were proposed by Persian scholars in the 17th century). Cardiac pump function is one of the main determinants of systemic BP. The amount of blood ejected by the heart's left ventricle per time unit (cardiac output) is determined by the heart rate and stroke volume. A simplified model of factors affecting cardiac output is presented in Figure 18.1. Stroke volume is the difference between the left ventricular volume at the end of the filling period (end-diastolic volume) and the volume of blood at the end of ventricular contraction (end-systolic volume). Left ventricular ejection fraction is a related measure of cardiac pump function and is defined by the proportion of end-diastolic volume ejected during ventricular contraction, with a normal range of 50–70% in healthy individuals. Both stroke volume and ejection fraction are determined by diastolic filling pressure (pre-load), cardiac contractility, and resistance to the pumping of the heart imposed by

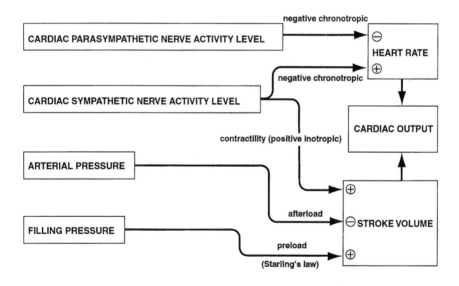

(From *Cardiovascular Physiology*, by L.J. Heller & D.E. Mohrman. Copyright © 1981 by McGraw-Hill. Reprinted with permission.)

Figure 18.1.    Influences on cardiac output.

arterial pressure (after-load or peripheral vascular resistance). The effects of SNS activation on cardiac pump function include: increased HR and related shorter diastolic and systolic intervals, elevated peak ventricular pressures, more forceful ventricular contraction and associated outflow velocity, and a shorter ejection period (Gottdiener et al., 1998). Furthermore, although stroke volume remains unaffected by SNS activation, ejection fraction increases due to smaller end-diastolic volume and more complete ventricular ejection (Rushmer, 1989). In contrast, PNS activation results in decreased heart rate and cardiac pump function.

The development of non-invasive techniques such as echocardiography and radionuclide imaging have made it possible to register stress-induced changes in cardiac pump function in humans. Impedance cardiography has been successfully used in psychophysiological research as an alternative to these cardiac imaging devices. The impedance cardiogram is based on electrocardiographic and auscultatory data and yields measures of cardiac output and the so-called pre-ejection period (a measure of SNS activity) (Wilson et al., 1989). Impedance cardiography is not frequently applied in investigations of patients with CAD because the aforementioned cardiac imaging techniques are easily accessible and have established clinical relevance in cardiac patients. In this chapter we limit our discussion of cardiac pump function to the application of this measure as an index of stress-induced cardiac ischemia.

BLOOD PRESSURE
Arterial BP is determined by cardiac output (see above) and the total peripheral resistance of the arterial network. Cardiac output determines the amount of blood ejected from the left ventricle into the aorta after which the blood is distributed throughout the arterial system at a speed of approximately 1 m/s. The arterial BP wave shows an initial sharp increase which reflects the increase in BP due to contraction of the left ventricle of the heart. During diastole, BP decreases gradually when arterial blood distributes in the peripheral circulation. The most commonly used BP measures are peak (SBP; systolic) and minimum (DBP; diastolic) BP. The main determinant of DBP is the total peripheral resistance, although several other factors (e.g., stroke volume and heart rate) affect DBP as well. Peripheral (or systemic) vascular resistance (PVR) can be estimated from the BP and cardiac output measurements (see below). Peripheral resistance is quite variable across the

various end-organs and is mainly determined by local metabolic demands, SNS activity, total blood volume (which is dependent on kidney function), and circulating hormones.

## AUTONOMIC NERVOUS SYSTEM ACTIVITY AND CATECHOLAMINES

The normal response of blood vessels to mental stress is vasodilation. However, blood pressure increases due to SNS activity result in part from peripheral vasoconstriction (i.e., increased PVR) of the smaller blood vessels (arterioles) in response to stress-induced norepinephrine release. Norepinephrine leads to increased PVR primarily via the $\alpha$-receptors located on the smooth muscle cells of the vascular bed. In larger blood vessels, these constrictive effects are opposed by endothelial release of nitric oxide elicited in response to increased blood flow and cholinergic stimulation (Broten et al., 1992; Dietz et al., 1994). The end result is that, under normal circumstances, mental arousal results in vasoconstriction in the skin and visceral organs, and vasodilation in the skeletal muscles as long as the endothelium is intact (Dietz et al., 1994; Yeung et al., 1991). $\beta$-receptors can be divided into those that predominantly affect the heart ($\beta_1$), and those that affect the lungs and blood vessels ($\beta_2$). In contrast to the SNS, evidence indicates that the PNS has little effect on the peripheral vascular circulation.

In addition to the neural innervation, HR and BP can be modulated indirectly via catecholamine release from the adrenal medulla into the blood circulation. Hormonal effects on the vascular bed include norepinephrine-related constriction, similar to the effects of SNS stimulation. Adrenal epinephrine causes vasoconstriction in most instances ($\alpha$ receptor mediated), but is known to produce pronounced vasodilation in specific organs such as the heart and skeletal muscles (via $\beta$ receptors). As mentioned above, the cardiovascular system consists of several afferent and efferent feedback loops. Catecholamines have pronounced increasing effects on HR, but in real-life situations this may be masked by the concomitant vasoconstrictive effects of norepinephrine which lead to BP elevation and substantial vagal discharge via baroreceptors, causing deceleration of HR. A detailed review of cardiovascular physiology can be found elsewhere (Guyton, 1991) and specific applications for behavioral medicine are discussed in Schneiderman et al. (1989), and Krantz and Falconer (1995).

# Measurement issues

The assessment of BP and HRV can be optimized by implementing practical procedures designed to reduce possible sources of measurement error. Measurement errors resulting from variations of actual BP and HR are differentiated here from errors due to invalid data collection resulting from inappropriate procedures or equipment. We will describe some of the technical issues involved in the measurement of BP and HRV, and review the most commonly-used measures derived from BP and HRV assessments. This section will conclude with a brief review of the issues involved in the assessment of mental stress-induced cardiovascular reactivity. Reactivity is defined as the increase from the resting level of a physiological measure induced by a specific challenge task such as exercise or mental arousal.

## BLOOD PRESSURE ASSESSMENT

Two main approaches are available to assess BP: intra-arterial and non-invasive assessments. The most accurate measure of BP is derived from intra-arterial assessments and therefore intra-arterial BP is used as the gold standard to which non-invasive assessments are compared. Experience in behavioral research has indicated, however, that minimally obstructive (i.e., non-invasive) techniques are preferable over more invasive techniques (Wilson et al., 1989). In addition to intra-arterial and non-invasive auscultatory methods, other (continuous) techniques are available to assess BP, such as plethysmography (volume assessment) and arterial tonometry (pressure detection).

Intra-arterial assessments are commonly obtained in the arm (brachial or radial artery) in most laboratory settings, whereas intra-aortic pressures can be obtained during cardiac catheterization. The method generally involves a wire filled with fluid that runs from the artery to a transducer which registers the beat-to-beat changes in pressure. Related to BP is blood flow. Using techniques based on the Doppler effect, invasive assessments of arterial flow velocity can now be made (Ofili et al., 1993). Coronary flow velocity is calculated from the Doppler frequency shift (which is the difference between the transmitted and returning frequency of a transducer placed in the artery) (Kop & Cohen, 2001). However, the necessary devices are generally too costly and invasive for wide-scale use in cardiovascular behavioral medicine research in humans.

Non-invasive BP assessments generally make use of a sphygmo-manometer which is used to determine the counter pressure in an inflatable cuff (i.e., the Riva Rocci method). For that purpose, the cuff is inflated around the upper arm at a higher pressure than the SBP. The cuff is connected to a mercury column which allows one to read the pressure in the cuff. After complete occlusion of the brachial artery, the air in the cuff is gradually released. Auscultation (using a stethoscope at the site of the inflated cuff) during release of the cuff pressure reveals the so-called Korotkoff sounds. The Korotkoff sounds result from pressure-induced changes in the arterial wall and/or turbulence in flow through the relatively narrow arteries. The first phase of the Korotkoff sounds is characterized by a clear tapping sound; the associated pressure reflects the SBP. Phase II is marked by a soft murmur which becomes louder in phase III and suddenly muffled in phase IV. When the cuff is further deflated, the Korotkoff sounds disappear (phase V) which is an index for the DBP. BP is commonly expressed in mmHg SBP / DBP. Normal SBP and DBP levels at rest vary from 100 to 140 mmHg, and from 70 to 90 mmHg, respectively; higher values indicate (borderline) hypertension. A more detailed review of BP assessment issues can be found in Pickering and Blank (1989). BP is often assessed using automatic BP monitors in psychophysiological laboratory studies. Automatic monitors generally use the Korotkoff sound detection or oscillatory procedures and have the clear advantage of not being subject to observer bias. A potential disadvantage of manual and automatic blood pressure assessments is that the obtained levels are essentially instantaneous, which may limit possibilities to examine fluctuations over short periods of time or beat-to-beat tracking of both HR and BP which is often used in studies investigating the baroreceptor response.

Non-invasive beat-to-beat assessments of arterial pressure can be obtained by finger cuff methods. In the early 1970s, the Czech physiol-ogist Penaz developed a procedure in which arterial pulsation is mea-sured using a photoplethysmograph located in a (finger) cuff. The plethysmograph feeds back on the finger cuff such that a 2/3 pressure is maintained, keeping the output constant. This system was commer-cially available under the name Finapress and at present under the name Portopress. The finger cuff methods have been demonstrated to yield valid assessments during a variety of experimental maneuvers such as hand grip, cold pressor, phenylephrine injections, and passive leg raising (Parati et al., 1989). The main advantages of this method are that it provides assessments of beat-to-beat variability in BP as well as continuous comparisons between HR and BP, which allows evaluation of the baroreceptor reflex (see below). Because these devices may interfere with daily activities, the finger pressure method is not recommended for ambulatory studies. Recent developments in tonometry for ambulatory BP assessments may prove useful in this respect.

### Blood pressure measurement: concerns and sources of error

Variability and errors in BP measurements may arise from two main sources: (1) factors inherent in variations of actual BP; and (2) variability resulting from the method used. Compared to aortic arterial BP, SBP levels increase somewhat (approximately 10 mmHg) as assessments are made more peripherally, whereas DBP drops slightly (approximately 4 mmHg) from aortic to peripheral. Several factors affect the actual BP. In supine position, the sympathetic tone is minimal, and considerably higher while standing. If a subject's position is changed from reclining to standing, DBP may increase slightly due to blood pooling to the legs and related decrease in cardiac stroke volume, whereas SBP remains unaltered due to reflex peripheral vasoconstriction. Somewhat lower pressures occur in the upright posture and during inspiration. A third determinant of BP concerns circadian fluctuations, although it has been argued that these fluctuations reflect changes in activities rather than an internal biological clock (Pickering et al., 1996). In addition, BP assessments are affected by the sex and professional status of the person who takes the BP. Physicians tend to have a bias of recording higher BP than nurses do, but in addition, the actual BP is generally higher when assessed by a physician, a phenomenon referred to as "white coat hypertension" (Pickering et al., 1990).

Equipment-based measurement errors can occur in case of non-invasive assessments where substantial artificial increases in SBP (up to 20 mmHg) may be recorded during exercise, or as a result of bending the arm to 90°. It is also important that the cuff size adequately fits the subject's arm because too small cuffs overestimate and too large cuffs underestimate actual BP. In addition, certain populations are more likely to require special attention in order to optimize hemodynamic assessments. For example, in children under 12 years, ultrasonographic (based on echographic techniques) rather than auscultatory procedures may prevent underestimation of actual BP. In elderly populations, stiffening of the arteries may artificially increase SBP assessment up to 30 mmHg. In these rare cases, valid assessments can only be obtained via the intra-arterial technique. BP assessments obtained with automatic monitors do not always correspond with assessments derived from manual assessments with error ranges of approximately 5 mmHg

(Pickering et al., 1989). In general, mercury sphygmomanometers reveal more reliable results than automatic BP monitors; the validity of the automatic assessments should be established using this manual procedure.

*Blood pressure indices*
In addition to SBP and DBP, other BP indices include: (1) mean arterial pressure (cycle length corrected area under the pressure wave) approximated as [SBP + (2 × DBP)/3]; (2) pulse pressure (SBP-DBP); and (3) rate pressure product (heart rate × SBP) which is a global index of cardiac demand. The total peripheral vascular resistance (PVR in dynes $s^{-1} m^{-7}$) can be calculated as: (mean arterial pressure × 80) / cardiac output. Therefore, to assess PVR, some measure of cardiac output must be obtained, either by impedance cardiography or cardiac imaging techniques such as echocardiography.

## HEART RATE AND SPECTRAL ANALYSIS OF HEART RATE VARIABILITY
Simple electrophysiologic equipment is sufficient to determine HR (i.e., the number of heart beats/minute). However, for more complex analyses of HR, especially measures of HRV, sophisticated electrocardiographic (ECG) sampling techniques are required. Two recent review articles have provided guidelines for assessing ANS activity based on HRV (Berntson et al., 1997; Task Force of the European Society of Cardiology and the North American Society of Pacing and Electrophysiology, 1996).

The ECG has a characteristic wave-pattern starting with the P wave (indicating the atrial contraction), followed by the QRS complex (the contraction of the left ventricle), and the T wave (repolarization of the left ventricle). Under normal conditions, the R wave peak is the most pronounced component of the ECG. It has been known for a long time that HR increases slightly during inspiration and decreases during expiration (e.g., Hales (1733); cited in Berntson et al., 1997), a phenomenon referred to as respiratory sinus arrhythmia. A functional relationship between the magnitude of respiratory sinus arrhythmia and vagal tone was purported by Hering (1910; cited in Berntson et al., 1997) and has been further documented in numerous studies since. We will outline below how the beat-to-beat variations in the HR can be used to estimate parasympathetic and possibly sympathetic activation. Measures of HRV have been used in cardiology and pediatrics as predictors of future sudden (infant) death. In psychophysiology, HRV has also been used as an index of cognitive effort and metabolic processes.

This chapter will focus on HRV measures relevant to the assessment of ANS activity. Two main analytical approaches are applied in the analysis of HRV: *time-domain* and *frequency-domain* analysis.

The time-domain approach assesses HRV by using standard statistical measures of the heart beats, such as standard deviation. This approach has proven to be useful clinically in the prediction of future cardiac death. However, in its basic application, time-domain analysis incorrectly assumes that the lengths of adjoining heart beats are unrelated phenomena. Various statistical (autoregressive) approaches are now available to adjust for this issue. Time-domain analysis of HRV provides descriptive statistics of the HR.

The frequency-domain analysis techniques are also based on the length of heart beat duration, referred to as the R-R interval. When each R-R interval is compared to the preceding R-R interval, a histogram can be obtained displaying the variations of subsequent differences between R-R intervals. These periodic components of HRV tend to cluster around certain frequency bands, and spectral density functions can be used to display the spectral power (vertical axis) plotted against the frequency (horizontal axis). Both autoregressive and fast Fourier transformation can be used to obtain these spectral density functions and generally reveal the same results (Berntson et al., 1997). The principle behind Fourier analysis is that a curve is assumed to be a composite of various sinus functions with specific frequencies; the autoregressive models make use of lagged correlations to correct for various potential statistical biases. The direct spectral analysis of successive R-R intervals is complicated by the fact that the unit of the spectral plot is cycles/beat and not cycles/second. Therefore, it has been recommended that a weighted average of the beats occurring within a fixed sample interval is used. Theoretically, the highest HRV frequency possible is 0.5 Hz because by definition the R-R interval represents a single sample per heart beat and has a maximum frequency of half the sampling frequency (0.5 cycles/beat).

*Measurement concerns and sources of error for HR and HRV*
Measurement errors in HR and HRV are generally attributable to changes in respiration rate, violations of the mathematical assumption underlying spectral analyses (stationarity), imprecise detection of the R wave (related to the detection method and sampling rate), and inadequate exclusion of artifacts or ectopic beats.

The rate and, to a lesser extent, the depth of inspiration affect the high frequency component of HRV. It is therefore preferable to obtain information regarding breathing frequency, especially in studies where this variable is likely to change. Rapid breathing is generally associated with a reduction rather than an increase in HRV (Hirsch & Bishop, 1981). It should be noted that even with statistical control for breathing frequency, the tasks under investigation may alter the coupling between respiration and vagal activity.

One important concern in time-domain and frequency-domain HRV analysis is the issue of stationarity. This assumption requires that the mean and covariance of the heart periods remain constant over time. For psychophysiological studies, this assumption is somewhat problematic because one generally examines task-induced changes in autonomic tone. In this respect it is suggested that epochs are selected such that heart period is constant within each phase of the task.

Artifacts and ectopic beats should be excluded from the analyses. It is therefore preferable to retain the original electrocardiograms (ECG) for post-hoc inspection of the heart period data. Careful inspection of the ECG tracings is essential since one missed R-wave in a 2-minute epoch can increase the HRV assessment as much as seven-fold (Berntson et al., 1997). If the ECG has many missing or abnormal beats, the analysis should be limited to time-domain statistics because frequency domain measures will be invalid.

The optimal storage of the digitized ECG is at a sampling rate of 500–1000 Hz. As a rule of thumb, a sampling rate of four times the target frequency is appropriate (Berntson et al., 1997). For example, to assess the high frequency component, a sample rate of 250 Hz will generally suffice. The optimal duration of a recording is generally ten times the lower wave-length of the frequency band under consideration. The standard use of analogue Holter monitors in cardiological research implies a digitization at 128 Hz which is not optimal and is associated with limitations, especially at the low and very low frequency bands. Various algorithms and template matching procedures may help to optimize data collected at a < 250 Hz sampling rate. Although HRV could in principle be derived from measures other than the ECG (e.g., via a finger cuff), these procedures are limited because the peak of the R wave cannot be detected precisely.

### Heart rate variability indices
Time-domain analysis yields several indices of HRV. For psychophysiological laboratory studies, the best time-domain measure for short-term periods of HRV is the root mean square of the successive beat differences (RMSSD). Other short-term time-domain measures have less

favorable statistical properties. For the long-term assessment of HRV, the standard deviation of the mean heart period over five minute intervals is recommended (SDANN), and time-domain measures of overall HRV also include the standard deviation of all R-R intervals (SDNN). The SDNN decreases with mental stress (Tuininga et al., 1995) and is predictive of future mortality in post-myocardial infarction patients (Task Force of the European Society of Cardiology and the North American Society of Pacing and Electrophysiology, 1996). Multivariate comparison of the predictive value of each of the time-domain HRV measures is complicated because these measures are mathematically dependent. The time-domain method of choice is therefore determined by the nature of the study question.

Using frequency-domain analysis, the most distinctive frequency band is the respiratory sinus arrhythmia band. This high frequency band ranges from 0.15 to 0.4 Hz (this is equivalent to 9 to 24 breaths/min). Respiratory sinus arrhythmia results from inhibition of the parasympathetic control of the heart. The low frequency band (0.05–0.15 Hz) is assumed to reflect both sympathetic and parasympathetic activity. Physiological correlates of other frequency bands are less well understood; these include the very low frequency band (0.003–0.05 Hz) possibly related to plasma renin and thermoregulation, and the ultra low frequency band (< 0.003 Hz) which may reflect circadian fluctuation of autonomic tone.

The high frequency component of HRV reflects respiratory sinus arrhythmia and hence parasympathetic tone. This notion is supported by evidence indicating that cholinergic blockade or surgical removal of the vagus will nearly eliminate the high frequency component, whereas sympathetic blockade with $\beta$-blocking agents has virtually no effect on this frequency band (Berntson et al., 1997). Respiratory sinus arrhythmia is a consequence of both central respiratory mechanisms as well as peripheral afferent information, and the rate of respiration may confound the inferential analysis of vagal activation.

The low frequency component is assumed to reflect sympathetic activity by some researchers (Pagani et al., 1991), but most evidence suggests that this frequency band reflects a combination of sympathetic and parasympathetic tone (Berntson et al., 1997; Task Force of the European Society of Cardiology and the North American Society of Pacing and Electrophysiology, 1996). This band includes the 0.1 Hz component (also referred to as Mayer wave or 10-s rhythm).[1] Increases in BP are projected to the brainstem via baro-receptor afferents.

Abrupt changes in BP are buffered by the afferent projection of the baroreceptor information to the vagal outflow to the heart. Therefore, the increases in BP following sympathetic activation may result in a vagal baroreceptor response which may become evident in the 0.1 Hz band. In addition, $\beta$-blockade does not always reduce the low frequency band, and exercise-induced increases in cardiac sympathetic activity are not accompanied by increases in the low frequency component (Kingwell et al., 1994). The ratio between the low and high frequency components has been suggested as an index for sympatho/vagal balance (Pagani et al., 1991), but this assertion has been challenged because the low frequency component includes different aspects of parasympathetic activation (baro-reflex) than the high frequency component (Berntson et al., 1997).

In sum, the PNS can modulate HR at all frequency bands ranging from 0–0.5 Hz. Because of the relatively slow action on the sinus node, the SNS will modulate heart rate at frequencies lower than 0.15 Hz. The most useful HRV measures for cardiovascular laboratory studies are probably the high and low frequency components. In addition to frequency-domain and time-domain analysis, other statistical and geometrical measures of HRV have been used in specific settings and, at present, no consensus exists as to the appropriate choice of methods. In general, time-domain analysis may not be very useful in psychophysiological research because it is suboptimal for analysis of short-term (within 10 minutes) changes in HRV, which is typically examined in task-induced responses of ANS activity. Short-term fluctuation in the high frequency component of HRV may prove useful in the assessment of parasympathetic responses to laboratory stress tasks.

## METHODOLOGICAL ISSUES IN THE ASSESSMENT OF STRESS-INDUCED REACTIVITY

To examine stress-induced reactivity, pre-task baseline measures are compared to measurements obtained during the task under consideration, e.g., mental stress. The duration of the resting period may vary from 10 to 30 minutes, depending on the nature of the study. Baseline levels of BP and HR can be assessed by averaging the measures at end-phase of the resting period. Several epidemiological studies in healthy individuals revealed support for the hypothesis that elevated cardiovascular reactivity is predictive of future adverse cardiac events (Alderman et al., 1990; Keys et al., 1971; Sparrow et al., 1984).

The optimal frequency of BP assessments depends on the nature of the research question. In the case of general screening, two or three assessments repeated on at least two occasions will reveal adequate estimates. For psychophysiological studies in which hemodynamic responses (reactivity) to experimental interventions are investigated, repeated automatic (generally every two minutes) assessments are preferable during rest periods and experimental tasks. If the frequency of cuff inflation is more than once per minute, interference with normal blood circulation may occur resulting in invalid assessments. For HRV analysis, the optimal duration of ECG recording is generally ten times the lower wave-length of the frequency band under consideration. This implies one minute for high frequency, two minutes for low frequency and overall a five-minute stationary epoch will be adequate to obtain high and low frequency data.

A task-induced hemodynamic response is defined as the difference between baseline and task levels. Both peak task levels as well as the average levels over the entire task have been used as indicators of the hemodynamic response. Three main approaches exist to calculate the magnitude of this response: (1) simple arithmetic difference (task—baseline); (2) percent change from baseline; and (3) residual (change) scores (Manuck et al., 1989). Residual scores have the advantage of specific control for the known association between baseline levels and levels during tasks, because scores are based on the regression of the task levels on the resting levels. Positive residual scores indicate higher reactivity than expected on the overall relationship between baseline and task levels, and negative values indicate relatively low responses. Alternatively, (4) repeated measures analyses of variance could be considered where the measures during rest are modeled as a within-subjects factor. The procedures to assess reactivity of HRV components are similar to those examining hemodynamic reactivity. The analysis of high frequency and low frequency domain responses have been sug-gested as most valid for short-term psychophysiological studies (Berntson et al., 1997; Task Force of the European Society of Cardiology and the North American Society of Pacing and Electrophysiology, 1996), but time-domain analysis has been success-fully applied as well (Tuininga et al., 1995). When multiple tasks are administered, an aggregated assessment of baseline hemodynamics is generally preferable over separate assessments (Kamarck et al., 1992). Also, the order of the tasks should be randomized whenever possible, to prevent bias from a specific task-sequence. The studies reviewed below have used several measures of cardiovascular reactivity in the prediction of short-term and long-term clinical manifestations of coronary disease.

## Implications and conclusions

Measures of cardiovascular reactivity to mental stress are increasingly used in pathophysiological studies of patients with CAD. Because it is not possible to obtain direct measures of ANS activation of the heart in human subjects, BP and HR are among the parameters used as surrogates to assess ANS responsiveness to mental stress. Accumulating evidence indicates that stress-induced ischemia is more likely due to increases in BP and PVR than to chronotropic and inotropic effects of ANS activation. In the conclusion of this chapter, three potential areas of research are discussed that may yield important new information in cardiovascular behavioral medicine: (1) the assessment of beat-to-beat variation of both BP and HR; (2) the role of catecholamines and other neurohormones in stress-induced cardiac events; and (3) alternative measures of ANS activity.

Ad (1). Although intra-arterial BP assessments are generally reliable indicators of the actual arterial pressure, non-invasive measures have been shown to correlate well with intra-arterial measures. Moreover, BP responses measured by non-invasive measures have proven useful in the prediction of future adverse cardiovascular outcome as well as concurrent ischemia in cardiac patients. New techniques on the beat-to-beat registration of BP as related to changes in HR are useful in the assessment of ANS activity, especially the baroreflex response. At present, there are no readily usable techniques for the ambulatory assessment of beat-to-beat BP variations that do not interfere with subjects' usual daily activities. Another topic for further study in this area involves the statistical data-reduction techniques of these beat-to-beat variations.

Ad (2). Most studies in cardiac patients have not found relationships between mental stress-induced increases in catecholamines and pathophysiological consequences of mental stress such as coronary vasomotion (Yeung et al., 1991) and myocardial ischemia (Goldberg et al., 1996). We did not discuss the possible role of task characteristics, sometimes referred to as $\alpha$-adrenergic (i.e., predominantly affecting BP through increased vascular resistance, such as the mirror trace task) and $\beta$-adrenergic tasks (i.e., predominantly affecting cardiac output, such as speech preparation) (Hurwitz et al., 1993). A few studies have examined both $\alpha$ and $\beta$ adrenergic tasks in the setting of stress-induced ischemia in cardiac patients (Blumenthal et al., 1995), but did not specifically document differences in the potency to induce ischemia between these two types of tasks. The distinction between $\alpha$ and $\beta$ adrenergic tasks is not without its problems (e.g., Allen et al., 1991). Studies using specific blockade provide preliminary evidence that $\alpha$-adrenergic mediation may play an important role in stress-induced ischemia (Dakak et al., 1995). Catecholamine responses are significantly correlated with hemodynamic factors that are known to predict ischemia, but do not seem to predict mental stress-induced ischemia; this apparent paradox requires further study.

Ad (3). Alternative approaches for the assessment of ANS activity, other than BP and HRV, include experimental manipulation of autonomic tone (e.g., vagal blockade by atropine, or selective SNS by $\beta$-blocking agents such as propranolol) or direct recordings of sympathetic activity (e.g., peroneal assessments). At present, direct measures of SNS nerve activity are quite prone to failure and inaccuracies, with a loss of data of up to 50% (Kingwell et al., 1994).

ANS tone and reactivity play an important role in the pathogenesis of cardiovascular disease progression and its clinical manifestations. We described how ANS activity can be assessed by using measures of HR, cardiac pump function, and BP, which are related to catecholamines and other neurohormones. More investigations are needed to examine the dissociation of stable ANS measures obtained during resting conditions and ANS responses to mental and other challenge tasks. Such studies will improve our understanding of the pathophysiological mechanisms involved in gradual cardiovascular disease progression and subsequent onset of activity triggered acute cardiac events. Furthermore, BP and HR variability are not necessarily the most optimal indirect indices of ANS activity and more targeted ANS markers are currently investigated as predictors of adverse health outcome in specific high-risk populations (e.g., QT-interval variability in patients with a high likelihood of cardiac arrhythmias). New devices are currently being developed to assess beat-to-beat variability in BP coupled with concurrent changes in HR. These new ANS measures, technological developments, and the increasingly sophisticated computer-assisted analysis techniques of digitized psychophysiological measures will reveal new opportunities in this field of research. Because of the indirect nature of most ANS indices, it will be important to investigate the interrelationships between the cardiovascular ANS measures described in this chapter with studies using cerebral imaging. Research targeted at optimization of ANS measures in laboratory and ambulatory settings, as well as specific pharmacological blockade studies, may prove useful in the further risk stratification of adverse cardiovascular health outcome, particularly in high risk populations.

## Acknowledgments

Preparation of this chapter was supported by a grant from the NIH (HL58638 and HL47337). The opinions and assertions expressed herein are those of the authors and are not to be construed as reflecting the views of the USUHS or the US Department of Defense.

## Notes

1.   Some researchers refer to this band as the mid-frequency band.

## References

Alderman, M.H., Ooi, W.L., Madhavan, S., & Cohen, H. (1990). Blood pressure reactivity predicts myocardial infarction among treated hypertensive patients. *Journal of Clinical Epidemiology, 43*, 859–866.

Allen, M.T., Boquet, A.J. Jr., & Shelley, K.S. (1991). Cluster analyses of cardiovascular responsivity to three laboratory stressors. *Psychosomatic Medicine, 53*, 272–288.

Berntson, G.G., Bigger, J.T., Eckberg, D.L., Grossman, P., Kaufman, P.G., Malik, M., Nagaraja, H.N., Porges, S.W., Saul, J.P., Stone, P.H., & Van der Molen, M.W. (1997). Heart rate variability: Origins, methods, and interpretive caveats. *Psychophysiology, 34*, 623–648.

Blumenthal, J.A., Jiang, W., Waugh, R.A., Frid, D.J., Morris, J.J., Coleman, R.E., Hanson, M., Babyak, M., Thyrum, E.T., & Krantz, D.S. (1995). Mental stress-induced ischemia in the laboratory and ambulatory ischemia during daily life. Association and hemodynamic features. *Circulation, 92*, 2102–2108.

Broten, T.P., Miyashiro, J.K., Moncada, S., & Feigl, E.O. (1992). Role of endothelium-derived relaxing factor in parasympathetic coronary vasodilation. *American Journal of Physiology, 262* (5 Pt 2), H1579–H1584.

Cannon, W.B. (1914). The interactions of emotions as suggested by recent physiological researches. *American Journal of Physiology, 25*, 256–282.

Dakak, N., Quyyumi, A.A., Eisenhofer, G., Goldstein, D.S., & Cannon, R.O. (1995). Sympathetically mediated effects of mental stress on the cardiac microcirculation of patients with coronary artery disease. *American Journal of Cardiology, 76*, 125–130.

Dietz, N.M., Rivera, J.M., Eggener, S.E., Fix, R.T., Warner, D.O., & Joyner, M.J. (1994). Nitric oxide contributes to the rise in forearm blood flow during mental stress in humans. *Journal of Physiology (London), 480*, 361–368.

Goldberg, A.D., Becker, L.C., Bonsall, R., Cohen, J.D., Ketterer, M.W., Kaufman, P.G., Krantz, D.S., Light, K.C., McMahon, R.P., Noreuil, T., Pepine, C.J., Raczynski, J., Stone, P.H., Strother, D., Taylor, H., & Sheps, D.S. (1996). Ischemic, hemodynamic, and neurohormonal responses to mental and exercise stress experience from the psychophysiological investigations of myocardial ischemia study (pimi). *Circulation, 94*, 2402–2409.

Gottdiener, J.S., Kop, W.J., & Krantz, D.S. (1998). Mental stress and silent myocardial ischemia: Evidence, mechanisms, and clinical implications. In: S. Stern (Ed.), *Silent myocardial ischemia* (pp. 175–199). London: Martin-Dunitz Ltd.

Guyton, A.C. (1991). *Textbook of medical physiology* (8th ed.). Philadelphia, London, Toronto: W.B. Saunders Company.

Hirsch, J.A., & Bishop, B. (1981). Respiratory sinus arrhythmia in humans: How breathing pattern modulates heart rate. *American Journal of Physiology, 241*, 620–629.

Hurwitz, B.E., Nelesen, R.A., Saab, P.G., Nagel, J.H., Spitzer, S.B., Gellman, M.D., McCabe, P.M., Phillips, D.J., & Schneiderman, N. (1993). Differential patterns of dynamic cardiovascular regulation as a function of task. *Biological Psychology, 36*, 75–95.

Kamarck, T.W., Jennings, J.R., Debski, T.T., Glickman-Weiss, E., Johnson, P.S., Eddy, M.J., & Manuck, S.B. (1992). Reliable measures of behaviorally-evoked cardiovascular reactivity from a PC-based test battery: Results from student and community samples. *Psychophysiology, 29*, 17–28.

Keys, A., Taylor, H.L., Blackburn, H., Brozek, J., Anderson, J.T., & Simonson, E. (1971). Mortality and coronary heart disease among men studied for 23 years. *Archives of Internal Medicine, 128*, 201–214.

Kingwell, B.A., Thompson, J.M., Kaye, D.M., McPherson, G.A., Jennings, G.L., & Esler, M.D. (1994). Heart rate spectral analysis, cardiac norepinephrine spillover, and muscle sympathetic nerve activity during human sympathetic nervous activation and failure. *Circulation, 90*, 234–240.

Kop, W.D. (1999). Chronic and acute psychological risk factors for clinical manifestations of coronary artery disease. *Psychosomatic medicine, 61*, 476–487.

Kop, W.J., Cohen, N. (2000) Psychological risk factors and immune system involvement in cardiovascular disease. In: R. Ader, D.L. Felten, & N. Cohen (Eds.), *Psychoneuroimmunology* (3rd ed.) (pp. 525–544). San Diego, CA: Academic Press.

Krantz, D.S., & Manuck, S.B. (1984). Acute psychophysiologic reactivity and risk or cardiovascular disease: A review and methodologic critique. *Psychology Bulletin, 96*, 435–464.

Krantz, D.S., & Falconer, J.J. (1995). Measurement of cardiovascular responses. In: S. Cohen, R.C. Kessler, & L. Underwood Gordon (Eds.), *Measuring stress* (pp. 193–212). New York: Oxford University Press.

Krantz, D.S., Kop, W.J., Santiago, H.T., & Gottdiener, J.S. (1996). Mental stress as a trigger of myocardial ischemia and infarction. *Cardiology Clinics, 14*, 271–287.

Manuck, S.B., Kasprowicz, A.L., Monroe, S.M., Larkin, K.T., & Kaplan, J.R. (1989). Psychophysiologic reactivity as a dimension of individual differences. In: N. Schneiderman, S.M. Weiss, & P.G. Kaufmann (Eds.), *Handbook of research methods in cardiovascular behavioral medicine* (pp. 365–382). New York: Plenum Press.

Ofili, E.O., Kern, M.J., Labovitz, A.J., St.Vrain, J.A., Segal, J., Aguirre, F.V., & Castello, R. (1993). Analysis of coronary blood flow velocity dynamics in angiographically normal and stenosed arteries before and after endolumen enlargement by angioplasty. *Journal of the American College of Cardiology, 21*, 308–316.

Pagani, M., Mazzuero, G., Ferrari, A., Liberati, D., Cerutti, S., Vaitl, D., Tavazzi, L., & Malliani, A. (1991). Sympathovagal interaction during mental stress. A study using spectral analysis of heart rate variability in healthy control subjects and patients with a prior myocardial infarction. *Circulation, 83*, 43–51.

Parati, G., Casadei, R., Groppelli, A., Di Rienzo, M., & Mancia, G. (1989). Comparison of finger and intra-arterial blood pressure monitoring at rest and during laboratory testing. *Hypertension, 13*, 647–655.

Pickering, T.G., & Blank, S.G. (1989). The measurement of blood pressure. In: N. Schneiderman, S.M. Weiss, & P.G. Kaufmann (Eds.), *Handbook of research methods in cardiovascular behavioral medicine* (pp. 69–79). New York: Plenum Press.

Pickering, T.G., Devereux, R.B., Gerin, W., James, G.D., Pieper, C., Schlussel, Y.R., & Schnall, P.L. (1990). The role of behavioral factors in white coat and sustained hypertension. *Journal of Hypertension, 8*, S141–S147.

Pickering, T.G., Schwartz, J.E., & Stone, A. (1996). Behavioral influences on diurnal blood pressure rhythms. *Annals of the New York Academy of Sciences, 783*, 132–140.

Rushmer, R.F. (1989). Structure and function of the cardiovascular system. In: N. Schneiderman, S.M. Weiss, & P.G. Kaufmann (Eds.), *Handbook of research methods in cardiovascular behavioral medicine* (pp. 5–22). New York: Plenum Press.

Schneiderman, N., Weiss, S.M., & Kaufman, P.G. (1989). *Handbook of research methods in cardiovascular behavioral medicine* (2nd ed.). New York: Plenum Press.

Sparrow, D., Tifft, C.P., Rosner, B., & Weiss, S.T. (1984). Postural changes in diastolic blood pressure and the risk of myocardial infarction: The Normative Aging Study. *Circulation, 70,* 533–537.

Task Force of the European Society of Cardiology and the North American Society of Pacing and Electrophysiology. (1996). Heart rate variability: Standards of measurement, physiological interpretation, and clinical use. *Circulation, 93,* 1043–1065.

Tuininga, Y.S., Crijns, H.J., Brouwer, J., van den Berg, M.P., Man in't Veld, A.J., Mulder, G., & Lie, K.I. (1995). Evaluation of importance of central effects of atenolol and metoprolol measured by heart rate variability during mental performance tasks, physical exercise, and daily life in stable postinfarct patients. *Circulation, 92,* 3415–3423.

Williams, R.B. Jr., Suarez, E.C., Kuhn, C.M., Zimmerman, E.A., & Schanberg, S.M. (1991). Biobehavioral basis of coronary-prone behavior in middle-aged men. Part I: Evidence for chronic SNS activation in Type As. *Psychosomatic Medicine, 53,* 517–527.

Wilson, M.F., Lovallo, W.R., & Pincomb, G.A. (1989). Noninvasive measurement of cardiac function. In: N. Schneiderman, S.M. Weiss, & P.G. Kaufmann (Eds.), *Handbook of research methods in cardiovascular behavioral medicine* (pp. 23–50). New York: Plenum Press.

Yeung, A.C., Vekshtein, V.I., Krantz, D.S., Vita, J.A., Ryan, T.J. Jr., Ganz, P., & Selwyn, A.P. (1991). The effect of atherosclerosis on the vasomotor response of coronary arteries to mental stress. *New England Journal of Medicine, 325,* 1551–1556.

# 19 ENDOCRINE ASSESSMENT IN BEHAVIORAL MEDICINE

Larry W. Hawk, Jr. and Andrew Baum

The endocrine system is one of the major control systems of the body. Hormones, the blood-borne messengers of the endocrine system, help to regulate an array of important processes, including digestion, metabolism, growth, and reproduction. In addition, the endocrine system, in conjunction with the nervous and immune systems, plays a strong role in generating, intensifying, and extending physiological responses to psychologically meaningful stimuli. In this light, it is not surprising that the endocrine system has long been of interest to researchers examining biopsychological aspects of health and illness. Early investigators focused on the "stress hormones" epinephrine (Cannon, 1914) and cortisol (Selye, 1936, 1976); to a large extent, contemporary models continue to focus on the sympatho-adrenal-medullary (SAM) axis, which produces epinephrine, and the hypothalamic-pituitary-adrenal (HPA) axis, which produces cortisol. However, it is increasingly clear that many other secreted substances, including some produced by the immune system, may be involved in emotion and stress processes (e.g., Weiner, 1992). Moreover, stress is only one biopsychological process, and research has shown that other aspects of endocrine function are related to health.

The purpose of this chapter is to assist investigators who are considering integrating endocrine measures into their research. The ever-growing possibilities for hormonal measurement and the broader array of potential questions that can be addressed necessitate that this not be a cookbook. Relatedly, the specific assays used to measure neuroendocrine products are only briefly reviewed (see Grunberg & Singer, 1990, for more details). Instead, a general framework focused on a series of questions is proposed to aid in decisions regarding inclusion of endocrine measures in behavioral medicine studies (see Table 19.1). After a review of the endocrine system, these questions are discussed.

Table 19.1. Questions to ask when considering inclusion of endocrine measures in behavioral medicine assessment

---

(a)  What is the rationale for using endocrine measures?
(b)  Which hormone(s) should be measured?
(c)  How should the measures be collected?
(d)  How should these measures be assayed, analyzed, and interpreted?

---

# A selective overview of the endocrine system

The endocrine system is important in many aspects of homeostasis and adaptation. Historically, it has been viewed as a "second nervous system," enhancing regulatory control over bodily activity. As such, endocrine function is critical to health and illness and serves as a potential mediator of relationships between psychological processes and aspects of physical health. We will discuss a few general points and provide more detailed coverage of cortisol and epinephrine, two hormones of historic and current interest in behavioral medicine (e.g., McEwen, 1998). More comprehensive coverage of the endocrine system is provided in a number of introductory physiology texts (e.g., Sherwood, 1997) and volumes dedicated specifically to endocrine physiology (e.g., Wilson & Foster, 1992).

## HYPOTHALAMIC-PITUITARY AXES

Endocrine system activity is regulated by the central nervous system, most notably by the hypothalamus. Although the pituitary has often been referred to as the master gland, the pituitary is actually regulated by centers in the hypothalamus, where numerous hormonal pathways, or *axes*, begin. In addition, the hypothalamus receives cognitive and affective input from neocortex and subcortical structures such as the hippocampus and amygdala. Thus, it is uniquely positioned to regulate autonomic and endocrine activity during threat, harm, stress and other psychological processes (see Lovallo, 1997, for a review). The hypothalamus causes the release of hormones from both the anterior and posterior pituitary.

The anterior pituitary is the target of multiple hypothalamic releasing factors, hormones that travel the short distance through an arterial portal. Releasing factors promote or inhibit the secretion of one of six hormones produced in the anterior pituitary. These systemic hormones may have direct effects on organs (e.g., prolactin stimulates milk secretion from mammary glands). More commonly, hormones released from the anterior pituitary cause the release of other hormones from peripheral endocrine glands. These hormones, which also enter systemic circulation, may have multiple effects on cells throughout the body by their interaction with receptors on/in target cells. Typically, activity in these axes is kept in check via negative feedback. That is, stimulation of receptors higher in the axis by the hormones produced by the pathway leads to a reduction of activity in the axis.

This process can be illustrated by considering production of cortisol in the HPA axis. The paraventricular nucleus of the hypothalamus produces and secretes corticotropin releasing hormone (CRH), which stimulates release of adrenocorticotropic hormone (ACTH) from the anterior pituitary. ACTH stimulates the outer layer, or cortex, of the adrenal gland to release corticosteriods. There are two general types of corticosteriods, mineralocorticoids and glucocorticoids. Among the glucocorticoids, cortisol is predominant in humans (corticosterone is the primary glucocorticoid in rats).

Cortisol crosses the cell membrane, binds with receptors in the nucleus, and alters protein synthesis. This produces a number of effects, including increased glucose availability (providing a ready supply of energy for cells), regulation of the immune system, and increased synthesis of catecholamines and sensitivity of adrenergic receptors (see e.g., Wilson & Foster, 1992). Cortisol is released in periodic bursts of activity and exhibits a diurnal rhythm, with a peak in the early morning and a nadir in the late evening. (A significant minority of the population does not exhibit this diurnal rhythm or does so inconsistently [Smyth et al., 1997]). Elevations in HPA function are counter-regulated: cortisol exerts negative feedback via inhibitory inputs to the hypothalamus, reducing CRH secretion, and to the anterior pituitary, inhibiting ACTH release.

In the short-term, HPA activity functions to increase availability of resources needed to assist in coping with stressors. However, the generally adaptive role of short-term cortisol elevations stands in contrast to that of prolonged heightened production of cortisol or to the exhaustion of corticoid production (Selye, 1976). In rats, prolonged overexposure of the hippocampus to glucocorticoids results in neuronal damage or even loss of neuronal mass, and this may be true in humans as well (e.g., Sapolsky, 1996). There is considerable interest in the implications of sustained elevations in cortisol for chronic stress and aging (e.g., Sapolsky et al., 1986). It should also be noted that receptor changes may alter the strength of the feedback system. For example, it has been hypothesized that chronic post-traumatic stress disorder (PTSD) is characterized by enhanced negative feedback of the HPA axis, with cortisol tonically suppressed but sensitized to acute challenge (see Yehuda, 1998).

A number of other hormones, including the sex hormones, growth hormone, and thyroid hormone, are products of hypothalamic-pituitary axes that are similar to that of cortisol. Although the role of most hormones in stress and related psychobiological processes has not been as widely studied as for cortisol, it is likely that many hormones are involved in these processes. In fact, it may be the pattern of endocrine activity that is most closely associated with particular states or traits (e.g., Mason, 1975; Mason et al., 1990).

Unlike the anterior pituitary, the posterior pituitary is an extension of the hypothalamus. Neurosecretory neurons in the hypothalamus produce oxytocin and arginine vasopressin (AVP). These hormones are transported down axons and stored in the posterior pituitary until they are released into systemic circulation. Oxytocin is best known for its role in stimulating uterine contractions during labor and promoting milk release for breast feeding. However, Taylor et al. (2000) recently reviewed evidence suggesting that oxytocin is an important component of a specifically female stress response, the "Tend-and-befriend" response (see also Light et al., 2000). AVP acts on kidney tubules to increase water retention (it is also referred to as antidieuretic hormone) and also exerts a vasoconstrictive action. Both effects can increase blood pressure. In addition, central AVP further affects blood pressure and may play a role in the development and/or maintenance of certain forms of hypertension (see Berecek & Swords, 1990), perhaps more so among African Americans than Caucasians (Bakris et al., 1997). The role of vasopressin in stress and depression, including an influence on HPA activity during such states, is currently being examined (e.g., Purba et al., 1996; Wotjak et al., 1996).

## SYMPATHO-ADRENO-MEDULLARY (SAM) AXIS
A second major class of neuroendocrine pathways that affect health and illness is derived from the CNS and adrenal medulla. The nervous system modulates endocrine function through autonomic innervation of endocrine organs. Perhaps nowhere is this clearer than in the SAM axis, which may be viewed as a melding of nervous and endocrine function. Most sympathetic nerves synapse in a chain of ganglia just outside the spinal cord, and post-synaptic neurons travel some distance to their organ targets. In the SAM axis, the presynaptic neuron

synapses in the inner portion of the adrenal gland, known as the adrenal medulla. Like the majority of postsynaptic sympathetic fibers, the adrenal medulla releases norepinephrine. However, the adrenal medulla differs from other post-synaptic neurons in two important respects. First, it also produces epinephrine, a key factor in endocrine regulation of emotional and stress-related processes. Whereas only a small amount of total norepinephrine is released from the adrenal, epinephrine is released primarily from the adrenal medulla. Second, the adrenal medulla secretes epinephrine and norepinephrine directly into the bloodstream as hormones, rather than synaptically as neurotransmitters. As a result, they circulate throughout the body.

Unlike cortisol and other steroids, catecholamines do not cross the cell membrane of target cells. Rather, they bind to receptors on cell membranes and cause changes in cell function via second messenger systems such as cyclic AMP. For example, epinephrine binds to $\beta_2$ adrenergic receptors on the surface of lymphocytes, causing apparent reductions in lymphocyte activity (Redwine et al., 1996).

SAM activity illustrates the manner in which endocrine activity can reinforce and extend nervous system activity. Like norepinephrine released from sympathetic terminals, norepinephrine and epinephrine bind to $\alpha$ and $\beta_1$ adrenergic receptors. This activity augments that of the sympathetic nervous system, including constriction of most arteries, increased heart rate and contractility, decreased digestive tract activity, and changes in other components of the so-called fight-or-flight response. Because it takes longer to clear hormone from blood than to clear neurotransmitter from synapses, SAM activity extends the duration of these effects. In addition, epinephrine has a much greater affinity than does norepinephrine for $\beta_2$ adrenergic receptors. This provides a mechanism for dilation of blood vessels in the heart and skeletal muscle, which need more oxygen during sympathetic activation, and dilation of the airway to allow maximal oxygen intake. Finally, epinephrine has several metabolic effects, most of which are aimed at releasing stored energy for immediate use.

Thus, the SAM axis plays a key role in response to challenges and stressors. Even mundane postural changes such as standing up increase circulating epinephrine and norepinephrine dramatically. In addition, both acute and chronic stress are associated with increased output of catecholamines by the adrenals (e.g., Dimsdale & Moss, 1980; Frankenhaeuser, 1975). The SAM axis also appears to be important in mediating health outcomes. For example, epinephrine exerts strong cardiovascular effects and also affects factors such as platelet activation (for a review, see Markovitz & Matthews, 1991) that may contribute to cardiovascular disease. Moreover, recent research documents the importance of catecholamines in regulation of the immune system (e.g., Bachen et al., 1995; Manuck et al., 1991; Sgoutas-Emch et al., 1994).

## Non-traditional endocrine measures

The hormones discussed so far represent only a fraction of the chemical messengers secreted into the body's fluids. Many substances secreted within the CNS are found in small amounts in the periphery. For example, endogenous opioid peptides, such as endorphin and met-enkephalin, can be assessed in tears, cerebrospinal fluid or plasma. In addition to their role in pain, these peptides may be important in studies of addictive drugs, eating behavior, and stress. Serotonin (5-HT), a neurotransmitter in the CNS, is also found in the bloodstream (e.g., in platelets) and in the intestinal mucosa. Although the functions of peripheral 5-HT are not clear, it has been suggested that platelet 5-HT can be used as a model for studying serotonergic activity at nerve terminals (e.g., Rotman, 1983).

To summarize, the endocrine system subserves multiple basic homeostatic processes. In addition, the HPA and SAM axes are central in mobilization of bodily resources, as during periods of stress. These and related endocrine parameters may be of interest to investigators in behavioral medicine for several related reasons, some of which are discussed in the following section.

## What is the rationale for using endocrine measures?

Given the complexity and cost that psychoendocrine measures add to a study, one should always first explicitly address the rationale for including them. We consider several potential uses of endocrines: (1) as an *indicator* of a physiological process; (2) as a *component* of a biopsychological process; (3) as a *mediator* of a biopsychological process; and (4) as an *objective indicator* of a biopsychological process.

### INDICATOR OF A PHYSIOLOGICAL PROCESS
Many physiological processes (e.g., blood glucose regulation, metabolism), and consequently many diseases (e.g., diabetes, thyroid disorders),

are fundamentally endocrine in nature. Therefore, endocrine measures may indicate the functional status of these processes (see also Grunberg & Singer, 1990). Within this general framework, endocrine measures may be useful selection/stratification variables, covariates, and/or dependent variables. We will provide examples of each of these possibilities.

There may be times when hormonal indices serve as important exclusion criteria. For example, it would be reasonable to screen for endocrine abnormalities in behavioral obesity-reduction trials, as inclusion of people with primary endocrine abnormalities could lead to an underestimation of the effect size of the treatment. However, it is also important to consider the base rates of endocrine disorders. For example, relatively common disorders that may be mistaken for depression (hypothyroidism) or anxiety (hyperthyroidism) may be more reasonably assessed than less likely endocrine problems like pheochromocytoma, a rare adrenal tumor involving hypersecretion of epinephrine.

In other situations, variations in endocrine status or function may be useful in establishing subsamples. For example, breast cancer cells may have receptors for estrogen, progesterone, or both, and the presence of these receptors is associated with differential treatment and outcome (e.g., Henderson, 1995). These sex hormone receptors might be used to select participants or to stratify a sample into subgroups (e.g., those with and without estrogen-sensitive tumors). Alternatively, an investigator might choose to use such variables as control variables in statistical analyses. This is most appropriate when measuring an endocrine factor that is thought to influence disease progression (or some other outcome) but is unrelated to the psychological processes under study.

Similarly, consider a study of the acute effects of stress or smoking on immune function among women. Because of the impact of estrogen and progesterone on immune function (McCruden & Stimson, 1991), stress responses (e.g., c.f., Litschauer et al., 1998; Sita & Miller, 1996), and the effects of nicotine (Pomerleau et al., 1991), obtaining measures of these hormones may be important in interpreting the findings of studies of any of these outcomes. Consistent with this, a recent study of immune responses during and after exposure to acute stress among women (Matthews et al., 1995) screened participants for oral contraceptive use and luteal phase progesterone levels, thereby eliminating these potential confounds.

The above examples focused on endocrine measures as means of refining samples and as predictors of varied outcomes. However, it is often the case that endocrine measures, as indices of disease severity or progression, may serve as important dependent variables. For example, basal cortisol response and response to pharmacologic challenge are critical in diagnosing adrenocortical insufficiency (Addison's disease) and excess (Cushing's syndrome). More generally, excesses or deficits in virtually all hormonal axes are associated with recognizable syndromes. Endocrine assessment is clearly important in these circumstances.

## COMPONENT OF A BIOPSYCHOLOGICAL PROCESS
Many investigators have called for a multi-systems operationalization of psychological constructs. The three-systems perspective (Lang, 1968) exemplifies this view, stating that psychological constructs cannot be directly observed but are inferred from data in three domains: self-report, physiological responding, and overt behavior. To the extent that data are consistent across these areas, an investigator can have greater confidence regarding the status of the construct. This is different from conceptualizing endocrine data as physiological "manipulation checks" of some psychological construct. It has become clear that, even under the best of circumstances, self-report does not necessarily offer a clear window upon mental processes (e.g., Nisbett & Wilson, 1977), much less the biopsychological processes that are often of interest in behavioral medicine research (e.g., the special issue of *Psychology and Health* on verbal reports, edited by Abraham & Hampson, 1996). Thus, it is important to take a multi-system approach to assessment.

Stress is clearly the most widely studied biopsychological process that involves integrated endocrine response. The endocrine system has played a central role in stress research since Cannon developed our modern-day use of the term. Numerous studies have demonstrated that a variety of acute laboratory stressors lead to increases in catecholamine and cortisol production (e.g., Baum et al., 1993; Dimsdale & Moss, 1980; Frankenhaeuser, 1975; Mason, 1975). However, there are clear individual differences in the magnitude of endocrine responses during acute stress (e.g., Cacioppo, 1994; Manuck et al., 1991). For example, there is evidence that gender (see Stoney et al., 1987), social support (Hellhammer et al., 1997; see also Seeman & McEwen, 1996; Uchino et al., 1996), and the interaction of gender and social processes (Kirschbaum et al., 1995) moderate endocrine aspects of the acute stress response. It has also been hypothesized that catecholamine response may be closely related to the effort required to cope with a stressor, whereas cortisol is more closely related to stressor-related dimensions such as distress or controllability (e.g., Lundberg & Frankenhaeuser, 1980; Peters et al., 1998; Pollard et al., 1996).

Like acute stress, chronic stress has also been reliably associated with increases in catecholamines and cortisol. For example, following a minor (the radiation was contained) but stressful accident at a US nuclear reactor, urinary catecholamine and cortisol levels were elevated among residents living near the reactor, relative to several control groups, for 15–58 months (see Baum et al., 1993). Interestingly, in cases of more extreme chronic stress, as in Post-traumatic Stress Disorder (PTSD), the HPA axis may become increasingly sensitive to negative feedback. This may explain why cortisol appears to be low among those with chronic PTSD (for a review, see Yehuda, 1998). Mason and his colleagues (1990) have further suggested that low cortisol may be specifically related to symptoms of emotional numbing. We (Hawk et al., 2000) recently found preliminary support for this hypothesis. Among persons who had been in motor vehicle accidents approximately six months earlier, greater numbing symptoms predicted lower 15-hour urinary cortisol excretion.

Changes in "stress hormones" are not always stress-related. Laboratory inductions of mood (sadness and elation) can increase cortisol (Brown et al., 1993; see also Futterman et al., 1994), and simple changes in posture may markedly alter circulating catecholamines. Exercise, diet, and other phenomena also affect these hormone levels. Thus, there are usually several possible interpretations of an endocrine difference among conditions or groups of people. Adequate interpretation of such differences requires careful consideration of measures of the hypothesized construct (from other response domains) as well as of alternative constructs.

In many cases, endocrine measures of processes such as stress are most useful when they are consistent with other measures. This convergence of measures increases confidence that one is tapping into an integrated, coherent process. However, divergence of responses may also be of interest. Inevitably, there are occasions when physiological data fail to converge with self-report or behavioral observation. Like most physiological systems, components of the endocrine system are multiply determined. For example, much of the variability in cortisol is not determined by psychological variables, but rather by processes such as infradian and circadian rhythms and genetic predispositions. Moreover, the primary "responsibility" of the endocrine system is to help maintain bodily systems within homeostatic limits. Psychoendocrine relationships may be evident only within certain portions of the range of possible endocrine values. Self-report and behavioral indices are likewise multiply determined and offer imperfect measures of any given construct. For these reasons, the correlations between physiological and self-report measures are generally low (see Öhman, 1987, for a cogent discussion of the limits on psychophysiological relations).

At first glance, this may seem discouraging. However, some of the most intriguing findings are situations in which changes occur in one response domain but not in another, or when changes occur but are in opposite directions. Although this may sometimes simply temper our conclusions about a given construct, divergence between response systems may indicate something more conceptually interesting. A good illustration of this is repressive coping, a tendency to avoid threat-related information and report minimal distress in situations that are typically viewed as distressing. Research on repressive coping has suggested a dissociation between verbal and psychophysiological reactivity, with repressive copers reporting minimal distress but exhibiting exaggerated physiological reactivity to laboratory stressors (e.g., Newton & Contrada, 1992; Weinberger et al., 1979). More recently, Brown and colleagues (1996) found higher resting salivary cortisol among repressive copers relative to participants low in self-reported anxiety and defensiveness. Important differences in how stimuli are experienced and how people respond to them can confound results or offer important new findings. They are best detected and studied with multi-system assessments of relevant constructs.

## MEDIATOR OF A BIOPSYCHOLOGICAL PROCESS

A related rationale for obtaining measures of endocrine function is to enable tests of mediational hypotheses. A mediator is a "generative mechanism through which the focal independent variable is able to influence the dependent variable of interest" (Baron & Kenny, 1986, p. 1173). The endocrine system is a potent mediator of the effects of psychological processes such as emotion, stress, depression, and repressive coping on physical health. According to the logic of mediational tests, it is necessary to demonstrate that: (1) psychological processes affect endocrine function; (2) endocrine function affects health-related variables; and (3) the effects of psychological processes on health are reduced or eliminated when the effects of the relevant endocrine parameters are removed. Despite the difficulties in testing such comprehensive models, evidence examining the mediational role of endocrine components of biobehavioral processes is steadily accumulating.

For example, both the HPA and SAM axes are important mediators of psychological influences on the immune system (e.g., Cohen & Herbert, 1996; Lovallo, 1997). First, cortisol assists in limiting immune responses; animal models of the inflammatory disease rheumatoid arthritis have demonstrated that normal HPA axis response to homeostatic and stress-related demands is instrumental in resistance to the disease (Sternberg et al., 1989). In humans, the evidence for immune regulation by cortisol is not as consistent. However, the association between depression and HPA axis hyperactivity (see Nemeroff, 1989) has led to the hypothesis that neuroendocrine activity mediates the relationships between depression and immunity (see Herbert & Cohen, 1993). Second, studies of acute laboratory stress in humans have demonstrated that stress-related immune changes are paralleled by increases in both cortisol and the adrenal catecholamines (e.g., Gerritsen et al., 1996; Sgoutas-Emch et al., 1994). Stronger evidence of sympathoadrenal mediation of acute stress-induced immune effects comes from a recent blockade study (Bachen et al., 1995): administration of the nonselective $\beta$-adrenoreceptor antagonist labetalol eliminated stress-related increases in natural killer cell number and decreases in blastogenic responses to two mitogens.

More preliminary evidence supports other mediational hypotheses. For example, the relationship between poor social support and increased mortality may be partially mediated by the inverse relationship between social support and catecholamine levels (see Uchino et al., 1996). Similarly, hostility is associated with increased risk of coronary heart disease, and perhaps even more strongly with all-cause mortality (see the meta-analytic review of Miller et al., 1996). Evidence that highly hostile individuals show exaggerated cardiovascular, norepinephrine, and cortisol responses to laboratory stress and concommitant harrassment by the experimenter (Suarez et al., 1998; see also Suls & Wan, 1993) is consistent with the hypothesis that increased autonomic and endocrine reactivity mediates the hostility-mortality relationship. However, firm conclusions await further work that directly tests these mediational hypotheses.

## "OBJECTIVE" INDICATOR OF A BIOPSYCHOLOGICAL PROCESS

For many, the allure of endocrine measures is in the objective nature of physiological assessment. It is as though the ability to assign scientific units, such as $\mu g/dL$, confers a higher status to such measures and reifies them as "true" indicators. Nothing could be further from the truth. Although it is the case that many biological measures are not as readily "faked" or biased as are self-report measures, endocrine measures cannot always be interpreted as reflecting any one construct. As mentioned earlier, hormonal indices are constrained in the degree to which they can vary with psychological processes. To make matters worse, there are many other variables (e.g., drug use, exercise, diet) that affect endocrine measures. Finally, assays used to quantify hormonal data are not without variability (reported as inter- and intra-assay coefficients of variation), though this is sometimes overlooked. As a result of all of these factors, it is unlikely that any one-to-one, invariant relationship exists between a single endocrine parameter and a specific psychological state or process (see Cacioppo & Tassinary, 1990). Endocrine measures may be quantifiable on a more objective scale, but that does not necessarily translate into a better or more objective measures of a particular process.

## Which hormone(s) should be measured?

Decisions about which endocrine parameter(s) to measure should reflect the purpose of the study and the rationale for including hormonal indices. This is most straightforward when considering endocrine measures as direct indicators of physiological processes. In this case, the process of interest largely determines the measures one might choose. The task is somewhat more complicated when considering multi-system assessment of biopsychological constructs such as stress. Similarly, mediational hypotheses, such as stress-endocrine-immune or stress-endocrine-health relationships, require careful consideration. Although cortisol, epinephrine, and norepinephrine are the most widely used endocrine measures of stress and related constructs, a growing number of alternative or additional hormones may be of interest (see, e.g., Mason, 1975; Weiner, 1992). Moreover, frequently overlooked theoretical and empirical considerations (see Vingerhoets & Assies, 1991) may lead to the selection of one measure over another.

Consider a typical finding: a stressor lasting only a few minutes is found to increase natural killer cell activity for the duration of the stressor (e.g., Bachen et al., 1995; Sgoutas-Emch et al., 1994). If one is interested in potential endocrine mediators of this effect, which hormones might be assessed? As noted above, both catecholamines and cortisol may mediate stress-immune relationships. However, in this example epinephrine would be a much better choice than cortisol. The reason is that cortisol responses, which take some time to be detectable and do not characterize immediate response, could not account for immune changes occurring more immediately after the introduction of the stressor.

It is also important to note that the best endocrine-related measure for a particular area may not be a hormone at all. Receptor number and function are equally important, but much less studied, aspects of endocrine processes. For example, stress may influence the immune system by altering $\beta$-adrenoreceptors on lymphocytes (e.g., Redwine et al., 1996). In addition, psychobiological models that are based on alterations in feedback mechanisms such as down-regulation or seques-tering of receptors may be more clearly tested by examining receptor activity. Unfortunately, discussion of receptor function and assessment is beyond the scope of this chapter. However, interested readers may wish to consider a number of comprehensive resources (e.g., Wilson & Foster, 1992), or focused reviews of the adrenergic/noradrenergic systems (e.g., Cameron, 1994; Mills & Dimsdale, 1988; 1993). Furthermore, indirect indicators of endocrine function may also be of interest. For example, glycosylated hemoglobin (HbA$_1$), not insulin, is often used as an index of long-term glucose control in diabetes (Karam, 1997).

# How should the measures be collected?

Because hormones are by definition blood-borne, plasma measures are obvious choices for examining endocrine function. Assessment of free hormone and/or hormone metabolites in urine is a frequently used alternative. There is also a growing literature on salivary cortisol, and recent evidence suggests that catecholamine levels may be determined from blood platelets. Each of these methods has relative advantages and disadvantages.

## BLOOD
Plasma sampling by venipuncture is frequently used to provide an index of acute catecholamine and cortisol levels. However, the cate-cholamines and cortisol differ in response latency. Plasma cate-cholamines increase immediately upon presentation of a relevant stimulus, while changes in plasma cortisol are not evident for at least several minutes. (Other hormones, such as thyroid hormone, achieve maximal response only after several days [Sherwood, 1997]). There are also differences in the duration of catecholamine and cortisol

responses. Both epinephrine and norepinephrine are largely unbound in plasma, making them accessible to enzymes that degrade them. Consequently, they have a short half-life (1–3 minutes; Berne & Levy, 1983). The same is true for the broad class of peptide hormones. However, cortisol and other cholesterol-derived steroid hormones (including progesterone, the estrogens, and testosterone) are more heavily bound to plasma proteins, with less rapid degradation and a correspondingly longer half-life (about 70 minutes for cortisol).

Thus, plasma measures of catecholamines and cortisol taken at the same point in time will reflect somewhat different processes. For example, the venipuncture itself may have a strong influence on catecholamine levels almost immediately, whereas this effect would not be evident right away in cortisol. By the time plasma cortisol changes are observed, there would be little or no residual impact on epinephrine or norepinephrine. This complicates the collection of "baseline" values. A blood draw immediately after catheter insertion is satisfactory for cortisol, but a resting period should precede the initial collection of epinephrine and norepinephrine. Thus, correct interpretation rests on an appreciation of the onset and offset properties of the relevant axis or axes.

Blood samples should be drawn directly into heparinized or EDTA-treated tubes, spun, and frozen at $-70°C$ without preservative as quickly as possible. (Some measures and assays may require the use of untreated or specialized collection vessels or preservatives.) Completing this process in a timely fashion reduces hormone loss due to oxidative and degradation processes.

## URINE

The relatively short half-lives of plasma catecholamines and cortisol, which make them useful for studying acute reactivity, render plasma measures less sensitive or useful for measuring more chronic processes. An alternative is to examine the levels of free hormone or hormone metabolites that are excreted in urine. A small but consistent fraction of hormone is excreted without being metabolized. By collecting urine over a prolonged period (typically 24 hours), an average estimate of activity in the endocrine axis of interest can be obtained. Multiple samples may be especially useful in studying ambient or chronic stress. Even in the case of intermittent processes (e.g., intrusive thoughts, daily hassles, anger episodes), urinary assessment may be advantageous. Although the effects of such processes are "diluted" in urine by periods of relative inactivity or benign mood, they may be missed completely by sampling procedures that are sensitive to only acute changes.

Conversely, urinary measures are not particularly useful for examining acute endocrine responsivity. The double-void technique was developed to enhance the sensitivity of urinary measures to relatively short-term changes. Using this procedure, a participant is asked to provide a urine sample before beginning a laboratory procedure and again at the end of the experiment. However, a number of conceptual and practical difficulties (e.g., poor temporal resolution for this technique and the fact that participants cannot always urinate on cue) are associated with this approach (see Grunberg & Singer, 1990).

There are two practical problems with traditional urine sampling. First, adherence to 24-hour urine collection may be problematic. As an alternative, investigators may wish to use an overnight sample (e.g., 6 p.m. to 9 a.m.). In addition to increasing adherence by avoiding collection during the work day, this procedure may also minimize differences in activity level, which may markedly influence catecholamine levels. Second, as in plasma samples, urinary catecholamines and cortisol are broken down if left at room temperature. Therefore, participants should be instructed to keep the sample refrigerated (a small cooler filled with ice is easily transported). Because participants may not always immediately refrigerate the sample, investigators may consider using a preservative. The antioxidant sodium metabisulfite appears to be particularly useful. It is easy to use (add 1 g to the collection bucket), noncaustic, and allows minimal oxidative loss in samples unrefrigerated for 24 hours. Upon receipt of the urine specimen, it should be stirred prior to aliquoting a smaller (e.g., 10 mL) sample, which should then be frozen at $-20°$ C for later analysis. Total urine volume should also be recorded.

SALIVA

There are times when acute reactivity is of interest but plasma sampling is contraindicated. A common logistic problem is the lack of an experienced phlebotomist. Alternatively, the study protocol may make it impossible to have a phlebotomist available (e.g., sampling just before bed or upon awakening in the morning). In addition, the aversive nature of blood draws may result in refusals to participate. Even among participants, the pain of venipuncture and discomfort of prolonged catheterization may affect the outcomes of interest (e.g., response to laboratory stressors or relaxation training) or present ethical concerns, particularly in some populations (e.g., young children). Fortunately, an alternative has been developed to allow the assessment of cortisol (and other steroid hormones) from saliva.

Early concerns that salivary cortisol does not parallel plasma cortisol values appear to have been unfounded. Although absolute levels of free cortisol in saliva are as much as 50% lower than in blood, salivary and plasma measures appear strongly related across individuals and time (for reviews, see Kirschbaum & Hellhammer, 1989, 1994).

Beyond reductions in logistic and ethical concerns with plasma sampling noted above, there are additional advantages of salivary cortisol measures. Salivary cortisol is less expensive and significantly easier to collect than is plasma cortisol. A simple plastic tube or container can be used to collect saliva samples at frequent intervals. Because some participants may find this unpleasant (possibly influencing cortisol levels and decreasing adherence), many studies ask participants to chew on a swab or roll of cotton for 30–60 seconds. Another advantage of salivary cortisol is its shelf-life. Saliva may be stored at room temperature for two weeks without significant cortisol degradation, and perhaps as long as 16 weeks when treated with citric acid (Kirschbaum & Hellhammer, 1994).

Interestingly, salivary cortisol may also be a reasonable alternative to urinary cortisol. Participants may be instructed to provide many samples per day (e.g., Smyth et al., 1997). Alternatively, the Oral Diffusion Sink (ODS; Wade & Haegele, 1991), a multi-cell device that fits inside the mouth without significant discomfort, may be used to measure salivary cortisol over periods of up to 8 hours. Although salivary cortisol using the ODS in two four-hour blocks was found to correspond well to urinary free cortisol in one study (Shipley et al., 1992), these results were not replicated in a similar paradigm (Kathol et al., 1995). Thus, it is not yet clear whether the ODS is a useful option for studying more chronic processes.

More generally, salivary cortisol is not without drawbacks. At present, many assays for salivary cortisol are developed "in house." Even minor differences in the assays make it difficult to compare across laboratories. This problem is made worse by the lack of reference standards for salivary cortisol (Kirschbaum & Hellhammer, 1989). Until these problems are addressed, plasma and urine are likely to continue to be the measures of choice in many situations.

## PLATELETS

Another alternative for measurement of catecholamines is to examine concentrations of epinephrine and norepinephrine in blood platelets, disk-shaped cells that circulate in the blood stream for 8–12 days before dying and being replaced by new platelets. Importantly for our purposes, platelets share some properties of sympathetic nerves, absorbing and transporting amino acids and accumulating catecholamines in the process (e.g., Zieve & Solomon, 1967). Accumulation of hormone in platelets can be measured and attributed to levels of plasma catecholamines over the life span of the individual platelet, suggesting that they reflect a week or more of sympathetic activity. Platelets cannot produce epinephrine, nor-epinephrine, or dopamine, so concentrations of these hormones in platelets must derive from circulating blood.

Platelets store catecholamines in dense granules located throughout the cell. Uptake can take place by passive diffusion of hormones through a series of openings in the platelet surface. Active transport may also occur across the cell membrane near adrenergic receptors on the surface of platelets (Born & Smith, 1970).

Because platelets live 8–12 days in circulation and are continuously accumulating catecholamines over this period, it is reasonable to assume that platelet concentrations of catecholamines will reflect plasma levels averaged over a week or more. This suggests that platelet catecholamine levels will reflect "ambient" or chronic situations and should provide stable estimates of long-term arousal of the SNS. However, several sources of bias exist. For example, variations in production of new platelets, or any events that might skew distributions of platelets towards very young or very old cells, could affect these measures.

In summary, investigators have a range of options for endocrine assessment. Indeed, beyond the samples discussed in depth, researchers may be interested in assaying tears (Frey, 1985), cerebrospinal fluid (e.g., Baker et al., 1997; Mulcahey et al., 2001), or other sources. The choice depends on a number of conceptual, ethical, and practical issues. Is the construct of interest transient, long-standing, or intermittent? Will the data likely be affected more by time requirements or the invasiveness of the procedure? Are within- or between-subjects comparisons of greatest interest? Are specially trained personnel available for drawing blood? Careful consideration of these and related questions will provide the information needed to make the most appropriate choice.

## Assessment of control variables

Given the integral role of the endocrine system in many bodily functions, it is not surprising that many factors affect hormonal measures.

Clearly, assessment of such factors is necessary to interpret endocrine data. A number of demographic variables, medications and other drugs, and health behaviors have been reliably associated with endocrine function. In fact, full coverage of these relationships goes well beyond the scope of this chapter. The examples provided below are selective.

*Demographic variables.* Gender is strongly related to many aspects of endocrine function. In addition to obvious differences in reproductive hormones, there are other notable gender differences. For example, men exhibit larger epinephrine responses to acute behavioral stress (see the meta-analysis by Stoney et al., 1987). Although some have suggested that both endogenous and exogenous estrogens reduce psychobiological reactivity, including endocrine reactivity, to stress (Sita & Miller, 1996), there are also failures to replicate such effects (Litschauer et al., 1998). Relatedly, even among women, endocrine function will vary with reproductive status. Age also influences endocrine function (see e.g., Sapolsky et al., 1986), and individual differences in catecholamines and cortisol among older adults may be important predictors of cognitive and physical function (McEwen, 1998).

*Drugs.* Many drugs are designed specifically to alter hormone levels or responsivity to hormones. Prominent examples include beta-blockers for hypertension, thyroid replacement supplements for hypothyroidism, and oral contraceptives and hormone replacement therapy. Many psychotropic drugs may also influence endocrine function (see, e.g., Guthrie, 1994, for a review of psychotropic medications effects on norepinephrine). More common drugs such as caffeine, nicotine, and alcohol, as well as many illicit drugs, can exert marked effects. For example, nicotine strongly increases HPA axis activity, and perhaps that of other hypothalamic-pituitary axes (see Matta et al., 1998, for a review). Even consumption of tyrosine-containing foods (i.e., most foods containing proteins) influences catecholamine production. Given the great number of possible confounds, investigators would be wise to use a combination of instructions regarding diet and medications and self-report and biochemical verification of drug use during the study period.

*Other aspects of health behavior and status.* As mentioned above, activity level markedly affects catecholamines. Investigators may wish to have participants self-monitor their activities or use more objective activity monitors (e.g., Actigraph, Ambulatory Monitoring, Inc., Ardsley, NY). Behavioral medicine researchers should also be aware that a number of psychological disorders are associated with alterations in endocrine function. Prominent examples, as noted above, include increased cortisol in depression and low basal cortisol in PTSD.

This portion of the review has been necessarily brief. It should be clear that there are numerous variables that may impact on any given endocrine parameter. Of course, only a few of them may be important for any given study. Investigators are urged to control, or at least measure, the subset that is most relevant to their particular research area.

# How should the measures be assayed, analyzed, and interpreted?

## ASSAYS

One of the great advances in psychoendocrine research has been the development of reliable and valid assays. At present, there are acceptable assays for virtually any endocrine parameter. Radioimmunoassay (RIA) is the measurement technique of choice for a variety of hormones, including cortisol. Radioenzymatic assay (REA) and high-performance liquid chromatography (HPLC) are techniques commonly employed for assessing catecholamines. All of these assays are relatively sensitive and specific, typically with intra- and inter-assay coefficients of variation less than 10%. Each of these procedures will be briefly described. Grunberg and Singer (1990) provide an excellent, more thorough overview and comparison of these procedures.

RIA, a general technique developed in the 1950s and 1960s (e.g., Yalow & Berson, 1959), has become the standard for assaying many physiological parameters, including cortisol levels in plasma, urine, and saliva (e.g., Walker et al., 1978). The target chemicals, such as cortisol, are combined with substances (antisera) that recognize the targets and bind to them. Radioisotopes are used to either label the target chemicals (single-antibody RIA) or to compete for binding with the target chemicals before quantification (competitive-binding RIA). Values are plotted against those obtained from standard concentrations of the target chemical to determine the amount of target present in the study sample.

REA, as the name implies, makes use of enzymes and radioactive labels. In the case of catecholamines, the enzyme catechol-O-methyltransferase (COMT) is combined with the catecholamine-containing fluid (see Durrett & Zeigler, 1980). As the catecholamines are metabolized, the primary metabolite of each catecholamine is radioactively tagged with a label donated by a compound (tritiated S-adenosylmethionine; SAM) added to the solution. After incubation, unbound radioactive molecules are rinsed away, leaving only radioactively tagged catecholamines. Following techniques to separate the catecholamines (epinephrine, norepinephrine, and dopamine), the concentration of each catecholamine can be determined by measuring the amount of radioactivity emitted from the sample and comparison with standard concentrations.

HPLC, unlike the techniques discussed so far, does not require radioactive isotopes. Instead, the fluid sample is exposed to extremely high pressure. Physical properties, such as molecular weight, or chemical properties, such as ionic or bonding characteristics, are used to separate different molecules within the sample. However, HPLC systems are expensive and require a highly-trained technician.

ANALYSES

As with any variable, endocrine data should be carefully screened prior to analysis. Because outliers may exert considerable statistical weight, screening for values more than 3 standard deviations from the mean may be useful. Depending upon the nature of the study, one may also wish to consider how the data compare to normal values (e.g., Stedman, 1995; Wilson & Foster, 1992). However, the "normal range" is often very broad, and somewhat different ranges are provided in different sources.

For urinary measures, urine volume and make-up should also be considered. For example, low volumes (< 250 mL in a 24-hour sample; Stedman, 1995) may indicate incomplete data collection. On the other hand, volumes in the normal range are not necessarily acceptable. Some nonadherent participants may add water to the sample to increase the appearance of compliance! Therefore, investigators may wish to examine creatinine levels in urine. In addition, creatinine in plasma or urine may be useful as a general indicator of kidney function.

Screened data may be converted to a number of formats. The most common metric for plasma and salivary measures is concentration per unit volume. Though estimates of total plasma hormone may be made from such measurements, total blood volume will not be precisely known. Rates of secretion into plasma are typically not provided due to the difficulty associated with drawing enough blood to provide a reliable estimate. Urinary hormones are not subject to these problems, allowing a broader range of possibilities. Total daily production can be easily estimated from a 24-hour sample. Consider an example in which norepinephrine concentration is 50 ng/mL and 24-hour urine output is 600 mL. Total daily production of norepinephrine would be estimated to be 50 ng/mL × 600 mL = 30,000 ng. In addition, an hourly rate of excretion can be computed: 30,000 ng ÷ 24 hours = 1250 ng/hr. If the total amount of norepinephrine had been obtained with a 15-hour sample, hourly excretion remains a straightforward computation (30,000 ng ÷ 15 hours = 2000 ng/hr). However, because rates of catecholamine release vary over the course of the day, rates of excretion based on different collection periods will not be comparable. Similarly, estimates of total daily production of hormone from 15-hour samples would be biased and are not recommended.

As noted above, a range of factors may influence endocrine indices. It is common to consider using one or more variables, such as age and nicotine intake, as covariates in the analysis of hormonal data. However, it is important to remember that no variable will reliably be related to a given endocrine measure in every circumstance. Investigators should first determine whether a potential covariate actually accounts for variance in a given hormone. Even when it does, the potential costs and benefits of including one or more covariates should be carefully weighed, and the smallest possible number of covariates should be used (e.g., Tabachnick & Fidell, 1997).

### INTERPRETATION

It has been repeatedly emphasized that interpretation of hormonal indices in biobehavioral research is complex. This is true in all psychophysiological research (e.g., Cacioppo & Tassinary, 1990). Consider an example. Frankenhaeuser and others have found support for the hypothesis that cortisol increases during distress and epinephrine increases during effort (e.g., Lundberg & Frankenhaeuser, 1980; Peters et al., 1998; Pollard et al., 1996). In a hypothetical study, researchers find that being informed of a cancer diagnosis leads to acute epinephrine increases among one subset of participants but cortisol increases among another subset. How strongly would this support a hypothesis regarding differences in coping styles? The answer to that question depends on a cogent discussion of other potential causes of epinephrine and cortisol increases, as well as data from other domains (overt behavior and self-report).

## Conclusion

Following the seminal work of Cannon and Selye, great strides have been made in our understanding of the role of the endocrine system in behavioral medicine. New techniques have made hormonal measures much less costly and more available. Advances in theory and empirical research have demonstrated the utility of including endocrine measures in behavioral medicine studies. In addition to serving as mediators of relationships between psychological processes and health outcomes, hormonal indices are an integral part of the assessment of biopsychological constructs such as stress. The question of whether to include such measures in research is increasingly replaced with questions regarding the most appropriate choices of measures, assays, and analyses. This chapter was designed to facilitate answering these questions.

# References

Abraham, C.S., & Hampson, S.E. (1996). The interpretation of verbal reports in health psychology; Editors' introduction. *Psychology & Health, 11*, 179–182.

Bachen, E.A., Manuck, S.B., Cohen, S., Muldoon, M.F., Raible, R., Herbert, T.B., & Rabin B.S. (1995). Adrenergic blockade ameliorates cellular immune responses to mental stress in humans. *Psychosomatic Medicine, 57*, 366–372.

Baker, D.G., West, S.A., Orth, D.N., Hill, K.K., Nicholson, W.E., Ekhator, N.N., Bruce, A.B., Wortman, M.D., Keck, P.E. Jr, Geracioti, T.D. Jr. (1997). Cerebrospinal fluid and plasma beta-endorphin in combat veterans with post-traumatic stress disorder. *Psychoneuroendocrinology, 22*, 517–529.

Bakris, G., Bursztyn, M., Gavras, I., Bresnahan, M., & Gavras, H. (1997). Role of vasopressin in essential hypertension: Racial differences. *Journal of Hypertension, 15*, 545–550.

Baron, R.M., & Kenny, D.A. (1986). The moderator-mediator variable distinction in social psychological research: Conceptual, strategic, and statistical considerations. *Journal of Personality and Social Psychology, 51*, 1173–1182.

Baum, A., Cohen, L., & Hall, M. (1993). Control and intrusive memories as possible determinants of chronic stress. *Psychosomatic Medicine, 55*, 274–286.

Berecek, K.H., & Swords, B.H. (1990). Central role for vasopressin in cardiovascular regulation and the pathogenesis of hypertension. *Hypertension, 16*, 213–224.

Berne, R.M., & Levy, M.N. (1983). *Physiology*. St. Louis: Mosby.

Born, G.V., & Smith, J.B. (1970). Uptake, metabolism and release of (3H)-adrenaline by human platelets. *British Journal of Pharmacology, 39*, 765–778.

Brown, L.L., Tomarken, A.J., Orth, D.N., Loosen, P.T., Kalin, N.H., & Davidson, R.J. (1996). Individual differences in repressive-defensiveness predict basal salivary cortisol levels. *Journal of Personality and Social Psychology, 70,* 362–371.

Brown, W.A., Sirota, A.D., Niaura, R., & Engebretson, T.O. (1993). Endocrine correlates of sadness and elation. *Psychosomatic Medicine, 55,* 458–467.

Cacioppo, J.T. (1994). Social neuroscience: Autonomic, neuroendocrine, and immune responses to stress. *Psychophysiology, 31,* 113–128.

Cacioppo, J.T., & Tassinary, L.G. (1990). Psychophysiology and psychophysiological inference. In: J.T. Cacioppo & L.G. Tassinary (Eds.), *Principles of psychophysiology: Physical, social, and inferential elements* (pp. 3–33). New York: Cambridge University Press.

Cameron, O.G. (Ed.) (1994). *Adrenergic dysfunction and psychobiology.* Washington, DC: American Psychiatric Association.

Cannon, W.B. (1914). The emergency function of the adrenal medulla in pain and the major emotions. *American Journal of Physiology, 33,* 356–372.

Cohen, S., & Herbert, T.B. (1996). Health psychology: Psychological factors and physical disease from the perspective of human psychoneuroimmunology. *Annual Review of Psychology, 47,* 113–142.

Dimsdale, J.E., & Moss, J. (1980). Short-term catecholamine response to psychological stress. *Psychosomatic Medicine, 42,* 493–497.

Durrett, L., & Zeigler, M. (1980). A sensitive radioenzymatic assay for catechol drugs. *Journal of Neuroscience Research, 5,* 587–598.

Frankenhaeuser, M. (1975). Sympathetic-adrenomedullary activity, behavior, and the psychosocial environment. In: P.H. Venables & M.J. Christie (Eds.), *Research in psychophysiology.* New York: Wiley.

Frey, W.H. (1985). *Crying: The mystery of tears.* Minneapolis, MN: Winston Press.

Futterman, A.D., Kemeny, M.E., Shapiro, D., & Fahey, J.L. (1994). Immunological and physiological changes associated with induced positive and negative mood. *Psychosomatic Medicine, 56,* 499–511.

Gerritsen, W., Heijnen, C.J., Wiegant, V.M., Bermond, B., & Frijda, N.H. (1996). Experimental social fear: Immunological, hormonal, and autonomic concomitants. *Psychosomatic Medicine, 58,* 273–286.

Grunberg, N.E., & Singer, J.E. (1990). Biochemical measurement. In: J.T. Cacioppo & L.G. Tassinary (Eds.), *Principles of psychophysiology: Physical, social, and inferential elements* (pp. 149–176). New York: Cambridge University Press.

Guthrie, S.K. (1994). Adrenergic effects of psychotropic drugs. In: O.G. Cameron (Ed.), *Adrenergic dysfunction and psychobiology* (pp. 89–130). Washington, DC: American Psychiatric Association.

Hawk, L.W. Jr., Liegey-Dougall, A., Ursano, R.J., & Baum, A. (2000). Urinary catecholamines and cortisol in recent-onset posttraumatic stress disorder following motor vehicle accidents. *Psychosomatic Medicine, 62,* 425–434.

Hellhammer, D.H., Buchtal, J., Gutberlet, I., & Kirschbaum, C. (1997). Social hierarchy and adrenocortical stress reactivity in men. *Psychoneuroendocrinology, 22*, 643–650.

Henderson, I.C. (1995). Breast cancer. In: G.P. Murphy, W. Lawrence, Jr., & R.E. Lenhard, Jr. (Eds.), *American Cancer Society textbook of clinical oncology* (2nd ed.) (pp. 198–219). Atlanta, GA: American Cancer Society.

Herbert, T.B., & Cohen, S. (1993). Depression and immunity: A meta-analytic review. *Psychological Bulletin, 113*, 472–486.

Karam, J.H. (1997). Diabetes mellitus and hypoglycemia. In: L.M. Tierney Jr., S.J. McPhee, & M.A. Papadakis (Eds.), *Current medical diagnosis and treatment* (36th ed.) (pp. 1069–1109). Stamford, CT: Appleton & Lange.

Kathol, R.G., Poland, R.E., Stokes, P.E., & Wade, S. (1995). Relationship of 24-hour urinary free cortisol to 4-hour salivary morning and afternoon cortisol and cortisone as measured by a time-integrated oral diffusion sink. *Journal of Endocrinological Investigation, 18*, 374–377.

Kirschbaum, C., & Hellhammer, D.H. (1989). Salivary cortisol in psychobiological research: An overview. *Neuropsychobiology, 22*, 150–169.

Kirschbaum, C., & Hellhammer, D.H. (1994). Salivary cortisol in psychoneuroendocrine research: Recent developments and applications. *Psychoneuroendocrinology, 19*, 313–333.

Kirschbaum, C., Klauer, T., Filipp, S.H., & Hellhammer, D.H. (1995). Sex-specific effects of social support on cortisol and subjective responses to acute psychological stress. *Psychosomatic Medicine, 57*, 23–31.

Lang, P.J. (1968). Fear reduction and fear behavior: Problems in treating a construct. In: J.M. Shlien (Ed.), *Research in psychotherapy: Volume 3* (pp. 90–102). Washington, DC: American Psychological Association.

Light, K.C., Smith, T.E., Johns, J.M., Brownley, K.A., Hofheimer, J.A., & Amico, J.A. (2000). Oxytocin responsivity in mothers of infants: A preliminary study of relationships with blood pressure during laboratory stress and normal ambulatory activity. *Health Psychology, 19*, 560–567.

Litschauer, B., Zauchner, S., Huemer, K.H., & Kaka-Lützow, A. (1998). Cardiovascular, endocrine, and receptor measures as related to sex and the menstrual cycle phase. *Psychosomatic Medicine, 60*, 219–226.

Lovallo, W.R. (1997). *Stress & health: Biological and psychological interactions*. Thousand Oaks, CA: Sage Publications.

Lundberg, U., & Frankenhaeuser, M. (1980). Pituitary-adrenal and sympathetic-adrenal correlates of distress and effort. *Journal of Psychosomatic Research, 24*, 455–476.

Manuck, S.B., Cohen, S.C., Rabin, B.S., Muldoon, M.F., & Bachen, E.A. (1991). Individual differences in cellular immune response to stress. *Psychological Science, 2*, 111–115.

Markovitz, J.H., & Matthews, K.A. (1991). Platelets and coronary heart disease: Potential psychophysiologic mechanisms. *Psychosomatic Medicine, 53*, 643–668.

Mason, J.W. (1975). Emotion as reflected in patterns of endocrine integration. In: L. Levi (Ed.), *Emotions: Their parameters and measurement* (pp. 143–182). New York: Raven Press.

Mason, J.W., Kosten, T.R., Southwick, S.M., & Giller, E.L. (1990). The use of psychoendocrine strategies in post-traumatic stress disorder. *Journal of Applied Social Psychology, 20,* 1822–1846.

Matta, S.G., Fu, Y., Valentine, J.D., & Sharp, B.M. (1998). Response of the hypothalamo-pituitary-adrenal axis to nicotine. *Psychoneuroendocrinology, 23,* 103–113.

Matthews, K.A., Caggiula, A.R., McAllister, C.G., Berga, S.L., Owens, J.F., Flory, J.D., & Miller, A.L. (1995). Sympathetic reactivity to acute stress and immune response in women. *Psychosomatic Medicine, 57,* 564–571.

McCruden, A.B., & Stimson,W.H. (1991). Sex hormones and immune function. In: R. Ader, D.L. Felten, & N. Cohen (Eds.), *Psychoneuroimmunology* (2nd ed., pp. 475–493). San Diego, CA: Academic Press.

McEwen, B.S. (1998). Seminars in medicine of the Beth Israel Deaconess Medical Center: Protective and damaging effects of stress mediators. *The New England Journal of Medicine, 338,* 171–179.

Miller, T.Q., Smith, T.W., Turner, C.W., Guijarro, M.L., & Hallet, A.J. (1996). A meta-analytic review of research on hostility and physical health. *Psychological Bulletin, 119,* 322–348.

Mills, P.J., & Dimsdale, J.E. (1988). The promise of receptor studies in psychophysiologic research. *Psychosomatic Medicine, 50,* 555–566.

Mills, P.J., & Dimsdale, J.E. (1993). The promise of adrenergic receptor studies in psychophysiologic research II: Applications, limitations, and progress. *Psychosomatic Medicine, 55,* 448–457.

Mulchahey, J.J., Ekhator, N.N., Zhang, H., Kaschkow, J.W., Baker, D.G., & Geracioti, T.D., Jr. (2001). Cerebrospinal fluid and plasma testosterone levels in post-traumatic stress disorder and tobacco dependence. *Psychoneuroendocrinology, 26,* 273–285.

Nemeroff, C.B. (1989). Clinical significance of psychoneuroendocrinology in psychiatry: Focus on the thyroid and adrenal. *Journal of Clinical Psychiatry, 50,* 13–20.

Newton, T.L., & Contrada, R.J. (1992). Repressive coping and verbal-autonomic response dissociation: The influence of social context. *Journal of Personality and Social Psychology, 62,* 159–167.

Nisbett, R.E., & Wilson, T.D. (1977). Telling more than we can know: Verbal reports on mental processes. *Psychological Review, 84,* 231–259.

Öhman, A. (1987). The psychophysiology of emotion: An evolutionary-cognitive perspective. In: P.K. Ackles, J.R. Jennings, & M.G.H. Coles (Eds.), *Advances in psychophysiology* (Vol. 2, pp. 79–127). New Greenwich, CT: JAI Press.

Peters, M.L., Godaert, G.L.R., Ballieux, R.E., van Vliet, M., Willemsen, J.J., Sweep, F.C.G.J., & Heijnen, C.J. (1998). Cardiovascular and endocrine responses to experimental stress: Effects of mental effort and controllability. *Psychoneuroendocrinology, 23*, 1–17.

Pollard, T.M., Ungpakorn, G., Harrison, G.A., & Parkes, K.R. (1996). Epinephrine and cortisol responses to work: A test of the models of Frankenhaeuser and Karasek. *Annals of Behavioral Medicine, 18*, 229–237.

Pomerleau, C.S., Pomerleau, O.F., & Garcia, A.W. (1991). Biobehavioral research on nicotine use in women. *British Journal of Addiction, 86*, 527–531.

Purba, J.S., Hoogendijk, W.J.G., Hofman, M.A., & Swaab, D.F. (1996). Increased number of vasopressin- and oxytocin-expressing neurons in the paraventricular nucleus of the hypothalamus in depression. *Archives of General Psychiatry, 53*, 137–143.

Redwine, L., Jenkins, F., & Baum, A. (1996). Relation between beta-adrenergic receptor density and lymphocyte proliferation associated with acute stress. *International Journal of Behavioral Medicine, 3*, 337–353.

Rotman, A. (1983). Blood platelets in psychopharmacological research. *Progress in Neuro-Psychopharmacology & Biological Psychiatry, 7*, 135–151.

Sapolsky, R.M. (1996). Why stress is bad for your brain. *Science, 273*, 749–750.

Sapolsky, R.M., Krey, L.C., & McEwen, B.S. (1986). The neuroendocrinology of stress and aging: The glucocorticoid hypothesis. *Endocrine Reviews, 7*, 284–301.

Seeman, T.E., & McEwen, B.S. (1996). Impact of social environment characteristics on neuroendocrine regulation. *Psychosomatic Medicine, 58*, 459–471.

Selye, H. (1936). A syndrome produced by diverse nocuous agents. *Nature, 138*, 32.

Selye, H. (1976). *The stress of life*. New York: McGraw-Hill.

Sgoutas-Emch, S.A., Cacioppo, J.T., Uchino, B.N., Malarkey, W., Pearl, D., Kiecolt-Glaser, J.K., & Glaser, R. (1994). The effects of an acute psychological stressor on cardiovascular, endocrine, and cellular immune response: A prospective study of individuals high and low in heart rate reactivity. *Psychophysiology, 31*, 264–271.

Sherwood, L. (1997). *Human physiology: From cells to systems* (3rd ed.). New York: Wadsworth.

Shipley, J.E., Alessi, N.E., Wade, S.E., Haegele, A.D., & Helmbold, B. (1992). Utility of an oral diffusion sink (ODS) device for quantification of saliva corticosteriods in human subjects. *Journal of Clinical Endocrinology & Metabolism, 74*, 698–700.

Sita, A., & Miller, S.B. (1996). Estradiol, progesterone, and cardiovascular response to stress. *Psychoneuroendocrinology, 21*, 339–346.

Smyth, J.M., Ockenfels, M.C., Gorin, A.A., Catley, D., Porter, L.S., Kirschbaum, C., Hellhammer, D.H., & Stone, A.A. (1997). Individual differences in the diurnal cycle of cortisol. *Psychoneuroendocrinology, 22*, 89–105.

Stedman, T.L. (1995). *Stedman's medical dictionary* (26th ed.). Baltimore, MD: Williams & Wilkins.

Sternberg, E.M., Hill, J.M, Chrousos, G.P, Kamilaris, T., Listwak, S.J., Gold, P.W., & Wilder, R.L. (1989). Inflammatory mediator-induced hypothalamic-pituitary-adrenal axis activation is defective in streptococcal cell wall arthritis susceptible Lewis rats. *Proceedings of the National Academy of Sciences, 86,* 2374–2378.

Stoney, C.M., Davis, M.C., & Matthews, K.A. (1987). Sex differences in physiological responses to stress and in coronary heart disease: A causal link? *Psychophysiology, 24,* 127–131.

Suarez, E.C., Kuhn, C.M., Schanberg, S.M., Williams, R.B., Jr., & Zimmermann, E.A. (1998). Neuroendocrine, cardiovascular, and emotional responses of hostile men: The role of interpersonal challenge. *Psychosomatic Medicine, 60,* 78–88.

Suls, J., & Wan, C.K. (1993). The relationship between trait hostility and cardiovascular reactivity: A quantitative review and analysis. *Psychophysiology, 30,* 615–626.

Tabachnick, B.G., & Fidell, L.S. (1997). *Using multivariate statistics* (3rd ed.). New York: HarperCollins.

Taylor, S.E., Klein, L.C., Lewis, B.P., Gruenewald, T.L., Gurung, R.A.R., & Updegraff, J.A. Biobehavioral responses to stress in females: Tend-and-befriend, not fight-or-flight. *Psychological Review, 107,* 411–429.

Uchino, B.N., Cacioppo, J.T., & Kiecolt-Glaser, J.K. (1996). The relationship between social support and physiological processes: A review with emphasis on underlying mechanisms and implications for health. *Psychological Bulletin, 119,* 488–531.

Vingerhoets, A.J.J.M., & Assies, J. (1991). Psychoneuroendocrinology of stress and emotions: Issues for future research. *Psychotherapy & Psychosomatics, 55,* 69–75.

Wade, S.E., & Haegele, A.D. (1991). Time-integrated measurement of corticosteriods in saliva by oral diffusion sink technology. *Clinical Chemistry, 37,* 1166–1172.

Walker, R.F., Riad-Fahmy, D., & Read, G.F. (1978). Adrenal status assessed by direct radioimmunoassay of cortisol in whole saliva or parotid saliva. *Clinical Chemistry, 24,* 1460–1463.

Weinberger, D.A., Schwartz, G.E., & Davidson, R.J. (1979). Low-anxious, high-anxious, and repressive coping-styles: Psychometric patterns and behavioral and physiological responses to stress. *Journal of Abnormal Psychology, 88,* 369–380.

Weiner, H. (1992). *Perturbing the organism: The biology of stressful experience.* Chicago: University of Chicago Press.

Wilson, J.D., & Foster, D.W. (Eds.) (1992). *Williams textbook of endocrinology.* Philadelphia: Saunders.

Wotjak, C.T., Kubota, M., Liebsch, G., Montkowski, A., Holsboer, F., Neumann, I., & Landgraf, R. (1996). Release of vasopressin within the rat paraventricular nucleus in response to emotional stress: A novel mechanism of regulating adrenocorticotropic hormone secretion? *The Journal of Neuroscience, 16,* 7725–7732.

Yalow, R.S., & Berson, S.A. (1959). Assay of plasma insulin in human subjects by immunological methods. *Nature, 184,* 1648–1649.

Yehuda, R. (1998). Psychoneuroendocrinology of post-traumatic stress disorder. *The Psychiatric Clinics of North America, 21,* 359–379.

Zieve, P.D., & Solomon, H.M. (1967). Accumulation of lipid-insoluble compounds by the human platelet. *American Journal of Physiology, 213,* 1275–1277.

# THE MEASUREMENT OF STRESS-RELATED IMMUNE DYSFUNCTION IN HUMANS: AN INTRODUCTION TO PSYCHONEUROIMMUNOLOGY

Kav Vedhara, Edward C.Y. Wang, Julie D. Fox, and Michael Irwin

Since Ader and Cohen's pioneering observations concerning the susceptibility of the immune system to behavioral conditioning (Ader & Cohen, 1975), there has been a dramatic increase in research dedicated to stress-neuroendocrine-immune interactions and their consequences for immunomodulation, i.e., the field of psychoneuroimmunology (PNI). Within this field, one area to have attracted considerable attention has been the phenomenon of stress-related immune impairment in humans. Multiple immunological changes have been reported. However, one of the major challenges to face human PNI research concerns the clinical significance of these immune alterations in people who experience psychological stress. In this regard, two main questions are evident:

1. What is the clinical significance of altered immunity, as measured by *in vitro*, *ex vivo* and *in vivo* humoral and cellular assays of immunity?; and
2. Is the magnitude of stress-associated immune changes sufficient to alter immunocompetence?

In this chapter we have aimed to review and evaluate some of the more frequently used *in vitro*, *in vivo* and *ex vivo* immunological techniques in the hope that a clearer understanding of what these assays can tell us will inform the discussion of the significance of stress-related immune impairment in humans. The chapter commences with a brief description of the immune system and this is followed by a review of the most commonly used *in vitro*, *in vivo* and *ex vivo* assays in PNI. The review of each assay includes: (1) a description of the rationale behind its use; (2) a commentary on the advantages and limitations of the assay; and (3), a consideration of their clinical relevance. The empirical work considered in this chapter has been conducted primarily with humans and, with the exception of the section on delayed hypersensitivity skin tests (DTH), focuses on sampling from peripheral blood.

## The immune system

Our immune systems are confronted with a rich variety of bacteria and infectious agents on a daily basis. However, for the most part, these are eradicated or contained long before they have an opportunity to result in symptoms. Two main features of the immune system have been identified: natural (innate) immunity and acquired immunity. The former system is the first to be encountered by an invading organism and consists of phagocytic cells that are already in circulation (e.g., monocytes, macrophages, granulocytes and natural killer (NK) cells) and which engulf and destroy microorganisms. These cells are assisted by the complement system which consists of serum proteins that are able to facilitate the destruction of the invading pathogen. When the defensive action of the natural immune system fails to contain or eradicate the pathogen, acquired immunity processes are brought into play. The activation of this aspect of the immune system produces a specific reaction to the pathogen which it subsequently "remembers" so that it can respond to the pathogen more efficiently during ensuing encounters. In this way, initial exposure to a disease such as diptheria or measles results in life-long immunity against reinfection.

The processes by which the immune system defends the host against disease have been described elsewhere (Brickman, 1994; Roitt et al., 1989). However, a diagrammatic summary of the principal features is presented in Figure 20. 1. This figure portrays the multiple arms of the specific immune system following a pathogenic challenge. Following contact with the pathogen, antigens are taken up and processed in antigen presenting cells (i) and presented to CD4+ T cells in the context of [1]major histocompatibility complex (MHC) II, and CD8+ T cells in the context of MHC I. CD4+ T cells supply cytokines (ii) which allow activation, differentiation and expansion (iii) of the cytotoxic CD8+ T cells (iv) and antibody-producing B cells. Antibodies are the soluble arm of the immune system and have a range of different functions, including direct inactivation of the pathogen, complexing with antigen to allow removal, activation of complement and acting as a recognition "bridge" for cell types which express antibody receptors, e.g., mast cells, NK cells, eosinophils (v). NK cells are another cytotoxic cell

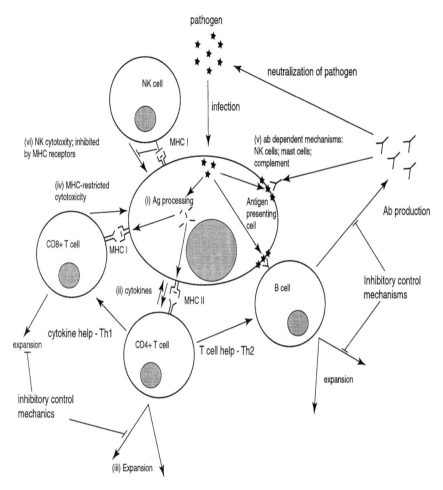

Figure 20.1.  Principles features of immune system activity.

subset, killing cells that do not express MHC I (vi)—thus they counter-act viral evasion mechanisms that reduce expression of MHC I.

It is evident, therefore, that the immune system is made up of several diverse yet interconnected components, and that the successful eradication of pathogens is dependent upon harmonious communication between these components. It is also clear that immune dysfunction could occur at the level of one or more of these components and, therefore, that the nature of the immune impairment is related to where the dysfunction occurs. The following sections of this chapter will explore the assays which have been used to assess the competence of the most frequently measured components of the human immune system in PNI research.

## Ex vivo measures

### LYMPHOCYTE SUBSETS

*Rationale*: The successful eradication of pathogens is dependent, in part, upon the existence of adequate numbers of immune cells and appropriate cell ratios. This is evident in diseases such as Human Immunodeficiency Virus (HIV) infection in which the loss of CD4+ cells disables the rest of the immune system thus, making the HIV infected patient vulnerable to a multitude of infections (Zunich & Lane, 1990). Similarly, immunity to herpes simplex virus I (HSVI) is known to be dependent upon NK cell activity (Fitzerald et al., 1985). Thus, a reduction in these cells leaves the host vulnerable to increased viral activity. The clinical relevance of cell counts has led, therefore, to the widespread use of total white blood cell (WBC) counts; WBC differentials (e.g., Fillion et al., 1996) and lymphocyte subset counts as indices of immune system efficacy (e.g., Egeler et al., 1996).

The systematic nomenclature of these immune cells has led to the identification of over 166 cluster designation (CD) markers and this number continues to increase. The CD nomenclature is related to phenotype and not necessarily function, although in some cases there is overlap. An overview of some of the most frequently measured cell subsets and markers, and those which may prove fruitful to examine, is presented in Table 20. 1.

*Advantages*: A cursory glance at the literature reveals that the enumerative assessment of cellular immunity in PNI research has traditionally focused on major cell subsets (e.g., Mills et al., 1996) and, more recently, on markers of T cell activation (e.g., Castle et al., 1995). Several advantages are accrued by such enumerative assessments. First, significant and selective changes have been reported in leukocyte subpopulations in response to acute stressors (Dhabhar et al., 1995). Thus, the measurement of cell counts would appear to be an effective way of assessing the effects of acute psychological challenges. Second, cell activation markers offer insight into the extent and nature of cellular activation and may, therefore, be more closely aligned with assessments of cell function. Indeed, the assessment of these markers can inform the debate on the ways in which stress may affect the immune system. This

Table 20.1.  The identity/function of some of the most frequently assessed lymphocyte sub-populations.

| ANTIGEN | IDENTITY/FUNCTION |
| --- | --- |
| CD3 | Present on all T cells. Molecular complex associated with the TCR and responsible for TCR-mediated transduction |
| CD4 | Present on T helper cells which direct the nature (i.e., cellular or humoral) of an immune response |
| CD8 | Present on suppressor and cytotoxic T cells |
| CD16/CD56 | Combined expression is a market for natural killer cells |
| CD19 & CD20 | Two primary B cell markers |
| CD57 | Found on a proportion of T and NK cells, present as a carbohydrate moiety on a variety of, as yet, unnamed glycoproteins |
| | MAKERS OF T CELL ACTIVATION |
| HLA-DR | This antigen is expressed on T cells, B cells and monocytes following activation |
| CD25 | The induction of CD25 on T cells occurs approximately 48 hours after activation, serving to increase the sensitivity of T cells to interleukin-2 (a T cell growth factor necessary for T cell proliferation). CD25 induction can, therefore, be used as a T cell activation marker |
| CD28 | T cell activation is dependent on T cell receptor signalling and co-stimulatory molecules. CD28 is one such molecule |
| CD38 | This antigen is expressed on T cells following activation, although its function is unknown |
| CD45RA(naive) & CD45RO (memory) | The CD45RA antigen is believed to indicate T cell "resting" status, i.e., the cell has not yet been activated. In contrast, CD45RO antigen is believed to indicate recent cell activation. The expression of these antigens is reversible |
| CD71 | This antigen is induced following T cell activation. However, it is expressed before CD25 and thus can be used as an earlier activation marker for T cells |

is clearly demonstrated in the results of a recent study which reported that caregivers of demented patients displayed an increase in CD8 cells but poorer T cell proliferation (Castle et al., 1995). However, an assessment of the numbers of cells exhibiting the CD38 activation marker revealed that both CD4 and CD8 cell subpopulations contained reduced percentages of CD38 cells. Thus, the poorer proliferation could be attributed to the reduction in activated T cells, as evidenced by CD38 percentages. The potential for activation markers to further elucidate the stress-immune system relationship would, therefore, appear to be considerable. Finally, when combined with functional assays, enumerative assessments of lymphocyte subpopulations allow one to ascertain whether observed alterations in cell numbers are of functional relevance, and conversely, whether apparent alterations in immune function are due to changes in the functional efficacy of the cells or simply changes in cell numbers.

*Limitations*: Several limitations do, however, also exist with the measurement of cell subsets. Firstly, cell numbers do not necessarily correlate well with cell function (Joseph et al., 1995). For example, Anesi and colleagues (1994) reported poorer T cell responses in subjects with major depression, but no evidence of a significant alteration in T cell numbers. Secondly, cell numbers fluctuate according to a number of factors unrelated to immune system activity (e.g., cell migration, circadian rhythms, etc; Pettingale, 1990). Thus, any apparent alterations in lymphocyte sub-populations may simply reflect physiological events, such as cell migration, rather than a stress-induced variation. Finally, there is often some overlap in lymphocyte subsets, many of which may have different functions. For example, CD8+ cells can be divided into several sub-populations (e.g., CD8+CD28+, CD8+CD28-, CD8+CD57+, CD8+CD57). Thus, unless the populations are defined precisely, the interpretation of lymphocyte counts can be problematic.

*Recommendations*: The above considerations would appear to advocate a reassessment of the way in which lymphocyte counts are used in PNI research. For example, we propose that the quantification of cell numbers is most informative when combined with functional assessments. In addition, the study of cell ratios may offer a more cogent index of immune system activity. For example, the normal ratio of CD4:CD8 cells is 2:1 and this ratio is known to be altered in the presence of some infections (Molback et al., 1996). It would be appropriate, therefore, to adopt the CD4:CD8 ratio as an outcome measure in investigations designed to explore issues such as the relationship between stress and viral infections. Finally, we contend that activation markers, used in conjunction with, or in isolation from, lymphocyte counts, may offer a more efficacious index of immune system activity for two main reasons. Firstly, they are more closely related to markers of cell function. Secondly, they can inform the debate on the ways in which stress may affect the immune system. For example, as described in Table 20.1, the assessment of both CD25 and CD71 would offer insight into the stage at which T cell activation may be affected.

*Clinical implications*: Immune cells travel through the bloodstream and between tissues and, as such, there is little doubt that the numbers and proportions of cells in circulation provide an indication of the state of leukocyte distribution and redistribution in the body. Thus, the enumerative assessment of cells informs us of the ability of the immune system to respond to potential or ongoing immune challenges.

## CYTOTOXICITY ASSAYS

*Rationale*: One of the major functions of the immune system is to remove foreign "non-self" cells such as those infected with virus, or those which are immortalized (i.e., cells which have lost the normal controls that inhibit perpetual cell division) or those which are tumorgenic. Active killing (i.e., cytotoxicity) of such targets can be carried out by both cytotoxic T lymphocytes (CTL) and NK cells and are measured by cytotoxicity assays. It is widely believed that the body regularly produces non-self cells and so the immune system's ability to identify and destroy these cells is an extremely important feature of its activity and, therefore, a highly relevant immune outcome measure.

The two subsets of effectors recognize their targets in different ways and thus different conclusions can be drawn from each assay. With regard to NK cell cytotoxicity, the typical assay involves the incubation of NK cells with a specific target known to be susceptible to NK cell killing. These targets are generally tumor cell lines such as K 562 or Molt 4 and cytokines such as interferon are often used to activate the NK cells beforehand. The serial dilution of effectors changes the effector to target ratio and thus provides a more accurate estimate of the number of NK cells needed to destroy a set number of targets. In contrast, T cell cytotoxicity assays involve coating a NK insensitive target cell line (usually a mouse B lymphoblastoid cell line such as JY) which expresses a receptor for antibodies, with a mouse anti-human CD3 monoclonal antibody (Phillips & Lanier, 1986). CD3 is a T cell specific marker, thus anti-CD3 antibodies serve to activate all T cells and hold the targets in close proximity allowing easy access for cytotoxic mechanisms to take place. This assay is considered to measure "total T cell cytotoxic capability". The final assay worthy of consideration is LAK (lymphokine activated killer) activity. This assay measures non-specific cytotoxicity against a wide range of targets following activation by high concentrations of IL-2, although the assay is most widely used in studies relating to tumor cells.

*Advantages*: Cytotoxicity assays inform us about the cytotoxic potential of the subsets in question, i.e., T or NK cells. A reduction in cytotoxicity would thus indicate a defect in the mounting of such a response, though it would not identify the mechanisms underlying this defect. The assays themselves are robust and relatively easy to perform. NK cytotoxic assays use effectors that are easy to stimulate in short-term culture against transformed cell lines targets that are straightforward to grow. This also applies to the anti-CD3 directed "total" T cell cytotoxicity assay mentioned above. In contrast, antigen-specific cytotoxic T cell lines and clones need long-term culture and are considerably more difficult to grow, but are very sensitive once established, with significant killing at effector:target ratios of <1. This allows the investigation of other cellular or cytokine-derived influences on the cytotoxicity. Furthermore, the targets (normally virally-infected, peptide-loaded or transformed cell lines) are generally well-defined and may allow clinical interpretations—e.g., malignant melanoma (MM) lines in patients with MM. Finally, because the mechanisms of cytotoxicity are relatively well understood, precise dissection of any defects is easier.

*Limitations*: Most investigations of NK cell cytotoxicity exhibit several methodological difficulties which make it difficult to conclude that the target lysis witnessed has been caused exclusively by NK cells. Firstly, some investigators use whole peripheral blood mononuclear cells (PBMC) as effectors (Goodkin et al., 1992). In such samples, NK cells constitute only a small and variable part. Secondly, PBMC samples clearly contain other cell subsets, some of which are capable of non-specific tumor line killing (e.g., CD3+, CD57+ T cells: Phillips & Lanier, 1986). Thirdly, some groups have examined NK cytotoxicity using only nonadherent cells (i.e., adherent cells are removed before the assay). However, adherent populations produce some cytotoxic activity and their removal can also result in alterations in cytokine release. Together, these factors clearly have implications for our evaluation of NK cytotoxic activity. Finally, cytotoxicity assays define NK cell activity according to the cells' ability to kill particular tumor lines. However, the extent to which responses to these lines (which have been transformed in culture for long periods) are indicative of a physiologically active cytotoxic response is not clear.

With regard to T cell cytotoxicity, it should be noted that anti-CD3 directed cellular cytotoxicity is known to generate false positives. This is believed to be due to the tendency for the anti-CD3 antibody to produce strong signals, which result in non-physiological T cell activation (Sette et al., 1994). In addition, the target cell line traditionally associated with such assays (P815) is known to be highly susceptible to lysis by a broad range of cell types including macrophages and T and NK cells (D'Angeac & Hale, 1980). Hence, this assay involves the use of a non-physiological stimulus against non-physiological targets. Similar physiological criticisms can also be directed against Lymphocyte Activated Killing (LAK) assays. While it can be argued that effector cells may encounter high concentrations of IL-2 in local microenvironments during an immune response (e.g., lymph nodes), the concentrations used to generate LAK cells are often 100-fold in excess of those capable of inducing a proliferative response. In addition, the constitution of LAK cells is not uniform, consisting of varying proportions of NK and T cells (depending on the subject) and the lack of target specificity (LAK cells kill both tumor and normal cells) would suggest non-physiological parameters.

*Recommendations*: It is clear from Figure 20.1 that an "end stage" event such as cytotoxicity can be affected in a number of ways, e.g., defects in antigen presentation, cytokine help, active suppression, defects in perforin release or just decreased proliferation of effectors. Thus, if an assay demonstrates reduced cytotoxicity and the assay has been conducted in isolation, information cannot be gleaned on the mechanisms that may be involved. The use of additional assays, such as cytokine or proliferation assays, would enable conclusions to be drawn regarding possible mechanisms.

With regard to NK cytotoxicity assays specifically, the methodological limitations described above suggest that future work with this assay would benefit from the use of either purified NK cells (using CD16 and CD56) or the depletion of NK cells from PBMC. Either approach would ensure that only NK cells were responsible for any cytotoxicity witnessed in the assay. Furthermore NK cytotoxicity assays should be combined with lymphocyte counts which identify the proportion of NK cells within a given sample. This would, in turn, allow conclusions to be made about the efficiency of cytotoxic activity within this subset.

*Clinical implications*: Cellular cytotoxicity is a major mechanism for removing virally- and bacterially-infected, or non-self, i.e., tumorgenic, cells, but a general defect is not necessarily lethal as shown by studies on perforin knockout mice (e.g., Lowin et al., 1994). The clinical importance of cytotoxicity is dependent on the pathogen. To date, no human disease is totally dependent on cytotoxicity for its clearance, although the absence of cytotoxic T lymphocytes is associated with the progression of a number of diseases (e.g., HIV, cervical carcinoma) indicating that these cells play a role in controlling these diseases. This is borne out by mouse studies where lymphocytic choriomeningitis virus (LCMV) infection is lethal (Kagi et al., 1996), and resistance to mouse AIDS reduced (Tang et al., 1997), in perforin knockout mice.

## LYMPHOCYTE PROLIFERATION

*Rationale*: Assays of lymphocyte proliferation are perhaps the most widespread functional *in vitro* assessment of the cellular arm of the immune system (Herbert & Cohen, 1993). These assays involve the measurement of lymphocyte division (i.e., proliferation) in response to any stimulus. Implicit in the performance of these assays is the assumption that the greater the proliferation the more effective the immune response, although it has not yet been determined whether or not such a linear relationship exists. Two main assays of proliferation have been reported: proliferation in response to non-specific stimuli or specific stimuli and blast transformation.

*(a) Proliferation to non-specific and specific stimuli*
*Advantages*: Proliferative responses to non-specific stimuli indicate whether there is a difference in the general responsiveness of lymphocytes. In addition, the use of different non-specific stimuli, or mitogens, can offer some insight into where in the proliferation process the impairment has occurred. For example, OKT3 antibodies specifically stimulate T cells in culture via the T cell receptor (TCR) so reduced responses would imply a fault in T cell responsiveness via TCR signaling. In combination, these assays can identify immune defects. Thus, lack of responsiveness to Con A (a monocyte dependent[2] polyclonal lymphocyte activator) but responsiveness to OKT3 would suggest the reduced proliferation was due to a monocyte defect.

In contrast, the advantage of using specific stimuli is that an examination of the immune response to a specific pathogen is possible. Any foreign antigen which has previously been met by the host's immune response can be tested. Furthermore, because one is examining a highly specific immune response (i.e., only those T cells which recognize the antigen in question), it is possible to undertake a more detailed analysis of specific T cell responses. Thus, any differences between individuals are more clearly defined.

*Limitations*: The principal limitation of proliferation assays using non-specific stimuli is their polyclonal nature (i.e., they stimulate multiple cell types). A great many investigations have employed this immune index as their outcome measure. However, the results from such investigations do not allow us to identify which subsets of lymphocytes are responding, nor do they inform us on the potential mechanisms involved. In addition, in studies where data on cell counts are not available, it is not possible to discount the possibility that differences in proliferation may simply be caused by alterations in the numbers and ratios of the different lymphocyte subsets in the sample of peripheral blood being tested. Finally, the synthetic nature of the stimuli used in such assays necessarily limits the scope of the conclusions that can be drawn regarding the efficacy of the immune system in the face of naturalistic pathogens.

Difficulties also exist with proliferation assays which use specific stimuli. Although specific stimuli provide data on the nature of the immune response to a naturalistic pathogen, they are essentially *ex vivo* assays from which conclusions regarding *in vivo* processes should be drawn with caution. In particular, it should be noted that the specific stimuli used in such assays tend to come in the form of soluble antigens derived from the pathogen under investigation. CD8+ cells typically have poor responses to such antigens and thus the proliferative responses that are witnessed are usually derived from CD4+ cells (Raychaudhuri & Morrow, 1993). CD8+ proliferative responses are only observed when intact cells (e.g., virus infected cells) are used as stimulators. A further difficulty with such assays is that the responses are strongly influenced by the recency of the last *in vivo* exposure to the antigen. As it is difficult to control for previous exposure, results from such assays can be confounded by this factor.

*Recommendations*: It is evident that proliferation assays involving non-specific stimuli are most informative when the stimulus is chosen with a view to identifying where in the proliferation process the immune dysfunction is occurring. In this regard, the use of multiple mitogens can help to delineate the causes of immune dysfunction. For example, Irwin and colleagues (1996) recently demonstrated, in a study with sleep deprived subjects, that the performance of several different tests, including proliferation assays, can help to determine which cell populations are affected. Specifically, they were able to evaluate whether deficits in T cells, monocytes or both contributed to the observed decline in interleukin-2 production. Thus, proliferation assays when used in conjunction with other assays can be instructive.

### (b) Blast transformation

Another method which has been used to assess lymphocyte activation is blast transformation (e.g., Lee et al., 1992). Actively proliferating lymphocytes, called blasts, are larger than their resting counterparts, and are identified by their larger and more granular physical characteristics.

*Advantages and limitations*: The measurement of blast transformation is relatively simple; however, it also lacks accuracy as the physical characteristics of cells vary with the point in the cell's cycle. In its simplest form, it measures only whether a cell can be activated and induced from a resting state with no reference to function.

*Recommendations*: A more subtle and definitive approach is available in the context of B cells and their antibody responses. Activated blasting B cells (before differentiation) produce IgM (resting cells do not; fully differentiated B cells produce other Ig classes) which can be measured, either using cytoplasmic staining of anti-$\mu$ chain monoclonal antibodies, or functionally by the ability of the blasts to fix complement and lyse sheep red blood cell in specially designed Cunningham-Szenberg chambers (referred to as plaque-forming cell assays; Cunningham & Szenberg, 1968). These assays can be modified with appropriate antibodies to investigate B cells secreting antibodies of any class. The assay measures the release of functional Ig and limiting dilution analysis (to be considered below) allows the quantification of the number of blasting B cells.

*Clinical implications*: Proliferation is an intrinsic part of immune responses, occurring in B and T lymphocytes following recognition of antigen by their respective antigen receptors and in the presence of the correct cytokines. The clinical implications are dependent on the magnitude of the defects. While a 50% reduction in proliferative responses may have little clinical effect, total abrogation would result in no immune response to an antigenic challenge and immunodeficiency, as seen in AIDS patients (Lane & Fauci, 1985). Less extreme examples come from reports of: (1) decreased specific proliferative responses to varicella zoster virus (VZV) in the elderly (Berger et al., 1981) (2) the higher frequency of VZV-specific T cells in elderly patients who have recently had herpes zoster (Hayward et al., 1991) and (3) a decline in VZV-specific T cell proliferative responses in depressed patients (Irwin et al., 1998). These data suggest a correlation between reduced T cell proliferation to a virus and clinical disease.

## LIMITING DILUTION ANALYSIS (LDA)

*Rationale*: T cell proliferation and cytotoxicity assays or B cell plaque-forming assays provide data on the levels of cellular responsiveness. These assays can not, however, tell us how many cells are responding. This can only be achieved through LDA. This assay measures the frequency of precursors for any given effector (e.g., NK cells, cytotoxic T cells, etc.) and thus allows estimates to be made of the actual numbers of a specific effector cell type.

*Advantages*: The principle advantage of this assay is that it enables one to examine whether any changes in responses are due to a change in frequency of cells deriving a particular immune response. The method is the only functional assay that gives a quantitative, as opposed to qualitative, result.

*Limitations*: The statistical nature of the assay is dependent on only one cell type generating the parameter being measured (single hit kinetics). When several cell types (e.g., suppressor T cells) influence the outcome, each growing out at their own frequencies, the semi-logarithmic plots become non-linear, making a frequency assessment impossible. The complicated nature of effector growth, manifestation and control often results in non-single hit kinetics, especially in the case of antigen-specific T cells. Furthermore, the assay is expensive and labor intensive as statistical errors are reduced by increasing the size of the test. Thus, while LDA is a very powerful assay it is not used extensively.

*Recommendations*: Ideally, LDA can be used to further define any differences seen in other gross assays. Thus, if a reduction in cytotoxicity is observed, LDA would identify whether this was due to a decrease in activity or a decrease in effector cell number. While use of LDA to define antigen-specific T cells (proliferative or cytotoxic) may be excessive in PNI research considering the difficulties in culturing these T cell subsets, its use for further defining changes in broader responses, e.g., to polyclonal, proliferative stimuli, would be recommended.

## CYTOKINE LEVELS

*Rationale*: Cytokines are soluble factors released by immune cells which control and direct the function of other immune effectors. Alterations in their concentration mediate the down-regulation and up-regulation of the immune system and thus offer insight into several aspects of immune system activity. The range of cytokines is extensive and is increasing continually (currently, 18 interleukins have been identified), with several sub-populations of other cytokines including interferons, colony stimulating factors, transforming growth factors and tumor necrosis factors. Hence, in Table 20.2, we describe the functions of only some of the important cytokines which have featured in investigations into the effects of stress on the immune system.

Two main classes of cytokines have been identified: Th1 and Th2. These have been defined as cytokines which stimulate the development of either cellular responses (Th1: e.g., $\gamma$-interferon, IL2, etc.) or humoral (antibody) responses (Th2: e.g., IL-4, IL-10, etc.). For a review, the reader is directed to Cohen and Cohen (1996) or Wardle (1993), but in brief, Th1 cytokines will activate CD8+ T cells, thus resulting in cytotoxic responses, while Th2 cytokines stimulate B cell activation resulting in antibody responses. However, Th1 and Th2 responses are opposing and will therefore inhibit each other.

A number of different systems are used to investigate cytokine levels, namely polyclonal mitogen stimulation, antigen-specific activation or broad measurements of cytokines in circulating plasma or serum. However, cytokines tend to act in the lymph node microenvironments where antigen presenting cells meet T and B cells (Liu et al., 1992). The *in vitro* systems, such as mitogen stimulation or antigen-specific stimulation are, therefore, just attempts to imitate a much more complex and subtle set of cellular interactions. Measurement of cytokine levels following mitogen stimulation is the least physiological investigation, as multiple cell subsets of different antigen specificities are activated. It is more a measure of the general ability of a group of cells, as a whole, to produce cytokines. Antigen-specific activation is a better defined system, as the stimulating antigen will only be presented to highly specific effectors. This is a closer scenario to *in vivo* events, though it is important to acknowledge that the organization and milieu of cells in peripheral blood, and those in lymph nodes, are very different. Thus, while *ex vivo* measurements of cytokines in circulation are the least contrived, such measurements are unlikely to reflect the events in lymph node microenvironments unless systemic infections are taking place.

Table 20.2. Cytokines and their functions

| Cytokine | Cell Expression | Function |
|---|---|---|
| IL-1 | Wide—nearly all immune cells | Wide—*in vivo* causes hypotension, fever, weight loss, acute phase responses |
| IL-2 | T cells | Stimulates growth and differentiation of T, B, NK, LAK cells, monocytes, macrophages |
| IL-3 | Activated T cells, mast cells, eosinophils | B cell growth factor; expands haematopoietic precursors; activates monocytes |
| IL-4 | T cells, mast cells | Multiple biological effects on B, T cells; stimulates IgG4/IgE secretion from B cells |
| IL-5 | T cells, mast cells, eosinophils | Eosinophil growth and differentiation factor |
| IL-6 | Wide—including non-lymphoid cells | Regulates B and T cell function, haematopoiesis and acute phase reactions |
| IL-7 | Bone marrow, thymic stromal and spleen | Proliferation and differentiation of B and T cells |
| IL-8 | Activated TH2 T cells | Neutrophil chemoattractant and activator; also attracts basophils and some lymphocytes |
| IL-9 | Wide—including non-lymphoid cells | Enhances proliferation of T cells, mast cells, erythroid precursors |
| IL-10 | Activated T cells, monocytes | Stimulates proliferation of B, thymocytes and mast cells; inhibits TH1 cytokine production |
| IL-11 | Bone marrow, stimulated fibroblasts | Growth factor for multipotential haemopoietic progenitors |

Table 20.2. Cytokines and their functions *(continued)*

| Cytokine | Cell Expression | Function |
|----------|-----------------|----------|
| IL-12 | B cells, monocytes/macrophages | Indices of proliferation and differentiation of TH1 cells; enhances NK killing |
| IL-13 | Activated T cells | Promotes B cell proliferation and IgM/IgE/IgG4 production |
| IL-14 | T cells | Enhances proliferation of activated B cells; inhibits Ig synthesis |
| IL-15 | Wide—more by monocytes/epithelial cells | Stimulates growth and differentiation of T and B cells |
| IFN-$\alpha$ | lymphocytes, monocytes, macrophages | Induce resistance to viruses; inhibits cell proliferation; enhances MHC 1 expression |
| IFN-$\beta$ | fibroblasts, epithelial cells | Similar to IFN-$\alpha$ |
| IFN-$\gamma$ | T and NK cells | Activates most immune cell types; potentiates antiviral effect of IFN-$\alpha$ and IFN-$\beta$ |

*Advantages and limitations*: Cytokine levels are able to inform us on a number of points in immune status. Firstly, the absence of certain cytokines offers potential mechanisms for any functional abnormalities recorded. For example, Kiecolt-Glaser and colleagues (1996) reported that stress in elderly caregivers was associated with a poorer antibody response to influenza vaccine. However, unlike previous investigations of this kind, they measured several cytokines (IL-2, IL-1β and IL-6) and thus were able to speculate on the possible mechanisms involved. Secondly, the level of Th1 and Th2 cytokines inform the researcher of the type of immune response being made to an antigen (i.e., cellular or humoral) and indicate the most active cell type involved.

Specific advantages are also conferred by each of the assays used to measure cytokines. For example, ELISAs provide information on the immunoreactivity of cytokines. Because monoclonal anticytokine antibodies are used in ELISAs, the investigator can be sure that the quantitative result is an accurate measure of the cytokine concentration. ELISAs do not inform on the actual activity of the cytokine; even if a cytokine is inactive, it may still be recognized by an antibody. In contrast, biological assays confer the advantage of informing the investigator of the bioactivity of the cytokines being measured. However, because cytokines are pleiotropic and can have very similar functions, e.g., IL-2 and IL-4 both induce T cell proliferation, biological assays should be carefully controlled. An example would be the cell line CT.4R, which can be used to estimate concentrations of both IL-2 and IL-4, but for definitive conclusions, such assays should be carried out in the presence of inhibitory antibodies to one or the other cytokine (Hu-Liu et al., 1989).

The advantage of the RT-PCR method is its incredible sensitivity— RT-PCR can now detect mRNA from a single cell. Unlike biological assays or ELISAs, the results from RT-PCRs are not confounded by the turnover of cytokines. Upon release, there is an active uptake of cytokines such that measures of cytokines in supernatant only reveal a proportion of the total cytokine released. Similarly, cytokines can bind to antagonists which also may interfere with their detection. Cytokine detection by RT-PCRs is not affected by physiological activity of this kind. However, intrinsic to RT-PCR is that it detects the level of messenger RNA and not protein itself. There are many intracellular processes that take place between the expression of mRNA and final release of a protein, any of which may be blocked or interfered with. Similarly, the lack of mRNA does not mean that there is not a stable, active cytokine present, that was previously released by the cell. Thus,

RT-PCR is in itself not a measure of actual cytokine levels, just a measure that a cell's machinery is ready to generate the cytokine. It is also, at best, semi-quantitative (unlike ELISAs), measuring levels of mRNA relative to those of a control housekeeping gene.

*Limitations*: Perhaps the most significant limitation impeding the widespread use of cytokine determination in PNI is the fact that only a very limited number of cytokines can be detected in the plasma of healthy individuals. Thus the measurement cytokines in plasma is ultimately of greater utility in diseased populations (e.g., HIV infected patients, individuals infected with influenza, etc.).

*Recommendations*: Despite some of the considerations outlined above, it is evident that the measurement of cytokine concentrations offer an exciting opportunity to explore in detail the potential mechanisms underlying stress-related immune dysfunction. It is for this reason that we advocate the more widespread assessment of multiple cytokines in PNI research where it has, hitherto, been limited.

*Clinical implications*: As with many biological systems, and as a recurring theme in this chapter, the clinical implications of changes in cytokine levels are dependent on the magnitude of the changes. Complete loss of a cytokine is often not immediately lethal, but the resultant immunodeficiency is likely to kill once a pathogen can take advantage of the defect (e.g., IL-7 knockout mice; von Freeden-Jeffry et al., 1995). Where the main role of the cytokine is immunoregulatory, removal can result in autoimmunity (i.e., the immune system attacks the host) as seen in IL-2 knockout mice (Horak et al., 1995). Partial loss often has no clinical significance, as many cytokines are partly redundant.

Changes in groups of cytokines, such as Th1 or Th2, give an indication of the type of immune response occurring (cellular vs. humoral). However, the dominance of Th1 or Th2 cytokines cannot in themselves be interpreted as being adaptive or maladaptive. Both cytokine subsets are essential features of the immune response and only in specific contexts is one or other dangerous to the host. For example, Decker and colleagues (1996) reported that surgical stress was associated with a shift in the Th1/Th2 balance in the favor of Th2 as shown by an increase in IL-4 production. However, the significance of this apparent down-regulation of cellular immunity and up-regulation of humoral immunity is unclear. This study clearly demonstrates that the immunological significance of cytokine concentrations should be interpreted in the context of the pathogen under investigation. For example, Th1 responses (cellular) are vital for the control of leprosy lesions (Modlin, 1994), while a Th2 response (antibody) is much more effective in controlling influenza infection (Kubiet et al., 1996).

## ANTIBODY ASSAYS

*Rationale*: Another popular assay in PNI research is the measurement of antibody levels (e.g., Shtarbova & Klein, 1995). Antibodies are proteins constructed from four polypeptide chains and are produced by B cells following exposure to antigens. They bind to the antigen which stimulated their development and, via a variety of mechanisms, counteract the pathogenic potential of the antigen. Hence, levels of circulating antibody offer some insight into the efficacy of the humoral arm of the immune system.

Five major classes of antibody (known as isotypes) have been identified and defined by their different heavy chains: IgA, IgG, IgM, IgD and IgE. IgG and IgA can be split further into 4 and 2 subclasses, respectively. The functions of the major isotypes are described in Table 20.3.

Table 20.3. Functions of the five classes of antibody found in the immune system.

| Antibody type | Function/description |
| --- | --- |
| Immunoglobulin A (IgA) | Secreted in body fluids like tears and saliva and therefore protects the mucosal surfaces |
| Immunoglobulin E (IgE) | Attaches to antigens and then to basophils and mast cells triggering the release of histamines |
| Immunoglobulin M (IgM) | Multiple functions including the triggering of complement-mediated lysis and the formation of antibody:antigen complexes which can be cleared by phagocytic cells of the liver |
| Immunoglobulin G (IgG) | Coat microorganisms making it possible for macrophages and neutrophils to recognize, engulf and destroy pathogens such as bacteria. This is the most abundant immunoglobulin consisting of multiple isotypes with different functions |
| Immunoglobulin D (IgD) | Little is known about the function of this antibody |

Each of these antibodies are ubiquitous, although certain classes tend to predominate in particular fluids. For example, IgA is found primarily in mucous secretions, while IgG predominates in serum. IgE is the antibody recognized by mast cells and basophils, and is the main pathogenic antibody in patients suffering from severe allergies. It is clear that the fluid in which the antibody predominates dictates the nature of the sample collected, and the isotype of the antibody dictates the type of immunity it confers.

*Advantages*: The assessment of total levels of antibody (e.g., Claussen, 1994) enables the investigator to detect gross immunodeficiency. Furthermore, the measurement of IgA in particular is especially attractive as its production in saliva makes it readily available for measurement. However, the quantification of antibody titers to a specific antigen (Glaser et al., 1994) is inherently superior. This approach is based on the premise that once antibodies are made in response to an antigen, the host retains a small proportion of these antibodies in circulation. It is possible, therefore, to assess the efficacy of humoral immunity to a specific pathogen with such assays; such data clearly have greater clinical relevance. Much of the work that has been conducted with antigen-specific antibody assays has involved the measurement of antibody titers to latent viruses, such as herpes simplex virus-1 (HSV-1) and Epstein Barr virus (EBV), which are known to be persistent and reactivating infections in humans (e.g., Esterling et al, 1994). Hence, unlike other antigens for which antibody presence is affected by the recency of the host's exposure to the antigen, moderate levels of antibody to the virus are always present in the host. Furthermore, these levels fluctuate in response to viral activity, with an increase in viral replication being associated with an increase in antibody titers. Thus, the assessment of antibody titers to latent viruses would appear to be ideally suited to investigations of the effects of stress on one virus-specific aspect of humoral immunity.

*Limitations*: Of all the antibody assays used in PNI research, the measurement of total antibody levels is perhaps the most limited. The antigen specificity of antibodies means that only a certain proportion of circulating antibody will respond to any particular antigen. Thus, total antibody is a poor index of the specific antibody response and can therefore provide only an imprecise measure of the immune system response. This is clearly evidenced by the predominance of data which fail to find a relationship between stress and total levels of antibody.

For example, Mouton et al., (1989) reported that they were only able to find a relationship between salivary IgA and examination stress when the highest and lowest stress periods were compared (i.e., final exam vs. end of summer vacation). These data led them to conclude that salivary IgA was a weak marker of the effects of stress on the immune system. In a more conclusive indictment of the utility of total antibody levels, Jabaaij and colleagues (1993) reported that there was no evidence of a relationship between daily hassles and serum IgG, IgA or IgM in their subjects. While data exist which have demonstrated stress-related alterations in total antibody levels (Farne et al., 1994), in general the literature is characterized by data which indicate that a consistent relationship does not exist.

The quantification of antibody titers to a specific antigen (e.g., Jenkins & Baum, 1995) is clearly more precise and clinically relevant. However, the antibody response can and does wane in the absence of the stimulating antigen. In addition, antibodies have a limited half-life. Thus, the assessment of antigen-specific antibodies is dependent, in part, upon ensuring recent exposure to the antigen. It is for this reason that several investigators have focused on antibody titers to latent viruses where moderate levels of antibody to the virus are always present in the host.

*Recommendations*: It is evident that, in isolation, differences in antibody titers can only inform us that there may be an impairment or increase in the production of antibodies *per se*. However, further information can be obtained on the processes involved by assessing antibody titers in conjunction with functional *in vitro* assays. For example, stimulation with pokeweed mitogen (a lectin which induces T cell dependent antibody production by B cells) can inform us whether T or B cells are involved in the altered process. In addition, the selection of different classes of antibody can help to determine which particular immune responses are altered. For example, IgM production is indicative of a primary immune response, i.e., a response to an antigen that has not previously been presented, or a response that has waned. Conversely, IgG is indicative of a more specific memory response, i.e., prior exposure to the antigen has occurred.

The process by which B cells change the isotype of the antibody they secrete is called isotype switching (Kataoka et al., 1980). This is regulated by cytokines released from T cells (Gauchat et al., 1990), and is accompanied by changes in the region which binds antigen (termed somatic hypermutation; Jacob et al., 1991), resulting in increased binding efficiency. This maturing of the antibody response helps, firstly, to fine tune the specificity of the antibody for its antigen, and secondly, to direct the humoral immune system to the areas where it is needed. Thus, multiple measures of antigen-specific antibodies of different isotypes can inform on the type of immune response taking place. Finally, as described earlier, it is important to acknowledge that immune responses can wane with time and thus a lack of IgG, for example, does not necessarily mean that immunological memory responses are impaired, but may simply represent an immune response that has waned.

One final issue concerns the measurement of neutralizing antibodies as an alternative to the total and specific antibody assays that have been described. Neutralizing antibody levels give a more specific measure of immunity to a particular virus by assessing sera for their ability to prevent replication of a known amount of virus. A susceptible cell line is inoculated with the target virus *in vitro* in the presence of a particular dilution of the test serum and the amount of virus replication is assessed by light microscopy or other standard tests for the presence of the virus or virion component. The antibody titer recorded is the reciprocal of the highest dilution that completely inhibits virus replication. In this way, the measurement of neutralizing antibody provides a more accurate measure of the effectiveness of a particular immune response in preventing virus infection or activation than gross measures of antibody levels. It would appear, however, that neutralizing antibody titers have not yet been used extensively as an index of stress-related immune impairment in PNI research. It is hoped that, in future, investigators will incorporate this parameter when examining the role of stress in compromising virus-specific immunity.

*Clinical implications*: It is widely agreed that an increase in antibody titers occurs as a consequence of an increase in viral activity. One of the many hypotheses that has been put forward to explain such increases is that the host has experienced some degree of immune disturbance which has resulted in infection, or in the case of latent viruses, virus reactivation (Jenkins & Baum, 1995). For example, Esterling and colleagues (1990) reported that students who displayed a repressive coping style when faced with a disclosure task were found to have the highest EBV viral capsid antigen titers. In investigations such as these, the increase in antibody titers is construed as a sign of underlying immune dysfunction. It could be argued, however, that elevations in antibody titers, far from being a sign of immunosuppression, are in fact characteristic of an effective humoral immune response to the antigen. Also, it should be recognized that alterations in antibody titers may reflect a virus-specific response and not a general humoral response. Furthermore, compared with other virus-directed methods (e.g., virus isolation) the significance of virus-specific antibody titers is limited by the fact that an increase in antibody titer occurs some time after virus activation and replication commences. Thus, while measurements of antibody levels are informative, clinical implications should be made with caution.

## IDENTIFICATION OF A VIRUS OR VIRAL COMPONENT

*Rationale*: It is evident from the previous discussion on the measurement of virus-specific antibody titers, that the immune system plays an important role in the control of virus infections. It is not surprising, therefore, that another index of stress-related immune impairment involves measurement of virus infection, activation or clearance (e.g., Cohen et al., 1991). In healthy individuals the acquisition and/or clearance of viruses may occur in the absence of symptoms, thus making clinically verifiable infection a poor outcome measure. However, a number of *in vitro* techniques are available to provide evidence of current or recent viral infection which may be utilized in the absence of identifiable clinical features. In the case of acute virus infections (such as influenza and the common cold) viruses are cleared after infection in the healthy individual but the time to clearance may give a measure of immune system efficiency. Detection of infectious virus particles (*in vitro* culture), visualization of virus particles (electron microscopy) or detection of virus particle (virion) components (tests for viral antigen or nucleic acid) can be used to confirm an acute (current) virus infection.

A number of viruses are not cleared after initial infection and persist for the life of the host. Herpes viruses exhibit a specialized form of persistence which is termed latency and is characterized by production of a few proteins but not infectious progeny. Herpes viruses can be activated from this latent stage (termed reactivation) when there is a switch to complete virus replication. Such reactivation may be associated with clinical symptoms (in which case this is termed recurrence) and a subsequent boost in specific immunity as measured indirectly by antibody or proliferation assays. Viruses are all obligate intracellular parasites and so have a requirement for a living cell to replicate. Detectable virion components or infectious particles outside a cell indicate current virus replication. Some assays allow a quantitative measure of the amount of viral nucleic acid or antigens which may allow the distinction between carriage of a virus and complete replication in cellular clinical samples. Below we will briefly describe the advantages and limitations of different approaches to virus identification.

## (1) Virus isolation

For those viruses which can be propagated *in vitro*, virus isolation is considered to be the gold standard for confirming the presence of infectious virus particles. It offers a more direct measure of replicating viruses than techniques which monitor total virus particles or virion components. However, the disadvantages of this approach include its relative insensitivity when compared with genome detection tests and the very significant limitation that some viruses are not easily cultured *in vitro*. The cytopathic effect produced by different viruses can look very similar and thus a virus isolate must be subjected to a further test to confirm its identity (e.g., antigen or neutralization test). This makes the procedure laborious and, for some viruses, very time consuming.

## (2) Electron microscopy for detection of viral particles

Electron microscopy is a quick method for identification of viruses but requires a high concentration of particles which also must have a characteristic appearance. In practice, this method is usually used where clinical symptoms are apparent (e.g., an obvious lesion) and the use in PNI is likely to be limited because of its lack of sensitivity in identification of asymptomatic infections. Although electron microscopy can provide relevant information for identification of current infection it does not give an indication of particle infectivity. In some circumstances it is useful for confirmation of the identity of a virus isolate but is of particular use for analysis of viruses which cannot be propagated *in vitro*.

## (3) Viral antigen detection

A virus-specific antigen test based on ELISA or particle-agglutination would be much quicker and more convenient for handling large numbers of samples than either virus isolation or electron microscopy. The only disadvantage of this approach is that the amount of viral antigen in a particular sample type may be low and only detectable after virus isolation and propagation *in vitro*. Suitable antibodies must be available for use in an antigen test and care must be taken that the antigen detected is not produced in significant amounts during latency. This method does not give an indication of infectivity but can be used for monitoring viruses which are not easily cultivated *in vitro*.

## (4) Viral genome detection

Molecular-based methods are very sensitive for detection of viral nucleic acid and allow assessment of virus infection and activation even where the amount of virus is low or where a "fastidious" virus (not culturable *in vitro*) is to be analyzed. If the sample-type is selected carefully and/or quantitative methods are used, it is possible to use molecular methods to assess immune control of persistent viruses. In addition to the detection of viral genomic nucleic acid, molecular-based assays can be used for identification of viral mRNA. Such assays are particularly suitable for the assessment of herpes viruses reactivation.

*Clinical relevance of virus-detection methods*: To date, the majority of studies of PNI have utilized virus isolation techniques or an indirect measure of virus activation using antibody tests. The development of assays for detection of viral antigen and nucleic acid will allow a more widespread use of assays relevant to virus infection and replication as a measure of immune function and control. Assays which detect the virus particle or virion component in a cell-free sample provide evidence of acute infection or recent activation (in the case of a latent virus). Providing care is taken to ensure that a particular viral antigen, mRNA or high level genomic sequence is only present during replication, cell-associated samples can also be used for the assessment of herpes virus activation.

## DNA REPAIR

*Rationale*: The DNA of immune cells, like other cells, can be damaged by carcinogens and other harmful substances. The host's ability to fully repair this DNA is considered to be crucial in reducing the incidence of cancer, cell death and alterations in cell growth and division (Hall & Johnson, 1996). Several techniques have been developed to assess the extent of DNA repair. However, we will offer a description of the only technique which has, to date, been used in PNI research, namely nucleoid sedimentation restoration rate (Kiecolt-Glaser et al., 1985). This approach involves exposing cells to irradiation and assessing the sedimentation restoration rate (DNA damage is associated with a reduction in the sedimentation restoration rate). Thus, DNA repair is measured by the time taken to return to baseline sedimentation rates (i.e., before DNA damage took place).

*Advantages and limitations*: This technique, while functionally interesting, has not been used widely in PNI research. Indeed, the only documented study at this time is by Kiecolt-Glaser and colleagues (1985) who observed that lymphocytes from subjects who reported high levels of distress displayed poorer DNA repair after exposure to X-irradiation. The limited use of this assay may be due, in part, to the limited conclusions one can draw from the data obtained. For example, although our DNA repair capability is of major importance, it is not clear what the relationship might be between DNA repair rates and the functional efficacy of cells. However, if DNA repair assays were conducted in conjunction with other functional assays of the immune system (e.g., cytotoxic or proliferation assays), they could offer some insight into whether stress-related impairments in cell function are due to cellular impairments inflicted at a molecular level.

## Integrated *in vivo* measures

Thus far, this chapter has provided an overview of many of the traditional *ex vivo* and *in vitro* assays. We hope this has served to illustrate the many levels at which immune impairment can occur, while also identifying the advantages and limitations inherent in these assays. We have not, however, explored the relationship between *in vitro/ex vivo* assays and *in vivo* functioning. This issue is, unfortunately, a perennial problem for all investigators of the human immune system as ethical considerations necessarily limit the scope for *in vivo* research in humans. It is not therefore possible to offer any informed discussion of the relationship between data from *in vitro/ex vivo* assays and *in vivo* functioning. Nonetheless, it is possible to contend that *in vivo* investigations of the immune system offer outcome measures of the greatest clinical relevance because they provide a measure of integrated immune responses. In recognition of this, consideration will be given to the limited number of *in vivo* approaches that have been utilized in this field.

### DELAYED HYPERSENSITIVITY TESTS
*Rationale*: Hypersensitivity is defined as an exaggerated or inappropriate form of an otherwise adaptive immune response that results in tissue damage. Four types of hypersensitivity have been described. Type I (immediate) is clinically observed in conditions such as hay fever, where an IgE response to pollen results in mast cell activation and the

release of chemical mediators that can result in asthma or rhinitis. Type II is caused by hypersensitivity of antibody-dependent cytotoxic mechanisms. Clinical examples of this type include hyperacute graft rejection, transfusion reactions following the introduction of incompatible blood types to a donor recipient and haemolytic disease in infants whose antibodies to the Rhesus antigen result in anemia. Type III is immune complex mediated, where large quantities of antibody-antigen complexes overwhelm the host's ability to clear them which results in serum sickness. Finally, type IV, delayed hypersensitivity occurs when the release of lymphokines, following a T cell-antigen interaction, results in an inflammatory response. Type IV delayed hypersensitivity will be the focus of this section as it has been adopted several times as an index of the functional efficacy of cell mediated immunity to antigenic stimulation (e.g., Vedhara & Nott, 1996).

*Advantages and limitations*: The advantage of delayed hypersensitivity tests of this kind is that they are symptomatic measurements of an *in vivo* process. Indeed, the tuberculin-type hypersensitivity reaction is a recognized measure of previous exposure to a specific antigen and is also considered a suitable assay for determining the presence of particular immunodeficiencies. However, complex mechanisms control the responses involved in DTH reactions and tests such as these do not allow us to determine where immune system impairment has taken place; nor is it possible to quantify easily the nature of the immune response generated. Finally, responses to the DTH antigens are also likely to be influenced by the recency of previous antigen exposure. Thus, this *in vivo* technique does also have some limitations.

## RESPONSES TO LIVE OR ATTENUATED VIRUS PREPARATIONS
*Rationale*: In such investigations healthy individuals are inoculated with a virus and a range of *in vivo* immunological responses to the virus or viral antigens contained in a vaccine, such as antibody responses, lymphocyte proliferation, etc., are examined. Two main approaches have been adopted: inoculation with a live virus (Cohen et al., 1991) and inoculation with a vaccine which contains inactivated or weakened virus preparations (e.g., Kiecolt-Glaser et al., 1996).

*Advantages*: The most significant advantage conferred by both live virus and vaccine challenge studies is that they enable the researcher to examine the relationship between stress and *in vivo* immunity in the face of a naturalistic pathogen. Thus, it is possible to conclude from investigations like that of Kiecolt-Glaser and colleagues (1996) that their elderly caregivers who produced a poor response to an influenza vaccine challenge may in fact be more susceptible to influenza infection. Such a conclusion could not have been reached if the immunological outcome measures had been any of the non-specific *in vitro* assays described previously (e.g., proliferative responses to non-specific stimuli, levels of total immunoglobulin, etc.).

A further advantage associated with live virus challenge studies in particular (and, to a lesser extent, live vaccine challenge studies) is that they enable the investigator to explore the relationship between stress and clinically verifiable disease. This is clearly demonstrated in the investigation described by Cohen and colleagues (1991) in which they reported that, after challenging subjects with one of five respiratory viruses, both respiratory infections and clinical colds increased in a dose-response manner with increases in psychological stress.

*Limitations*: It is evident from these data that live virus challenge studies represent the gold standard of the field. However, there is one caveat which deserves consideration which is of relevance to all *in vivo* work and virus and vaccine challenge studies in particular. This concerns the relationship between *in vivo* challenges and *ex vivo* responses. Data exist which indicate that the immunological history of the host (e.g., previous exposure to pathogens, vaccinations, etc.) can influence immunological responses to subsequent challenges. For example, it has been shown that, in mice, CD8 cell responses to viruses are determined by previous exposure to other viruses and the responses mounted to them (Selin et al., 1996). Data such as these demonstrate that an individual's immunological responses to an *in vivo* challenge do not occur in isolation, but are in fact modulated by previous challenges. This should be taken into consideration when interpreting data from *in vivo* investigations.

## Additional methodological considerations

In addition to the methodological issues that have been identified thus far, there are several other factors, the majority of which are external to the assay but intrinsic to the host, which may also confound the results from PNI investigations. These factors, or health related behaviors, include nutritional status, exercise, alcohol/drug use, etc., and serve to add to the confusion surrounding the nature of the relationship between stress and the immune system in three main ways. First, each of these behaviors are known to have immunomodulatory effects and so should be controlled for in investigations into the effects of stress on immune function. Second, alterations in these behaviors rarely occur in isolation. For example, an increase in alcohol consumption is likely to affect an individual's nutritional status and quality of sleep. Thus, a range of behaviors need to be examined to ensure that their confounding effects are minimized. Finally, and perhaps of most significance to this discussion, many of these behaviors are known to change as a consequence of exposure to stressful situations. Thus, it could be argued that any apparent effects of stress on the immune system may not be a direct consequence of exposure to a stressor, but rather a secondary effect caused by changes in health behaviors (e.g., smoking, alcohol consumption, etc.). All of these considerations strongly advocate that the measurement of health related behaviors should be an integral feature of PNI research. We will, therefore, conclude this chapter with a brief review of some of these behaviors and the evidence pertaining to their immunomodulatory effects. For a discussion of some of the measurement issues surrounding these behaviors the reader is directed to Kiecolt-Glaser and Glaser (1988).

## ALCOHOL AND/OR NON-PRESCRIPTION AND PRESCRIPTION DRUG USE

Several investigations have reported that the frequency of alcohol and non-prescription drug use is increased during periods of chronic psychological distress (Barnet et al., 1995; Pavis et al., 1997). The evidence pertaining to the effects of these substances on the immune system is, however, equally compelling. Investigators have reported a multitude of immune effects including disrupted cytokine production (Wang et al., 1997), poorer delayed hypersensitivity responses (Mendall et al., 1997), and impaired lymphocyte proliferation (Nair et al., 1997).

A related confounding behavior is the use of prescription drugs. Many of the individuals who are the focus of PNI investigations receive pharmacological treatments for co-existing diseases, such as, spousal carers of dementia patients (Kiecolt-Glaser et al., 1996) or individuals with chronic and/or terminal illnesses such as HIV infected individuals (Vedhara et al., 1997). Individuals in both groups are often treated concurrently with several different drugs for the treatment of a variety of conditions. It is likely that, for some individuals, adherence to a treatment regime can be an additional source of stress, and that some of the drugs themselves may have immunomodulatory properties (Pastores et al., 1996). These considerations, and those outlined above, demonstrate the importance of assessing alcohol and prescription and non-prescription drug use when evaluating the effects of stress on the immune system.

## SLEEP DISTURBANCE

Insomnia is one of the most common complaints reported by individuals experiencing distress, although its role in moderating and/or mediating immune alterations has been relatively unexplored. Recent research from the depression literature has, however, demonstrated that subjective insomnia correlates with NK activity (Cover & Irwin, 1994). This has led to the hypothesis that, certainly in depression, disordered sleep may account for some of the immune alterations observed. A series of studies have now been conducted by Irwin and colleagues to test more carefully the role of sleep in the modulation of multiple aspects of the immune system and to determine the moderating effects of sleep disturbance on immune measures in depressed subjects. Although a detailed review of this literature is outside of the scope of this chapter (the interested reader is directed to: Benca et al., 1992; Hall et al., 1998; Irwin & Gillin, 1998; Irwin et al., 1992, 1994, 1996).

## EXERCISE

The influence of exercise on immune function has traditionally been investigated in two main ways: the measurement of immune activity following a period of vigorous exercise, or an exploration into the relationship between immune activity and an objective measure of fitness (e.g., oxygen consumption levels during exercise). Both approaches have demonstrated a positive association between exercise/fitness and immunity (e.g., Brandon et al., 1991; Simon, 1991). However, two caveats should be acknowledged. First, although moderate levels of exercise are associated with immune enhancement, the clinical significance of exercise induced immune changes are not clear. Indeed, some investigators have reported that exercise-related immune changes are short-lived (Simon, 1991). Second, there is evidence to suggest that over-exercising, as seen in high intensity athletes, can result in immune impairment (Gleeson et al., 1995). Thus, while a relationship between exercise and immunity exists, it is evident that it is not a linear relationship and that we should be circumspect when considering the stability and clinical relevance of exercise associated immune changes.

## NUTRITION

Nutrition, like many of the other factors considered in this section, is known to affect the immune system, both directly and indirectly, through stress related changes in eating behavior. For example, considerable evidence exists to suggest that malnourished individuals have significantly poorer immune function across a variety of immune parameters (e.g., Gogos & Kalfarentzoz, 1995). Similarly, there has been substantial interest in the effects of emotions on eating patterns (e.g., Ganley, 1989) and data suggesting that periods of depression can contribute to poor appetite and thus, malnutrition (Kerstetter et al., 1992). This relationship between stress, nutrition and immunity is further complicated by evidence that the presence of infections can also alter the individual's nutritional status. For example, infections which result in increases in pro-inflammatory cytokines can adversely affect nutrition by impairing metabolic activity and inducing anorexia (Muñoz et al., 1995). Similarly, the use of dietary supplements has also been associated with immune alterations (Muñoz et al., 1995). It is evident, therefore, that the interactions between stress, nutrition and immunity are complex and warrant detailed consideration in PNI research.

## SMOKING

In view of the prevalence of tobacco use in chronically stressed and depressed subjects (Breslau et al., 1998) and the possible influence of cigarette smoking on immune function (Ferson et al., 1979), it is important to explore whether cigarette smoking is another moderator of the relationship between mood disorder and immunity. However, few studies conducted within PNI have examined this issue. One exception is the recent study by Jung and Irwin (1998) who examined the influence of current cigarette smoking on total white blood cells, numbers of major immune cell classes, and NK activity in depressed subjects and in controls. Their findings showed that depressed subjects had higher numbers of total cells than controls, and that smokers had elevated total white blood cell counts as compared to non-smokers. In addition, there was a significant interaction between depression and smoking on total cell counts. Depressed smokers had higher numbers of white blood cells than depressed non-smokers and control non-smokers and smokers. They concluded that the immunologic changes found in depressed smokers were not due to the simple effects of smoking. Controls who were current smokers showed white blood cell counts and levels of NK activity that were similar to those found in control non-smokers. Furthermore, there was no correlation between amount of smoking and NK activity in either the control or depressed smokers, a finding consistent with previous studies of smoking populations (Meliska et al., 1995).

## Conclusion

We have aimed in this review to alert the reader to some of the limitations and strengths of existing *in vitro/ex vivo* and *in vivo* assessments of the immune system. Our discussion has focused on the rationale behind the various assays and the methodological issues which limit the interpretability of the data obtained. Several key considerations for future research are apparent from this discussion. The first of these concerns the selection of immunological outcome measures. Many investigations into the effects of stressor exposure on the immune system adopt a single outcome measure and then attempt to draw conclusions on the basis of the enumerative or functional status of this single parameter. The machinery of the immune system is, however, highly complex and intimately interconnected and, therefore, warrants the assessment of multiple parameters. In the same way that a single trait does not provide an adequate description of an individual's personality, a single immunological index should not be regarded as an adequate marker of the immune system.

A second related issue concerns the choice of immunological parameters. It is evident from this review that the various assays are able to inform us about various features of the immune system. The selection of assays should, therefore, be closely aligned with the research question that is being asked and, if relevant, the disease process under investigation. For example, the selection of immune measures relevant for investigations into stress-associated immune changes in inflammatory disorders would differ substantially from those required to evaluate the role of immune mechanisms in viral disease. Indeed, even with viral disease, consideration of what immune measures would be important in primary vs. secondary infection would be required. Such issues necessarily introduce another layer of complexity into this debate which is beyond the scope of this review. Suffice to say that we hope that the isolated use of non-specific immunological outcome measures (e.g., non-specific lymphocyte proliferation) will become increasingly obsolete.

Thirdly, caution should always be exerted when interpreting immunological data. The complex interactions between the various facets of the immune system mean that immunological impairment at one level does not translate into impairment at all other levels. This issue is clearly illustrated by fluctuations in T cell numbers. An increase in T cell numbers may indicate the presence of infection and thus, at one level, indicates a lapse in the functional efficacy of the immune system. However, it also indicates that a cellular response has been mounted.

We hope that it is evident from the assays reviewed in this chapter that the measurement of stress-related immune impairment is an incredibly complex issue. However, if adequate consideration is given to the strengths and weaknesses of the various assays available, it is possible to delineate the consequences of stress for the immune system and further our understanding of stress immune interactions.

## Acknowledgment

This chapter is based upon and has been reprinted from *NEURO-SCIENCE & BIOBEHAVIORAL REVIEWS*, Vol 23, 699–715, Vedhara, K., Fox, J.D. & Wang, E.C.Y., "The measurement of stress-related immune dysfunction: An introduction to psychoneuroimmunology", 1999, with permission from Elsevier Science.

## Notes

1. The MHC system represents a cluster of genes which facilitate immune recognition and signaling between cells of the immune system.
2. Polyclonal stimuli non-specifically activate lymphocytes in general.

## References

Ader, R., & Cohen, N. (1975). Behaviorally conditioned immunosuppression. *Psychosomatic Medicine, 37*, 333–340.

Anesi, A., Franciotta, D., Di Paolo, E., Zardini, E., Melzi, D., Eril, G., & Zerbi, F. (1994). PHA-stimulated cellular immune function and T-lymphocyte subsets in major depressive disorders. *Functional Neurology, 9*, 17–22.

Barnet, B., Duggan, A.K., Wilson, M.D., & Joffe, A. (1995). Association between postpartum substance use and depressive symptoms, stress, and social support in adolescent mothers. *Pediatrics, 96*, 659–666.

Benca, R.M., Obermeyer, W.H., Thisted, R.A., & Gillin, J.C. (1992). Sleep and psychiatric disorders: A meta-analysis. *Archives of General Psychiatry, 49*, 651–668.

Berger, R., Florent, G., & Just, M. (1981). Decrease of the lymphoproliferative response to varicella-zoster virus antigen in the aged. *Infection, 32*, 24–27.

Brandon, J.E., Loftin, J.M., & Curry, J. (1991). The role of fitness in mediating stress: A correlational exploration of stress reactivity. *Perceptual and Motor Skills, 73*, 1171–1180.

Breslau, N., Peterson, E.L., Schultz, L.R., Chilcoat, H.D., & Andreski, P. (1998). Major depression and stages of smoking. A longitudinal investigation. *Archives of General Psychiatry, 55*, 161–166.

Brickman, C.M. (1994). The molecular basis of the human immune system. *Journal of Clinical Immunoassay, 17*, 85–91.

Castle, S., Wilkins, S., Heck, E., Tanzy, K., & Fahey, J. (1995). Depression in caregivers of demented patients is associated with altered immunity: Impaired proliferative capacity, increased CD8+, and a decline in lymphocytes with surface signal transduction molecules (CD38+) and a cytotoxicity marker (CD56+ CD8+). *Clinical and Experimental Immunology, 101*, 487–493.

Claussen, B. (1994). Psychologically and biochemically assessed stress in a follow-up study of long-term unemployed. *Work and Stress, 8*, 4–18.

Cohen, M.C., & Cohen, S. (1996). Cytokine function: A study in biologic diversity. *American Journal of Clinical Pathology, 105*, 589–598.

Cohen, S., Tyrrell, D.A.J., & Smith, A.P. (1991). Psychological stress and susceptibility to the common cold. *New England Journal of Medicine, 325*, 606–612.

Cover, H., & Irwin, M. (1994). Immunity and depression: Insomnia, retardation and reduction of natural killer cell activity. *Journal of Behavioral Medicine, 17*, 217–223.

Cunningham, A.J., & Szenberg, A. (1968). Further improvements in the plaque technique for detecting single antibody forming cells. *Immunology, 14*, 599–600.

D'Angeac, A.D., & Hale, A.H. (1980). Pretreatment of P815 mastocytoma cells with inhibitors of protein synthesis reduces their susceptibility to lysis by cytotoxic thymus-derived lymphocytes. *Cellular Immunology, 55*, 342–354.

Decker, D., Schondorf, M., Bidlingmaier, F., Hirner, A., & Von Ruecker, A.A. (1996). Surgical stress induces a shift in the type1-type2 T helper cell balance, suggesting down regulation of cell-mediated and up-regulation of antibody-mediated immunity commensurate to the trauma. *Surgery, 119*, 316–325.

Dhabhar, F.S., Miller, A.H., McEwen, B.S., & Spencer R.L. (1995). Effects of stress on immune cell distribution: Dynamics and hormonal mechanisms. *Journal of Immunology, 154*, 5511–5527.

Egeler, R.M., Shapiro, R., Loechelt, B., & Filipovich, A. (1996). Characteristic immune abnormalities in hemophagocytic lymphohistiocytosis. *Journal of Pediatrics in Haematology/Oncology, 18*, 340–345.

Esterling, B.A., Antoni, M.H., Fletcher, M.A., Margulies, S., & Schneiderman, N. (1994). Emotional disclosure through writing or speaking modulates latent Epstein-Barr virus antibody titers. *Journal of Consulting and Clinical Psychology, 62,* 130–140.

Esterling, B.A., Antoni, M.H., Kumar, M., & Schneiderman, N. (1990). Emotional repression, stress disclosure responses and Epstein-Barr viral capsid antigen titers. *Psychosomatic Medicine, 52,* 397–410.

Farne, M.A., Boni, P., Corallo, A., Gnugnoli, D., & Sacco, F.L. (1994). Personality variables as moderators between hassles and objective indications of distress (S-IgA). *Stress Medicine, 10,* 15–20.

Ferson, I., Edwards, A., Lind, A., Milton, G.W., & Hersey, P. (1979). Low natural killer cell activity and immunoglobulin levels associated with smoking in human subjects. *British Journal of Cancer, 23,* 603–609.

Fillion, L., Lemyre, L., Mandeville, R., & Piche R. (1996). Cognitive appraisal, stress state, and cellular immunity responses before and after diagnosis of breast tumor. *International Journal of Rehabilitation & Health, 2,* 169–187.

Fitzerald, P.A., Mendelsohn, M., & Lopez, C. (1985). Human natural killer cells limit replication of herpes simplex virus type 1 in vitro. *Journal of Immunology, 134,* 1665–1672.

Ganley, R.M. (1989). Emotion and eating in obesity: A review of the literature. *International Journal of Eating Disorders, 8,* 343–361.

Gauchat, J.F., Lebman, D.A., Coffman, R.L., Gascan, H., & De Vries, J.E. (1990). Structure and expression of germline ε transcripts in human B cells induced by interleukin 4 to switch to IgE production. *Journal of Experimental Medicine, 172,* 463–473.

Glaser, R., Pearl, D.K., Kiecolt-Glaser, J.K., & Malarkey, W.B. (1994). Plasma cortisol levels and reactivation of latent Epstein-Barr virus in response to examination stress. *Psychoneuroendocrinology, 19,* 765–772.

Gleeson, M., McDonald, W.A., Cripps, A.W., Pyne, D.B., Clancy, R.L., & Fricker, P.A. (1995). The effect on immunity of long-term intensive training in elite swimmers. *Clinical and Experimental Immunology, 102,* 210–216.

Gogos, C.A., & Kalfarentzoz, F. (1995). Total parental nutrition and immune system activity: A review. *Nutrition, 11,* 339–344.

Goodkin, K., Blaney, N., Feaster, D., Fletcher, M.A., Baum, M.K., Mentero-Atineza, E., Klimas, N.G., Millon, C., Szapocznik, J., & Eisdorfer, C. (1992). Active coping style is associated with natural killer cell cytotoxicity in asymptomatic HIV-1 seropositive homosexual men. *Journal of Psychosomatic Research, 36,* 635–650.

Hall, M., Baum, A., Buysse, D.J., Prigerson, H.G., Kupfer, D.J., & Reynolds, C.F. (1998). Sleep as a mediator of the stress-immune relationship. *Psychosomatic Medicine, 60,* 48–51.

Hall, M., & Johnson, R.T. (1996). The role of DNA repair in the prevention of cancer. *Molecular Aspects of Medicine, 17,* 235–383.

Hayward, A., Levin, M., Wolf, W., Angelova, G., & Gilden, D. (1991). Varicella-zoster virus-specific immunity after herpes zoster. *Journal of Infection, 163,* 873–875.

Herbert, T.B., & Cohen, S. (1993). Stress and immunity in humans—A meta-analytic review. *Psychosomatic Medicine, 55,* 364–379.

Horak, I., Lohler, J., Ma, A., & Smith, K.A. (1995). Interleukin-2 deficient mice: A new model to study autoimmunity and self-tolerance. *Immunology Review, 148,* 35–44.

Hu-Liu, J., Ohara, J., Watyson, C., Tsang, W., & Paul, W.E. (1989). Derivation of a T cell line that is highly responsive to IL-4 and IL-2 (CT.4R) and of an IL-2 hyporesponsive mutant of that line (CT.4S). *Journal of Immunology, 142,* 800–907.

Irwin, M., & Gillin, J.C. (1998). The neuroimmunology of normal and disturbed sleep. *Journal of Sleep Research, 7,* 126.

Irwin, M., Smith, T.L., & Gillin, J.C. (1992). Electroencephalographic sleep and natural killer activity in depressed patients and control subjects. *Psychosomatic Medicine, 54,* 107–126.

Irwin, M., Mascovich, A., Gillin, J.C., Willoughby, R., Pike, J., & Smith, T.L. (1994). Partial sleep deprivation reduces natural killer cell activity in humans. *Psychosomatic Medicine, 56,* 493–498.

Irwin, M., McClintick, J., Costlow, C., Fortner, M., White, J., & Gillin, J.C. (1996). Partial night sleep deprivation reduces natural killer and cellular immune responses in humans. *FASEB Journal, 10,* 643–653.

Irwin, M., Costlow, C., Williams, H., Artin, K.H., Levin, M.J., Hayward, A.R., & Oxman, M.N. (1998). Cellular immunity to varicella-zoster virus in depression. *Journal of Infectious Disease, 178 (Suppl. 1),* 104–108.

Jabaaij, L., Benschop, R.J., Vingerhoets, A.J.J.M., Kirschbaum-Buske, A., Duivenvoorden, H.J., Oostveen, F.G., & Ballieux, R.E. (1993). Daily hassles and symptoms: Their relationship to enumerative immunologic measures. *Stress Medicine, 9,* 259–269.

Jacob, J., Kelsoe, G., Rajewsky, K., & Weiss, U. (1991). Intraclonal generation of antibody mutants in germinal centres. *Nature, 354,* 389–392.

Jenkins, F.J., & Baum, A. (1995). Stress and reactivation of latent herpes simplex virus: A fusion of behavioral medicine and molecular biology. *Annals of Behavioral Medicine, 17,* 116–123.

Joseph, B.Z., Beam, R., Martin, R.J., & Borish, L. (1995). Prednisone inhibits leukocyte granule secretion into the asthmatic airway. *International Journal of Immunopathology and Pharcololology, 8,* 23–30.

Jung, W., & Irwin, M. (1999). Reduction of natural killer cytotoxic activity in major depression: Interaction. *Psychosomatic Medicine, 61,* 263–270.

Kagi, D., Ledermann, B., Burki, K., Zinkernagel, R.M., & Hengartner, H. (1996). Molecular mechanisms of lymphocyte-mediated cytotoxicity and their role in immunological protection and pathogenesis in vivo. *Annual Review of Immunology, 14,* 207–232.

Kataoka, T., Kawamaki, T., Takahashi, N., & Honjo, T. (1980). Rearrangement of immunoglobulin $\gamma$1-chain gene and mechanism for heavy chain class switch. *Proceedings of the National Academy of Sciences, 77,* 919–923.

Kerstetter, J.E., Holthausen, B.A., & Fitz, P.A. (1992). Malnutrition in the institutionalized older adult. *Journal of the American Dietetic Association, 92*, 1109–1116.

Kiecolt-Glaser, J.K., & Glaser, R. (1988). Methodological issues in behavioural immunology research with humans. *Brain, Behavior and Immunity, 2*, 67–78.

Kiecolt-Glaser, J.K., Stephens, R.E., Lipetz, P.D., Speicher, C.E., & Glaser, R. (1985). Distress and DNA repair in human lymphocytes. *Journal of Behavioral Medicine, 8*, 311–320.

Kiecolt-Glaser, J.K., Glaser, R., Gravenstein, S., Malarkey, W.B., & Sheridan, J. (1996). Chronic stress alters the immune response to influenza virus vaccine in older adults. *Proceedings of the National Academy of Sciences, 93*, 3043–3047.

Kubiet, M.A., Gonzales-Rothi, R.J., Cottey, R,. & Bender, B.S. (1996). Serum antibody response to influenza vaccine in pulmonary patients receiving corticosteroids. *Chest, 110*, 367–370.

Lane, H.C., & Fauci, A.S. (1985). Immunologic abnormalities in the acquired immunodeficiency syndrome. *Annual Review of Immunology, 3*, 477–500.

Lee, D.J., Meehan, R.T., Robinson, C., Mabry, T.R., & Smith, M.L. (1992). Immune responsiveness and risk of illness in U.S. air force academy cadets during basic cadet training. *Aviation, Space, & Environmental Medicine, 63*, 517–523.

Liu, Y.J., Johnson, G.D., Gordon, J., MacLennan, I.C.M. (1992). Germinal centres in T-cell dependent antibody response. *Immunology Today, 13*, 17–21.

Lowin, B., Beermann, F., Schmidt, A., & Tschopp, J. (1994). A null mutation in the perforin gene impairs cytolytic T lymphocyte and natural killer cell-mediated cytotoxicity. *Proceedings of the National Academy of Sciences, 91*, 11571–11575.

Meliska, C.J., Stunkard, M.E., Gilbert, D.G., Jensen, R.A., & Martinko, J.M. (1995). Immune function in cigarette smokers who quit smoking for 31 days. *Journal of Allergy & Clinical Immunology, 95*, 901–910.

Mendall, M.A., Patel, P., Asante, M., Ballam, L., Morris, J., Strachan, D.P., Camm, A.J., & Northfield, T.C. (1997). Relation of serum cytokine concentrations to cardiovascular risk factors and coronary heart disease. *Heart, 78*, 273–277.

Mills, P.J., Dimsdale, J.E., Nelesen, R.A., & Dillon, E. (1996). Psychologic characteristics associated with acute stressor-induced leukocyte subset redistribution. *Journal of Psychosomatic Research, 40*, 417–423.

Modlin, R.L. (1994). Th1-Th2 paradigm: Insights from leprosy. *Journal of Investigative Dermatology, 102*, 828–832.

Molbak, K., Lisse, I.M., & Aaby, P.T. (1996). Lymphocyte subsets and prolonged diarrhea in young children from Guinea-Bissau. *American Journal of Epidemiology, 143*, 79–84.

Mouton, C., Fillion, L., Tawadros, E., & Tessier, R. (1989). Salivary IgA is a weak stress marker. *Behavioral Medicine, 15*, 179–185.

Muñoz, C., Schlesinger, L., & Cavaillon, J-M. (1995). Interaction between cytokines, nutrition and infection. *Nutrition Research, 15*, 1815–1844.

Nair, M.P.N., Schwartz, S.A., Polasani, R., Hou, J., Sweet, A., & Chadha, K.C. (1997). Immunoregulatory effects of morphine on human lymphocytes. *Clinical and Diagnostic Laboratory Immunology, 4*, 127–132.

Pastores, S.M., Hasko, G., Vizi, E.S., & Kvetan, V. (1996). Cytokine production and its manipulation by vasoactive drugs. *New Horizons, 4*, 252–264.

Pavis, S., Cunningham-Burley, S., & Amos, A. (1997). Alcohol consumption and young people: Exploring meaning and social context. *Health Education Research, 12*, 311–322.

Pettingale, K.W. (1990) Is stress immunosuppressive? In: L.J. Whalley and M.L. Page (Eds.), *Current approaches: Stress, immunity and disease.* (pp. 10–22). Southampton, UK: Duphar.

Phillips, J.H., & Lanier, L.L. (1986). Lectin-dependent and anti-CD3 induced cytotoxicity are preferentially mediated by peripheral blood cytotoxic T lymphocytes expressing Leu-7 antigen. *Journal of Immunology, 136*, 1579–1585.

Raychaudhuri, S., & Morrow, W.J.W. (1993). Can soluble antigens induce CD8+ cytotoxic T-cell responses? A paradox revisited. *Immunology Today, 14*, 344–348.

Roitt, I.M., Brostoff, J., & Male, D.K. (1989). *Immunology (2nd Ed.).* Churchill Livingstone: London .

Selin, L.K., Vergilis, K., Welsh, R.M., & Nahill, S.R. (1996). Reduction of otherwise remarkably stable virus-specific cytotoxic T lymphocyte memory by heterologous viral infections. *Journal of Experimental Medicine, 183*, 2489–2499.

Sette, A., Alexander, J., Ruppert, J., Snoke, K., Franco, A., Ishioka, G., & Grey, H.M. (1994). Antigen analogs/MHC complexes as specific T cell receptor antagonists. *Annual Review of Immunology, 12*, 413–431.

Shtarbova, M., & Klein, S. (1995). Assessment of immunoglobulins after hip replacement. *International Orthopaedics, 19*, 51–54. 1995.

Simon, H.B. (1991). Exercise and immune function. In: R. Ader, D.L. Felten, & N. Cohen (Eds.), *Psychoneuroimmunology (2nd Ed.)* (pp. 869–895). San Diego, CA: Academic Press Inc.

Tang, Y., Hugin, A.W., Giese, N.A., Gabriele, L., Chattopadhyay, S.K., Fredrickson, T.N., Kagi, D., Hartley, J.W., & Morse, H.C. 3rd (1997). Control of immunodeficiency and lymphoproliferation in mouse AIDS: Studies of mice deficient in CD8+ T cells or perforin. *Journal of Virology, 71*, 1808–1813.

Vedhara, K., & Nott, K.H. (1996). The assessment of the emotional and immunological consequences of examination stress. *Journal of Behavioural Medicine, 19*, 467–468.

Vedhara, K., Nott, K.H., Bradbeer, C.S., Davidson, E.A.F., Ong, E.L.C., Snow, M.H., Palmer, D., & Nayagam, A.T. (1997). Greater emotional distress is associated with accelerated CD4+ cell decline in HIV infection. *Journal of Psychosomatic Research, 42*, 379–390.

von Freeden-Jeffrey, U., Vieira, P., Lucian, L.A., McNeil, T., Burdach, S.E., & Murray, R. (1995). Lymphopenia in interleukin (IL)-7 gene-deleted mice identifies IL-7 as a nonredundant cytokine. *Journal of Experimental Medicine, 181,* 1519–1526.

Wang, J.Y., Liang, B., & Watson, R.R. (1997). Alcohol consumption alters cytokine release during murine AIDS. *Alcohol, 14,* 155–159.

Wardle, E.N. (1993). Cytokines: An overview. *European Journal of Medicine, 2,* 417–423.

Zunich, K.M., & Lane, H.C. (1990) The immunology of HIV infection. *Journal of the American Academy of Dermatology, 22* (Suppl. II), 1202–1205.

# Index

Note: Page references in **bold** refer to Tables; those in *italics* refer to Figures

For Product Safety Concerns and Information please contact our EU
representative GPSR@taylorandfrancis.com
Taylor & Francis Verlag GmbH, Kaufingerstraße 24, 80331 München, Germany

www.ingramcontent.com/pod-product-compliance
Ingram Content Group UK Ltd.
Pitfield, Milton Keynes, MK11 3LW, UK
UKHW020936180425
457613UK00019B/427